# AGARWAL'S
# Principles of
# Optics and Refraction
### Fifth Edition

Under the auspices of
'Sankalp'
(A charitable trust)
and
Federation of Ophthalmic Research
and Education Centres, India

# AGARWAL'S
# Principles of
# Optics and Refraction

### Fifth Edition

**Prof. (Dr.) Lalit P. Agarwal**

MBBS (Luck.), DOMS, R.C.P. & S. (Eng.), D.O. (Oxon),
M.S. (Luck.), F.A.M.S. (India), F.O.R.C.E. (India), F.S.E.S. (USA)

Formerly :
Director : All India Institute of Medical Sciences, New Delhi
Founder & Chief Organiser : Dr. Rajendra Prasad Centre for
Ophthalmic Sciences, A.I.I.M.S., New Delhi
Chief and Principal Eye Surgeon : A.I.I.M.S., New Delhi
Adviser Ophthalmology : Government of India
Examiner : National Board of Examinations
and
Formulator : National Programme for Prevention of
Visual Impairment and Control of Blindness

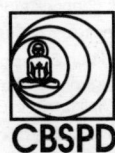

CBSPD

# CBS Publishers & Distributors Pvt Ltd

New Delhi • Bengaluru • Chennai • Kochi • Kolkata • Lucknow • Mumbai
Hyderabad • Jharkhand • Nagpur • Patna • Pune • Uttarakhand

Agarwal's Principles
of Optics &
Refraction
Fifth Edition

**ISBN:** 978-81-239-0604-1

Copyright © Author

**First Edition:** 1961

**Second Edition:** 1985

**Third Edition:** 1988
**Fourth Edition:** 1995
**Fifth Edition:** 1998
**Reprint:** 1999, 2003, 2004, 2005, 2006, 2008, 2009, 2010, 2012, 2013, 2015, 2016, 2019, 2023, 2024

Published by Satish Kumar Jain and produced by Varun Jain for

**CBS Publishers & Distributors** Pvt Ltd

4819/XI Prahlad Street, 24 Ansari Road, Daryaganj, New Delhi 110 002, India
Ph: 011-23289259, 23266861     Website: www.cbspd.com
                               e-mail: delhi@cbspd.com
*Corporate Office:* 204 FIE, Industrial Area, Patparganj, Delhi 110 092
Ph: 011-4934 4934     Fax: 011-4934 4935     e-mail: publishing@cbspd.com
                                              publicity@cbspd.com

**Branches**

• **Bengaluru:** Seema House 2975, 17th Cross, KR Road, Banasankari 2nd Stage, Bengaluru 560 070, Karnataka, India
  Ph: +91-80-26771678/79     Fax: +91-80-26771680     e-mail: bangalore@cbspd.com
• **Chennai:** 7, Subbaraya Street, Shenoy Nagar, Chennai 600 030, Tamil Nadu, India
  Ph: +91-44-26680620, 26681266     Fax: +91-44-42032115     e-mail: chennai@cbspd.com
• **Kochi:** 42/1325, 1326, Power House Road, Opp KSEB, Power House, Ernakulam 682 018, India
  Ph: +91-484-4059061–65     Fax: +91-484-4059065     e-mail: kochi@cbspd.com
• **Kolkata:** 147, Hind Ceramics Compound, 1st Floor, Nilgunj Road, Belghoria, Kolkata 700 056, West Bengal, India
  Ph: +91-9096713055/56     e-mail: kolkata@cbspd.com
• **Lucknow:** Basement, Khushnuma Complex, 7-Meerabai Marg (behind Jawahar Bhawan), Lucknow 226 001, India
  Ph: +91-522-4000032     e-mail: tiwari.lucknow@cbspd.com
• **Mumbai:** PWD Shed. Gala no. 25/26, Ramchandra Bhatt Marg, Next to JJ Hospital Gate no. 2, Opp. Union Bank of India Noorbaug Mumbai 400 009, Maharashtra, India
  Ph: +91-22-66661880/89     e-mail: mumbai@cbspd.com

*Representatives*

• **Hyderabad** 0-9885175004  • **Jharkhand** 0-9811541605  • **Nagpur** 0-8692091830
• **Patna** 0-9334159340  • **Pune** 0-9664372571  • **Uttarakhand** 0-9716462459

*Printed at* Glorious Printers, Delhi, India

*Respectfully dedicated to my father*

*Madhoram*

*whose sacrifice and guidance inspired me all through*
*and who is no more amongst us to inspire and guide*

*and to my mother*

*Smt. Kalavati*

*to whom I owe my very existence.*

# Preface to the Fifth Edition

The fourth edition of the book was published in 1995 and the fifth edition is coming out in 1998. The fifth edition is being renamed as 'Agarwal's Principles of Optics and Refraction'.

The book has been revised with addition of material on lasers, elaborating descriptions on several optical principles adding new diagrams to make the written matter more understandable. Use of cross cylinders and its optics have been given in greater details to enable the student to put them in practical use. Use of keratometers, their principles and optics have been revised. To the description of auto-refractors has been added some relevant material.

Some classifications have been tabulated before their descriptions, e.g., classification of aniso-metropia, aniseikonia, anomalies of accommodation, components of convergence. Convergence in-sufficiency has also been tabulated.

At several places in ocular motility diseases, convergence, accommodation, etc. more details have been added including anatomical and physiological. Classification of squint has been tabulated.

Material has been added in the chapter of contact lenses to make it more lucid.

Low vision aid still poses a problem. Considerably more material has been added in this chapter. Malingering is becoming more common with increasing industrialisation of the country. In view of this, information with regard to malingering tests is included in this edition.

The book has been so thoroughly revised that it has become quite comprehensive; though the style of presentation has been preserved.

Lalit P. Agarwal

Several illustrations have been reproduced from other books and these are gratefully acknowledged.

1. Phyllis L Rakow : Contact Lenses
2. Sanders and Goldberg : Peyman's Principles and Practice of Ophthalmology
3. Stein HA, Slatt BJ, Stein RM : The Ophthalmic Assistant
4. Berliner ML, Miller SJH : Biomicroscopy of the Eye, vol. II
5. Parsons' Diseases of the Eye, 17th ed.
6. Abrams I David : Duke-Elder's Practice of Refraction
7. Duke-Elder's Systems of Ophthalmology, vol. V, Optics & Refraction

# Preface to the First Edition

Often I felt a great need for a simple book on the principles of optics and refraction during my student career and later as a teacher of postgraduate students. There are several books on the subject. There are some books which are simple but do not deal with the subject fully and there are others which are rather elaborate and complex for the purpose. In some of these, the mathematical calculations are more subjective than objective which makes it difficult to understand the fundamentals and to make logical deductions therefrom. The reader is, therefore, at a loss to understand the subject and its underlying meaning. Complex mathematical calculations, in others, overawe a postgraduate student. In India and several other countries, where students enter the medical faculty with an inadequate knowledge of the elementary principles of trigonometry and other equally important sections of mathematics, it becomes difficult for the students to grasp fully the mathematical processes. An effort has, therefore, been made in this book to clearly explain the elementary principles of optics and to introduce adequate, though not complex, mathematical calculations in such a way that they are easy to follow for an average postgraduate medical student and permit him to understand the derivations without taxing his memory.

The book is primarily meant for students going in for a postgraduate degree or diploma. Many students in the Asian countries find it difficult to understand and follow the books written by Western authors. The book has according been written in simple English as it is spoken and understood by the people in these countries. It is an amplification of the class notes and lectures the author delivers to the graduate students. The subject has been simplified and practical hints have been added to make the book useful for a practitioner in ophthalmology. Refraction is not only a science but it is also an art in its practice which requires tact and patience in execution. An attempt has been made to present the subject in this perspective in this book.

The book has been divided into seven sections and 27 chapters. It has been adequately illustrated. Some of the illustrations, though elementary, have been included in the book to make the subject lucid and understandable. A chapter each on 'contact lenses' and 'aids to the visually handicapped' has been included in this book to indicate to the practitioners and students that much can be done to alleviate human suffering in cases which are seemingly hopeless.

A section on 'muscular anomalies' and 'orthoptics and pleoptics' has been added as the author feels that refraction work is incomplete without an assessment of muscular balance and uniocular and binocular functions. The short note on the therapy of muscular imbalance will give the students an insight into the principles of tackling problems of muscular imbalances. The general principles of the fascinating subject of pleoptics have also been described. This will give the readers an idea of the hope that the future holds for the improvement of visual functions in those who were so far considered to be incurable.

The book is not a complete treatise but only enunciates the principles of the subject. It may be said that the art of refraction and its theory and practice cannot be learnt by any treatise on the subject but can only be acquired by long and patient practice. If the book helps in making the principles involved in the art and science of the refraction simple to understand to the readers it would have served its purpose.

I acknowledge with thanks the kind courtesy of Dr. B.B. Dikshit, Director and other authorities of the All India Institute of Medical Sciences for according me permission to publish this book. I am grateful to Dr. S.R.K. Malik for writing the chapters on 'contact lenses' and 'visual aids for the visually handicapped', Dr. Madan Mohan for writing the chapter on 'principles of therapy of squint' and Dr. Prem Khosla for assisting me in writing the chapters on 'accommodation' and 'convergence'. These chapters have been fully edited and parts rewritten by me. I am grateful to Drs. S.P. Dhir, A.K. Gupta and P.R. Karwal for helping me in many other ways. I express my appreciation for the work of M/s Hylite Halftone Corporation, Delhi in the excellent preparation of the blocks. I take this opportunity of expressing my gratitude to my artist Mr. Umashankar for his untiring work in the preparation of the drawings of this book. My publishers deserve all the gratitude for their ungrudging cooperation and manifold guidance besides technical excellence in publishing this book. I also thank M/s Albion Press, Delhi for the printing of this book.

I wish to record my grateful thanks to my junior colleagues in the department for their cooperation and help.

I wish also to place on record my deep sense of gratitude to Mr. R.C. Davenport and Dr. Dukhan Ram who have always inspired and guided me.

I am grateful to Mr. K.P. Agarwal for his excellent suggestions in improving the language of the manuscript.

Last but not the least I am thankful to my wife Dr. (Mrs.) Savitri Agarwal who always encouraged me whenever I felt despondent.

15th October, 1961                                                                                    Lalit P. Agarwal

# Contributing Author

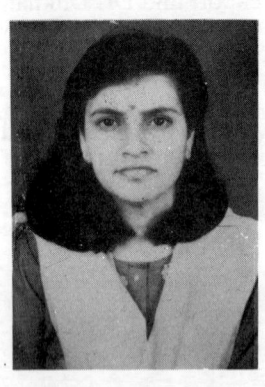

**Dr. Namrata Sharma**

She passed her M.D. examination in December 1992 and Diplomate National Board in May 1993. She joined the speciality of Cornea as a post-doctoral fellow (Senior Resident) in 1993 for three years and acquired experience in cornea and lens surgery.

She demonstrated an extraordinary skill and purpose towards the patient care and actively participated in various eye surgery camps. She has successfully completed numerous research projects and has published papers, reviews and chapters in various journals and books. She has exhibited particular interest in optics and refraction. She has published over 50 articles, review papers and original research papers in various national and international journals.

She received Col. Rangachari Award for best paper presentation at All India Ophthalmic Society (AIOS) in 1993. The American Society of Contemporary Ophthalmology conferred upon her the CME credit award of the year 1995. Dr. Namrata is a life-member of AIOS. She was admitted to the Council as a member of National Academy of Medical Sciences (India) in 1993. She had attended and participated in the World Congress on Cornea, held in Orlando, Florida, USA in April 1996.

Dr. Namrata has a keen interest in academic ophthalmology and has demonstrated in-depth knowledge and extraordinary understanding of optics and refraction.

She has contributed as author the material on the autorefractors and the keratometers.

# Contents

# SECTION I

# Physical Optics

# CHAPTER 1

# Properties of Light

Light is a form of energy. It has a dual nature—particle and wave. Light can pass through media as well as vacuum. It behaves like a corpuscle (photon) and can, therefore, pass through vacuum and behaves like a wave when it passes through media.

The media through which light passes totally and almost undisturbed are termed transparent. Those which cause hindrance in its passage are called translucent and those which do not allow it to pass are called opaque.

It behaves like a particle (photon) as an individual characteristic when it is created or destroyed and like an electromagnetic wave when as a group it propagates through space. A series of waves makes up the energy spectrum consisting of cosmic rays, electronic rays, gamma rays, x-rays, ultraviolet rays, the visible rays (consisting of violet, indigo, blue, green, yellow, orange and red), the infrared rays, the wireless rays (short and long), and the slow electromagnetic oscillations (Fig. 1.1 and Table 1.1).

The electromagnetic spectrum of visible light has wavelengths varying roughly between 400 and 800 nanometres (a nanometre is a billionth, i.e., 1/1,000,000,000 of a metre). Light is a very special form of electromagnetic energy. When it falls on retina it causes reactions included under the term of photobiology.

**Table 1.1. Wavelength of different rays**

| Type of rays | Wavelength |
|---|---|
| 1. Cosmic rays | $4 \times 10^{-5}$ nm |
| 2. Electronic rays | $2.7 \times 10^{-4}$ nm |
| 3. Gamma rays | $6 \times 10^{-3}$ nm to 0.14 nm |
| 4. X-rays | 0.14 to 13.6 nm |
| 5. Ultraviolet rays | 13.6 to 379 nm |
| 6. Visible rays | 397 to 723 nm |
| (a) Violet | 397 to 424 nm |
| (b) Indigo | 424 to 455 nm |
| (c) Blue | 455 to 492 nm |
| (d) Green | 492 to 575 nm |
| (e) Yellow | 575 to 585 nm |
| (f) Orange | 585 to 647 nm |
| (g) Red | 647 to 723 nm |
| 7. Infrared rays | 723 to $1 \times 10^5$ nm |
| 8. Wireless rays (Hertzian rays) | $1 \times 10^5$ to $3 \times 10^{13}$ nm |
| (a) Short | $1 \times 10^5$ to $1 \times 10^{10}$ nm |
| (b) Long | $1 \times 10^{10}$ to $3 \times 10^{13}$ nm |
| 9. Electromagnetic oscillations | Over $3 \times 10^{13}$ nm |

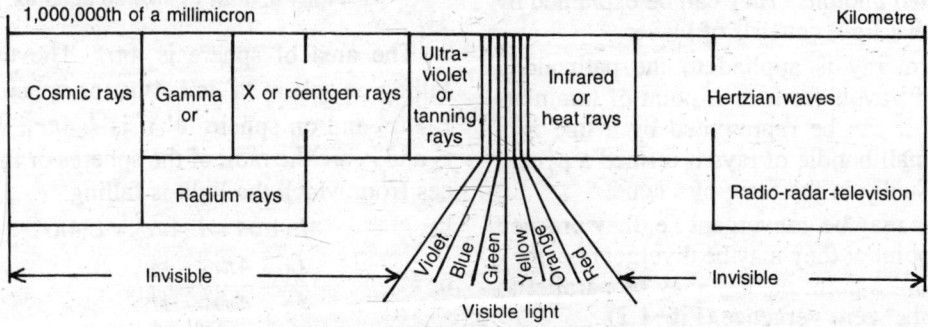

**Fig. 1.1.** Electromagnetic spectrum.

Photobiological process occurs when light is absorbed by certain chemicals in the retina. It produces mechanical, chemical and electrical changes.

These changes stimulate certain highly specialised cells which produce nerve impulses. These produce perception of light, colour, form, size and motion.

Visible light is an agent which by its action on the retina excites a sensation of vision. When some objects are visible in the absence of all sources of light, they are called self-luminous, e.g., a luminous paint, glowworm, a lighted match-stick, a lighted candle, the sun, etc. There are other objects which are nonluminous and can only become visible by the light received from luminous objects and returned to the eyes.

## Propagation of light

There are several theories to explain the propagation of light amongst which the wave theory is the most satisfactory. It envisages that from the propagating source there are set in motion waves of light which pass in various directions. Thus the light emitted from a luminous body is supposed to travel in a homogeneous medium in all directions and in straight lines.

## Photon

Light may, therefore, be considered to be a stream of particles when it interacts with matter. An example is the liberation of photons from a metal surface by light, called the photoelectric effect. For a complete explanation it should be assumed that light consists of small bundles of energy called photons. They can be explained by assuming that light consists of waves.

The term ray is applied to the path along which light travels from each point of luminous object and it can be represented by a line in a plane. A small bundle of rays is termed a pencil, which is usually in the form of a cone.

The rays may be convergent i.e. they proceed towards a point or they may be divergent i.e. proceed from a point or they may be parallel to each other i.e. zero vergence (Fig. 1.2).

The light travels in all directions and as such the intensity of light rapidly diminishes as the

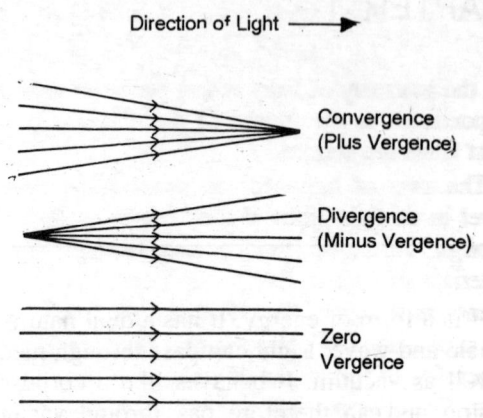

Direction of Light ⟶

Convergence (Plus Vergence)

Divergence (Minus Vergence)

Zero Vergence

**Fig. 1.2.** Vergence of rays.

distance of the point from the source increases. The intensity obeys the *Law of Inverse Squares*.

In Fig. 1.3, let $L_1$, $L_2$ and $L_3$ be the amount of light falling per second on unit area of each sphere. The total light falling on each sphere is equal.

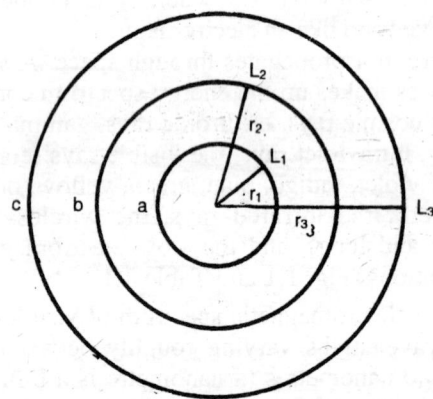

**Fig. 1.3.** Law of inverse squares.

The area of sphere is $4\pi r^2$. The total light falling on sphere 'a' is $L_1 4\pi r_1^2$, on sphere 'b' it is $L_2 4\pi r_2^2$ and on sphere 'c' it is $L_3 4\pi r_3^2$, where $r_1$, $r_2$ and $r_3$ are the radii of the spheres or the distances from which the light is falling.

i.e.
$$L_1 4\pi r_1^2 = L_2 4\pi r_2^2 = L_3 4\pi r_3^2$$

or
$$\frac{L_1}{L_2} = \frac{4\pi r_2^2}{4\pi r_1^2} = \frac{r_2^2}{r_1^2}$$

or
$$\frac{L_1}{L_3} = \frac{4\pi r_3^2}{4\pi r_1^2} = \frac{r_3^2}{r_1^2}$$

or
$$\frac{L_2}{L_3} = \frac{4\pi r_3^2}{4\pi r_2^2} = \frac{r_3^2}{r_2^2}$$

i.e., the intensity of light at any point is inversely proportional to the square of the distance of the point from the source.

The rays of light, for all practical purposes, travel in straight lines if they travel in space or through isotropic media and non-absorbing materials like glass. Every point on each ray represents an image of the point of light from which it is propagated. We have in this phenomenon the principles of formation of images of various objects. The commonest way to indicate it is the pinhole box camera. The image formed is an inverted image.

Take a cardboard box which can be opened from above. In one of its panels make a pinpoint hole and place a burning candle in front of it at some distance.

A dim and inverted image of the flame (Fig. 1.4) of this candle can be seen on the opposite panel. All the rays except those passing through the pinpoint hole are cut off. The rays passing

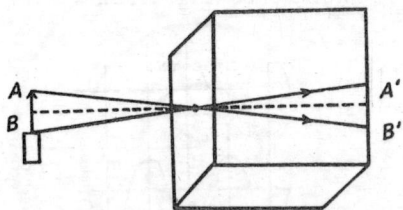

**Fig. 1.4.** Rectilinear propagation of light (one hole).

from the bottom of the flame only reach the top portion of the panel where the image is formed, the rays from the top only reach the bottom and the intermediate rays occupy the intermediate area thus forming the whole image which is inverted. If several holes are made away from each other, several such images can be obtained (Fig. 1.5).

If the holes are near each other the images overlap and the final picture is blurred (Fig. 1.6) but if the hole is very large many rays pass into the box and illuminate it without forming any definite image.

If an opaque object comes in the path of the rays, coming from a luminous source of a small

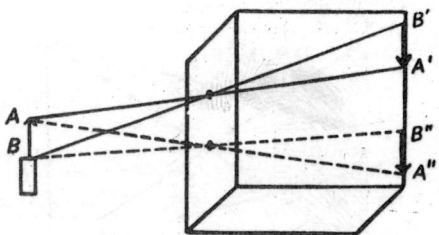

**Fig. 1.5.** Rectilinear propagation of light (two holes wide apart).

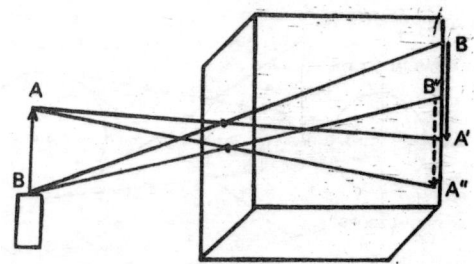

**Fig. 1.6.** Rectilinear propagation of light (two holes near each other).

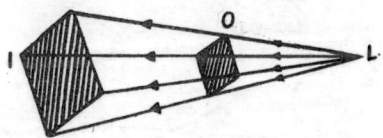

**Fig. 1.7.** Formation of shadow.

size, a shadow is formed. In Fig. 1.7, L is the small luminous source and O an opaque object. The rays emanating from L are intercepted at O. I is the shadow of O at the screen placed here. If the source of light is bigger than the opaque object each point of source throws a shadow cone. The area common to each shadow cone is entirely free from light. The conical space which receives no light is termed the umbra. The surrounding area which is partially in shadow is termed the penumbra.

In Fig. 1.8, LL′ is the big source of illumination, OO′ the opaque object and XY the screen. II′ is the area where no light falls on the screen and is termed the umbra, while areas XI and YI′ receive part of the light and are called penumbra.

The observation of solar and lunar eclipse is based on the same principle (Figs. 1.9 and 1.10).

## Interference

One of the most dramatic phenomena in physical

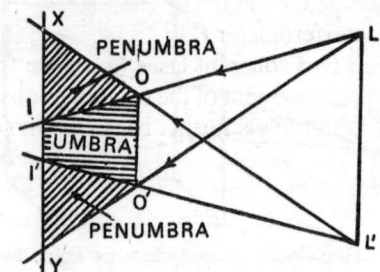

**Fig. 1.8.** Umbra and penumbra.

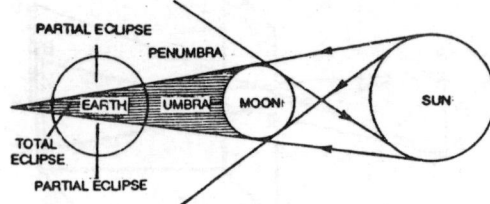

**Fig. 1.9.** Solar eclipse.

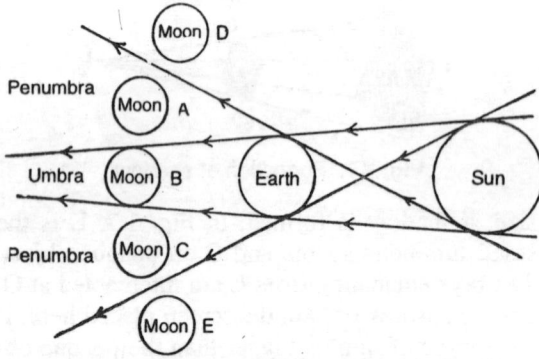

**Fig. 1.10.** Lunar eclipse.

optics is interference. It is governed by Huygens' principle. When waves pass through an aperture or past the edge of an obstacle, they always spread to some extent into the region which is not directly exposed to the oncoming waves. The phenomenon is called diffraction. In order to explain the phenomenon, Huygens proposed the rule that each point on wavefront may be regarded as a new source of waves. When two waves of the same wavelength interact, one of the three things may happen :

1. Summation of the two waves if their maxima and minima correspond with each other, i.e., zero or full wavelength of phase difference.

This is termed as constructive interference, where the resulting amplitude is the sum of amplitudes of the two waves (Fig. 1.11).

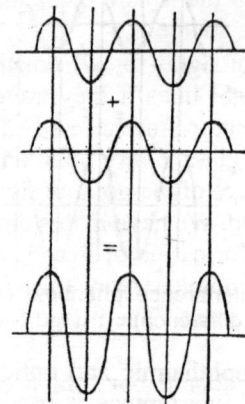

**Fig. 1.11.** Interference phenomenon in light waves (full wavelength difference—constructive interference).

2. When the maxima of one correspond with the minima of the other (half-phase difference) the amplitude of the resulting wave in this case is zero. This is termed as destructive interference (Fig. 1.12).

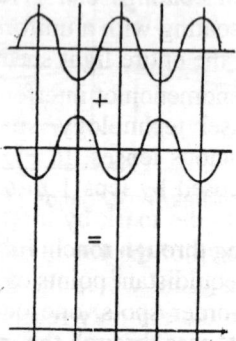

**Fig. 1.12.** Interference phenomenon in light waves (half phase difference—destructive interference).

3. When there is 1/8th phase difference the sum is a wave of the same wavelength but different phase and amplitude (Fig. 1.13).

Whenever two rays vibrate with a constant phase difference, a stationary interference pattern is produced. Two sources which vibrate with a fixed phase difference between them are said to be coherent.

These optical phenomena are now being used

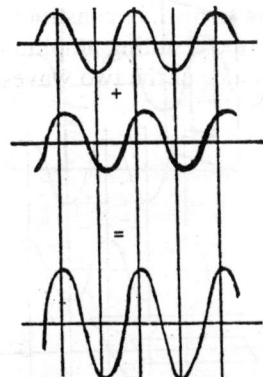

**Fig. 1.13.** Interference phenomenon in light waves (1/8th phase difference).

in various ophthalmic and optical devices. The principle of interference is used to design anti-reflection coatings for good quality lenses to decrease unwanted reflections. The coating materials available are all imperfect in as much as the index of refraction of the coating material required does not match with the index of refraction of material used for lenses to be coated. To obviate this difficulty multiple coating of different coating materials is employed. Systematic use of such coatings can give rise to an anti-reflection coating with a uniform and low reflection across the entire light spectrum.

The phenomenon of interference is used clinically in laser technology, specially in patients with cataractous lenses. In Fig. 1.14, light from laser is focused by lens 1 through pinhole, then imaged onto the mask by a second lens (lens 2) after passing through ronchi ruling, which creates numerous equidistant points of light on the mask. Only first-order spots, one on each side of the centre spot, pass through the mask through dove prism and are focused onto the eye by a third lens (lens 3). The dove prism rotates image to check

whether patient can tell orientation of stripes. Laser interferometer (Fig. 1.14) is an instrument in which two coherent laser lights are focused in the anterior segment of the eye under observation. As the light travels further back into the eye these points diverge and interfere with each other resulting in alternating light and dark fringe pattern falling on the retina of the observed eye. The fringe thickness and the separation between the fringes are both inversely proportional to the distance between the two pinpoints of light. These are altered as the distances between the points are changed. By judiciously altering these one can produce fringes separated by distance equivalent to standard visual acuities directly on the observed retina.

With its use it may be possible to predict the post-operative visual expectancy of the patient of cataract.

The second important use of the knowledge is in holography. It is a highly technical method and is used to take pictures of living eye. The image of eye at various levels can be seen.

## POLARIZATION

### Polarization of transverse waves

Let a rope AB be passed through two parallel slits $S_1$ and $S_2$. The rope is attached to a fixed point at B (Fig. 1.15). Hold the end A and move the rope up and down perpendicular to AB. A wave emerges along CD and it is due to transverse vibrations parallel to $S_1$. It is observed that the slit $S_2$ does not allow the wave to pass through it when it is at right angles to the slit $S_1$ (Fig. 1.16).

If the end A is moved in a circular manner the rope will show circular motion up to the slit $S_1$. Beyond $S_1$, it will show only linear vibrations parallel to slit $S_1$ because the slit $S_1$ will stop the other components. If $S_1$ and $S_2$ are at right angles

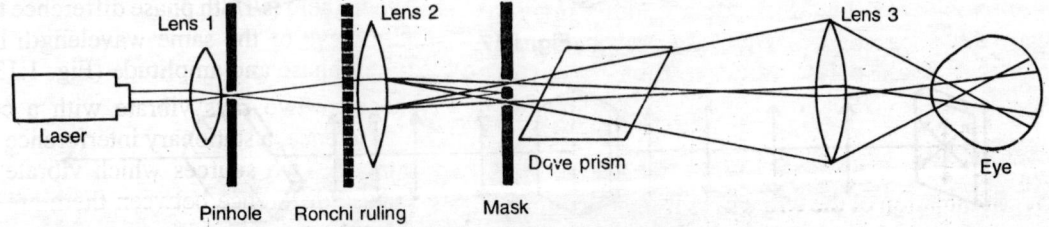

**Fig. 1.14.** Laser interferometer.

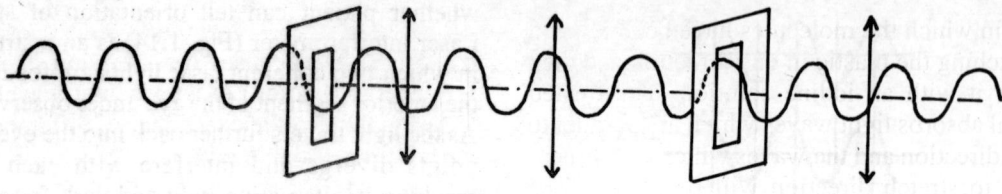

Fig. 1.15.

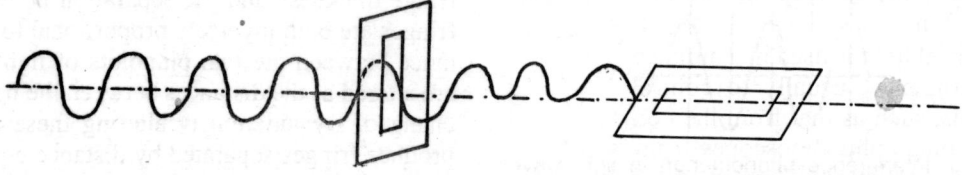

Fig. 1.16.

to each other the rope will not show any vibration beyond S₂.

If longitudinal waves are set up by moving the rope forward and backward along the string, the waves will pass through $S_1$ and $S_2$ irrespective of their position. A similar phenomenon has been observed in light when it passes through a tourmaline crystal.

Let light from a source S fall on a tourmaline crystal A which is cut parallel to its axis (Figs. 1.17 and 1.18). The crystal A will act as slit $S_1$. On rotating the crystal A, no remarkable change is noticed. Now place the crystal B parallel to A.

1. Rotate both crystals together so that their axes are parallel. No change is observed in the light coming out at B (Fig. 1.17).

2. Keep crystal A fixed and rotate crystal B. The light transmitted through B becomes dimmer and dimmer. When B is at right angles to A no light emerges out of B (Fig. 1.18).

3. If the crystal B is further rotated, the intensity of light coming out of it gradually increases and is maximum again when two crystals are parallel.

The light coming out of crystal A is said to be polarized because it has acquired the property of one-sidedness.

If a number of light waves are travelling in the same direction their electric fields may or may not be parallel to each other. If there is a random mixture of orientations of the electric field, the light is non-polarized. However, if all the electric fields are in the same direction the light is linearly polarized. This can be easily achieved by passing the unpolarized light through a sheet of polarizing material.

The principle of this mechanism is to use a

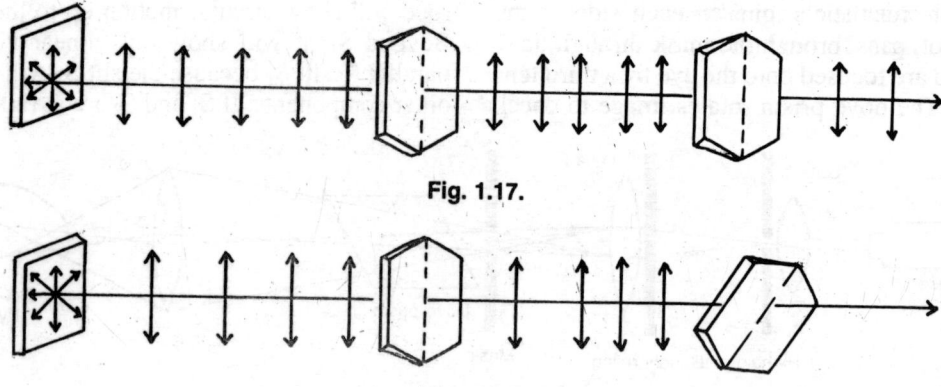

Fig. 1.17.

Fig. 1.18.

plastic in which the molecules have been aligned by stretching the plastic in one direction and then treating it with an iodine solution. The treated material absorbs light waves which are parallel to stretch direction and the waves which are perpendicular to stretch direction will be passed. The transmitted beam, therefore, becomes plane polarized. This is seen in Haidinger's brush phenomenon.

Polarized light is used in a number of ophthalmic instruments, usually to control unwanted reflections, such as that from the cornea. This is used in some ophthalmoscopes from which disturbing corneal image is removed.

## LASER

Laser is a device which converts electric energy to light energy emerging as a monochromatic coherent light that can be directed to a desired target. The emitted light is a radiational energy in the nature of monochromatic light, the colour and wavelength of which depends upon the substance in which the electric energy is passed.

The basic principle of laser is that molecules of any substance oscillate and emit light at a certain frequency. A highly concentrated form of light can be coaxed out if the substance is stimulated with energy. The coaxed light is laser. The classical theory on atomic energy elucidates that each electronic orbital is spaced by a definite energy interval. Substance which has the ability to lase has the unique property of transferring electrons from one orbital of lower energy to a second metastable orbit of higher energy (Fig. 1.15), they may suddenly jump to a lower energy level which was their original energy level. This jump from original orbital (lower energy level) to

metastable orbital (higher energy level) and back to original level causes the emission of a new light energy (photon) of a particular wavelength corresponding to the exact energy difference between the metastable orbital to the original orbital. It is coherent because all electrons jump at the same time and thus form a light wave which begins at the same time and is, therefore, at the same place. The light then oscillates back and forth within the laser cavity [tube with a mirror at either end; one mirror is highly reflective and the other mirror allows source laser light to pass through for use (in the eye)]. Because the light is oscillating back and forth within a long tube, it tends to produce a beam of almost parallel rays of light and hardly any or low divergence (collimated).

The need in laser therapy is to further concentrate the laser light into a small time interval such as by quality switching (Q-switching) which may be active (Q-switching) or passive (Mode-locking). The active Q-switching is performed by an acoustic-optical crystal (Fig. 1.16).

The commonly used lasers are classified in Table 1.2.

**Table 1.2. Commonly used ophthalmic lasers**

| Type | Material | Wavelength (nm) |
|---|---|---|
| Thermal photocoagulative | Argon | 488-514 |
| | Argon/Krypton | 488-514 |
| | Krypton | 647 |
| | Dye lasers | 575 |
| Photodisruptive | Nd-YAG | 1064 |
| | Erbium-YAG | 2940 |
| Photoablators | Excimer | 193 |

# CHAPTER 2

# Principles of Reflection of Light

When a ray of light meets any surface, a part of the incident light is absorbed, a part is refracted and a part is reflected back. If the surface is smooth and polished most of the incident light is reflected back. The reflection of light obeys certain laws.

### Laws of reflection

1. The incident ray, the normal to the surface at the point of incidence and the reflected ray lie in one plane.
2. The incident ray and the reflected ray are equally inclined to and lie on the opposite sides of the normal (Fig. 2.1). This implies that the angle which the incident ray makes with the normal (angle INO) is equal to the angle which the reflected ray makes at the same point with the normal (angle of reflection ONR).

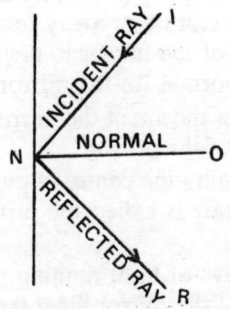

**Fig. 2.1.** Laws of reflection.

Generally three types of mirrors can be used in optical instruments—plane, concave and convex.

### Plane mirrors

The plane mirrors reflect the light in a way that the reflected rays are divergent, hence, they do not form a real image.

In Fig. 2.2, let I be an object situated in front of a plane mirror AB. The incident ray IN, obeying the laws of reflection, is reflected along NR. The incident ray IN' is likewise reflected along

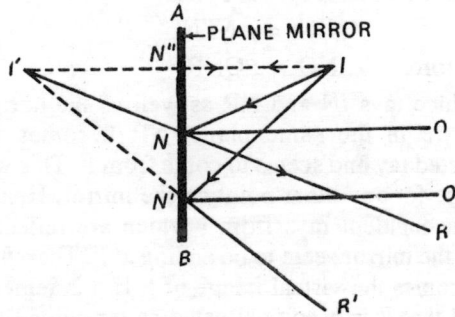

**Fig. 2.2.** Image of the object in plane mirror.

N'R'. The reflected rays NR and N'R' are divergent, hence, they cannot meet in front of the mirror. The rays seem to emanate from a virtual point I' situated behind the mirror. IN" is normal at N". The distance N"I is equal to the distance N"I'. This shows that the image in a plane mirror is virtual and is situated as far behind the mirror as the object is in front of it. This can also be geometrically proved.

In Fig. 2.3, let I be the object and I' a point as far behind the mirror as the object is in front, i.e., I'N' = IN', the line II' being perpendicular to AB. Let IN be the incident ray at N and ON be the normal. Join I'N and produce it to R. By construction, IN, NR and ON are in the same plane.

In two triangles IN'N and I'N'N, IN' = I'N'. Angles IN'N and I'N'N are equal both being right angles and the side NN' is common. The two triangles are, therefore, congruent i.e., equal in all

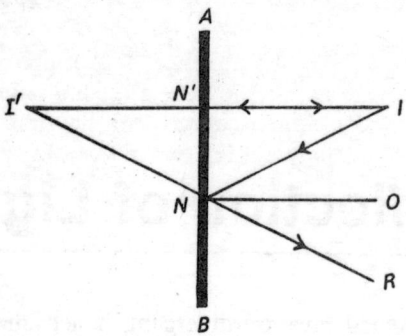

**Fig. 2.3.** Proving that I' is the image of object I.

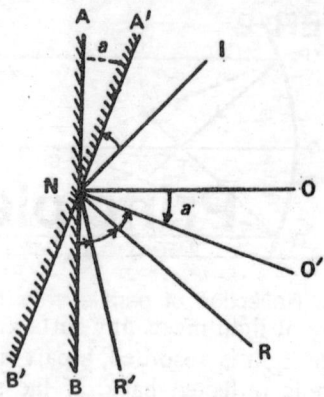

**Fig. 2.4.** Deflection of reflected ray with movement of plane mirror.

respects. Therefore, angle NIN' is equal to angle NI'N'. Since IN' is parallel to ON, $\angle$NIN' = $\angle$INO.

| | |
|---|---|
| Since | $\angle$NI'N = $\angle$ONR |
| and | $\angle$NIN' = $\angle$NI'N' |
| therefore, | $\angle$INO = $\angle$ONR. |

Since rays IN and NR as well as the normal ON are in the same plane, NR becomes the reflected ray and seems to come from I'. This will be true for any other point on the mirror. Hence, all the incident rays from I which are reflected from the mirror seem to be ending at I'. Therefore I' becomes the virtual image of I. If it is remembered that I' is a point situated as far behind the mirror as I is in front, it can be surmised that in plane mirrors the image is situated as far behind as the object is in front. It would be proved later that the size of the image is calculated by the formula :

$$I = \frac{v}{u}$$

where $v$ is the distance of the image from reflecting surface, $u$ is the distance of the object from the reflecting surface and $I$ is the size of the image. By this formula the size of the image in plane mirrors is equal to the size of the object, since the distance of the image from the mirror is the same as the distance of the object.

It may be concluded that in plane mirrors the image is virtual, equal in size and is situated as far behind as the object is in front of it.

If the mirror is turned through an angle, the reflected ray also turns, but it turns through twice that angle (Fig. 2.4). The reflected ray is turned through angle RNR'.

$$\angle RNR' = \angle INR' - \angle INR$$
$$= 2\angle INO' - 2\angle INO$$
$$= 2\angle(INO' - INO)$$
$$= 2\angle(ONO' \text{ or } ANA')$$
$$= 2a.$$

where 'a' is the angle through which the mirror turns.

**Special mirrors**

The laws of reflection are equally applicable to polished surfaces having the form of a portion of a sphere. These mirrors are termed spherical mirrors. They may be concave or convex depending upon whether the polished surface is towards the centre of curvature or away from it. Any line joining the arc of the mirror to the centre of curvatures is the normal for the mirror.

The centre of the arc of the mirror is called the pole or vertex of the mirror.

The line joining the centre of curvature to the pole of the mirror is called the principal axis of the mirror.

When the rays of light running parallel to the principal axis of the mirror meet the mirror, they are reflected back or seem to be reflected back on the same point on the principal axis (Figs. 2.5 and 2.6).

In Fig. 2.5, which deals with the reflection of light in concave mirrors, O is the pole of the mirror, C the centre of curvature and CO is the principal axis. Rays AP and BQ, which are parallel to CO, meet the surface of the mirror at P and Q, respectively. CP and CQ are normals to the

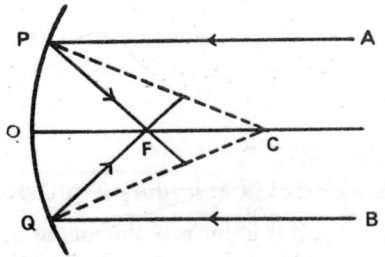

**Fig. 2.5.** Reflection of parallel rays in a concave mirror.

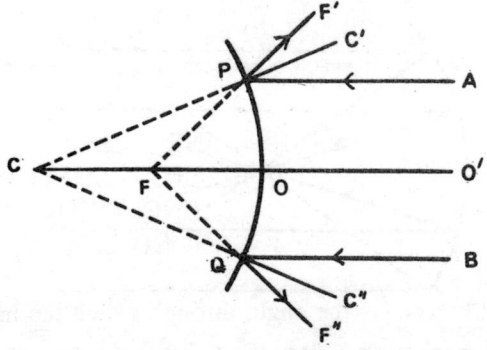

**Fig. 2.6.** Reflection of parallel rays in a convex mirror.

concave mirror at P and Q. Ray AP forms an angle of incidence APC and is reflected along PF making the angle of reflection CPF which is equal to angle APC. Similarly the ray BQ forms an angle of incidence BQC and is reflected along QF making an equal angle of reflection CQF. Both the reflected rays meet at F. If other rays parallel to CO are examined they will show similar behaviour. The point F at which these reflected rays will meet, when the incident rays are parallel to the principal axis CO, is called the focal point. This point is situated on the principal axis.

In convex mirrors the reflected rays do not actually meet at the focal point but seem to meet there (Fig. 2.6).

In Fig. 2.6, a ray parallel to the principal axis COO' of the convex mirror meets it at P forming an angle of incidence APC'. It is reflected along C'PF' since CPC' is normal. Similarly the ray BQ is reflected along QF''. The rays PF' and QF'' are divergent and seem to meet at F which is then the focus of the convex mirror.

The distance of the focal point from the pole of the mirror is termed the focal length of the mirror.

A pencil of rays diverging from a point on the principal axis of a spherical mirror converges to or appears to diverge from a second point on the axis is the geometrical image of the first. A point and its geometrical image are interchangeable in position and are spoken of as *conjugate foci*.

When distances are measured in a direction opposite to the incident ray they are termed positive and when they are measured in the same direction they are designated as negative. The pole of the mirror is the fixed point used for all these measurements. The focal length and the radius of curvature are positive in concave mirrors (Fig. 2.7) and are negative in convex mirrors (Fig. 2.8).

In Fig. 2.7, AC which is the radius of curvature is measured in opposite direction to the incident ray; hence, it is positive ($+r$), while in Fig. 2.8 it is measured in the direction of the incident

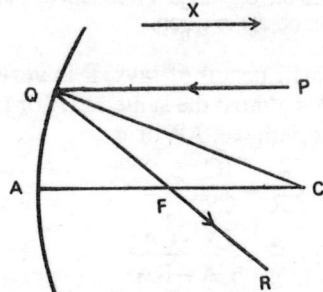

**Fig. 2.7.** Measurement of various distances from the concave mirror in the direction of the arrow (X) i.e. opposite to the direction of incident ray.

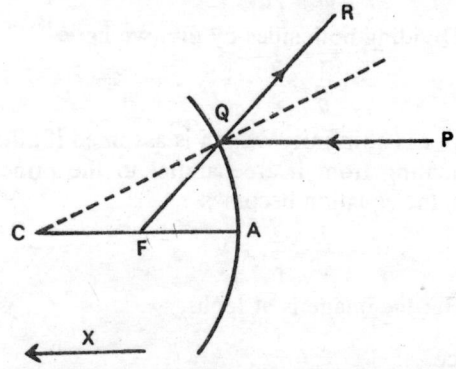

**Fig. 2.8.** Measurement of various distances from the convex mirror in the direction of the arrow (X) i.e., in the direction of the incident ray.

ray, hence, it is negative (–r). Similarly the focal length f in Fig. 2.7 is positive (+f) and in Fig. 2.8 it is negative (–f).

## Position of image

In Fig. 2.9, I is the object and R is the image, C is the centre of curvature, the distance IA = u, RA = v and CA = r. In this figure ∠IPC = ∠CPR according to the theorem of proportions.

$$\frac{IP}{PR} = \frac{IC}{CR}$$

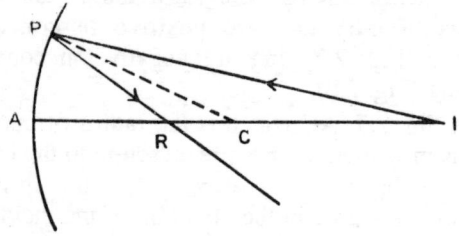

**Fig. 2.9.** Position of image in concave mirror if the position of the object is given.

But in small pencil of rays, P is very near to A so that IP is almost the same as IA or u and PR is almost the same as AR or v.

Hence,  $\dfrac{IA}{AR} = \dfrac{IC}{CR}$

or  $\dfrac{u}{v} = \dfrac{IA - CA}{CA - RA}$

or  $\dfrac{u}{v} = \dfrac{u - r}{r - v}$

or  $ur - uv = uv - vr$

or  $ur + vr = 2uv$

Dividing both sides by uvr, we have

$$\frac{1}{v} + \frac{1}{u} = \frac{2}{r}$$

If u is at infinity, which is assumed if all rays emanating from it are parallel to the principal axis, the equation becomes

$$\frac{1}{v} = \frac{2}{r}$$

But the image is at focus,

hence  $\dfrac{1}{v} = \dfrac{1}{f}$

or  $\dfrac{1}{f} = \dfrac{2}{r}$

i.e., the focal length is half of the radius of curvature. With the enunciation of these principles geometrical construction of images is not difficult.

## Images in concave mirrors

### When the object is at infinity (Fig. 2.10)

When the object is at infinity the image is formed at the focus. The rays coming from infinity are supposed to run parallel to the axis of the mirror. The image is real and pinpoint.

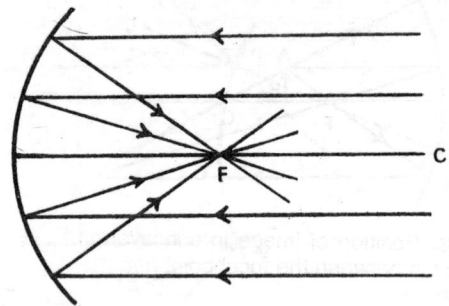

**Fig. 2.10.** Position of image in concave mirror when the object is at infinity.

### When the object is between the centre of curvature and infinity (Fig. 2.11)

In Fig. 2.11, the object is AB. The ray AP, parallel to the principal axis, is reflected back as PA′ passing through the focal point at F and ray AQ passing through the centre of curvature C strikes the surface as normal and is reflected back along its own path. The ray AR passing through the focal point F is reflected back parallel to the principal axis as RA′. Thus A′ is the image of A. Similarly B′ is the image of B so that A′B′ becomes the image of AB. The image is seen to be situated between the focal point and the centre of curvature. It is real, inverted and is diminished in

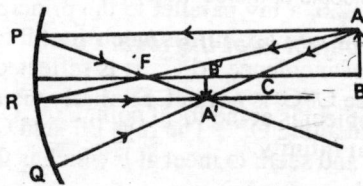

**Fig. 2.11.** Position of image in concave mirror when the object is between the centre of curvature and infinity.

size. In this case, $u$ is greater than $v$ and the magnification of an image is determined by the formula $v/u = I$, where $I$ represents the size of the image.

### When the object is between the centre of curvature and the focal point (Fig. 2.12)

The image formed is between the centre of curvature and infinity. It is real, inverted and magnified since $u$ is less than $v$.

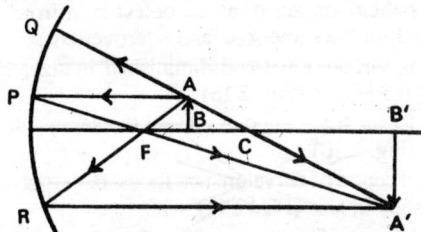

**Fig. 2.12.** Position of image in concave mirror when the object is between the focal point and the centre of curvature.

### When the object is at the centre of curvature (Fig. 2.13)

When the object is at the centre of curvature the image is formed at the same place but inverted. It is real and of equal size since $u$ is equal to $v$.

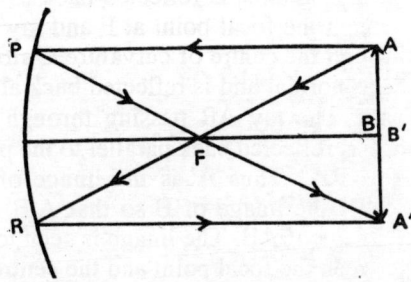

**Fig. 2.13.** Position of the image in concave mirror when the object is at the centre of curvature.

### When the object is at the focal point (Fig. 2.14)

When the object is at the focal point F, real image is formed at infinity.

### When the object is between the pole of the mirror and the focal point (Fig. 2.15)

The image is virtual, erect and magnified. It is

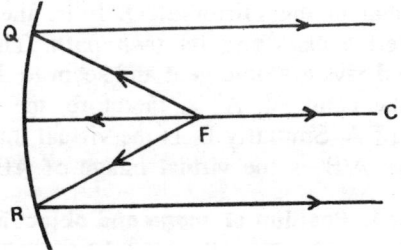

**Fig. 2.14.** Position of image in concave mirror when the object is at the focal point.

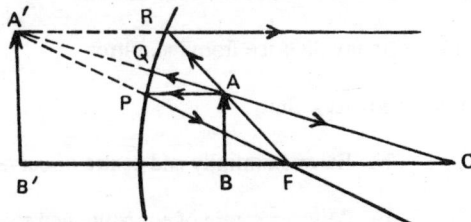

**Fig. 2.15.** Position of image in concave mirror when the object is between the focal point and the pole of mirror.

located behind the mirror. In this case, the reflected rays are divergent and cannot really meat but seem to meet.

### Convex mirrors

In case of convex mirror the image formed is virtual and erect and is diminished in size irrespective of the place of the object (Fig. 2.16).

In Fig. 2.16, AP is a ray running parallel to the principal axis. The ray is reflected along PF' and it seems as if this reflected ray is passing through the focal point F. AQ is the ray which seems to pass through the centre of curvature and

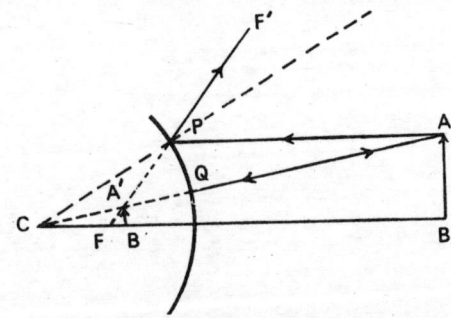

**Fig. 2.16.** Position of image of the object in convex mirror.

is normal to the mirror at Q. It is, therefore, reflected back along its own path. The two reflected rays are divergent and seem to diverge from the point A'. A' is, therefore, the virtual image of A. Similarly B' is the virtual image of B. Thus A'B' is the virtual image of AB. It is always diminished in size, $u$ is always greater than $v$. It is for this reason that convex mirrors are not used for ophthalmoscopic work.

Position of image with reference to the position of object in different types of mirrors is summarised in Table 2.1.

**Table 2.1. Position of image and object in different types of mirrors**

| Type of mirror | Object | | Image |
|---|---|---|---|
| Plane | At any distance from the mirror | | As far behind the mirror as the object is in front of it; it is virtual, of the same size, and lateroverted |
| Convex | At any distance from the mirror | | Image is virtual, erect and diminished in size; situated behind the mirror (Fig. 2.16) |
| Concave | (a) | At infinity | At the focus, real, pinpoint and on the same side of the mirror (Fig. 2.10) |
| | (b) | Between infinity and centre of curvature | Between centre of curvature and focus, real, inverted and diminished in size (Fig. 2.11) |
| | (c) | Between centre of curvature and focus | Beyond centre of curvature, on same side, real, inverted and enlarged (Fig. 2.12) |
| | (d) | At centre of curvature | At centre of curvature, same side, real, inverted and equal in size to the object (Fig. 2.13) |
| | (e) | At focus | At infinity, real (Fig. 2.14) |
| | (f) | Between focus and pole of mirror | Behind the mirror, virtual, magnified and erect (Fig. 2.15) |

# Principles of Refraction of Light

When a ray of light meets a denser medium even normally i.e. perpendicular to the surface, it meets with resistance and the velocity gets reduced. It emerges in the same direction (Fig. 3.1).

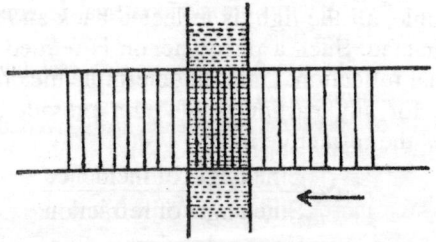

**Fig. 3.1.** Passage of light through a glass plate when the light strikes normally.

As already stated in Chapter 2 the undeviating straight line character of light rays in a homogeneous medium is altered when the rays strike an interface. If the ray continues its journey from one medium to another bending of this ray takes place, so that the new direction differs from the old. If the second medium is rarer than the first, the refracted ray is bent away from the normal and if the second medium is denser than the first it is bent towards the normal. Thus in the former case the angle of incidence is smaller than the angle of refraction i.e., the angle the bent ray makes with the normal (Fig. 3.2). In the latter case the angle of incidence is larger than the angle of refraction.

In Fig. 3.2, XY represents the interface between a rarer and a denser medium. AB is the normal to this interface. CD represents a ray of light travelling from the denser to the rarer medium. The refracted ray DE bends away from the normal. In the same figure FD represents a

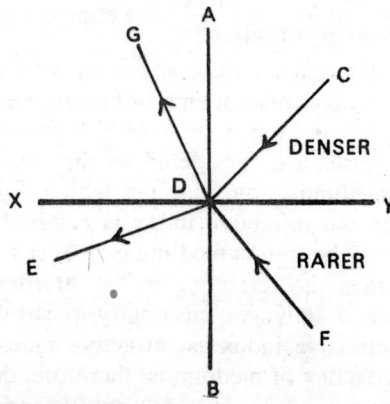

**Fig. 3.2.** Refraction of rays while passing from one medium to another.

ray travelling from rarer to the denser medium. The refracted ray DG bends towards the normal. Thus, in Fig. 3.2, angle ADC, i.e., angle of incidence, is smaller than angle BDE, i.e., angle of refraction when the light is travelling from the denser to a rarer medium. In the same figure angle BDF, i.e., the angle of incidence is larger than the angle ADG, i.e., the angle of refraction when the light is travelling from a rarer to a denser medium. If the surface XY is perpendicular to the paper then the incident rays CD and FD, the refracted rays DR and DG and the normal AB are all in the same plane. The behaviour of the incident ray while passing from one medium to another obeys certain laws which can be enunciated as under.

## Laws of refraction

1. The incident ray, the normal to the surface on the point of incidence and the refracted ray lie in one plane.
2. Sine angle of refraction at an optical surface

is proportional to the sine angle of incidence and to the ratio of the indices of refraction on either side of the surface.

This can also be expressed as a constant ratio which the sine of angle of incidence bears to the sine of angle of refraction. This ratio depends firstly on the nature of light and secondly on the nature of the two media. This can be mathematically represented as :

$$\frac{\text{Sine angle of incidence}}{\text{Sine angle of refraction}} = \text{a constant } (\mu)$$

This constant is termed as the refractive index which is a ratio and not an absolute figure. If the first medium is vacuum or air (which for all practical purposes are considered as the same) and second medium is one through which light can pass then the refractive index is referred to as absolute. If the former medium is neither vacuum nor air then the refractive index referred to is relative. It is, however, customary to call the absolute refractive index as refractive index. The refractive index of medium is, therefore, defined as the ratio between the sine angle of incidence in air or vacuum to the sine angle of refraction in the medium.

The bending of these rays is essentially dependent upon the resistance that the light meets in the other medium while traversing it or in other words, the refraction depends upon the change in velocity of light while travelling from one medium to another. The higher the velocity of light in a particular medium as compared to air or vacuum the lower is the refractive index. The refractive index is inversely proportional to the velocity of light in that medium.

When the light travels from a denser to a rarer medium then the refractive index from denser medium (B) to rarer medium (A) is reciprocal of the refractive index when the light travels from a rarer medium (A) to the denser medium (B). Let $\mu$ be the refractive index of B when light travels from A to B, then when light travels from B to A the refractive index of A will be $1/\mu$.

When the light travels from the denser to rarer medium (Fig. 3.2) the refracted ray DE bends towards the surface (XY) and away from the normal (ADB).

In Fig. 3.3, it can be seen that the incident ray

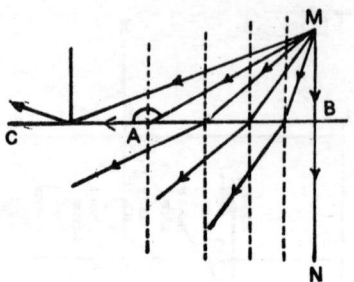

**Fig. 3.3.** Critical angle

MA makes an angle of incidence for which the angle of refraction is 90° and the refracted ray AC just grazes the surface of the medium. This angle of incidence is called the critical angle.

If the angle of incidence is more than the critical angle, all the light is reflected back and none is refracted. Such a phenomenon is termed total internal reflection. One can determine the critical angle for any particular medium provided one knows the refractive index.

$$\mu = \frac{\text{Sine angle of incidence}}{\text{Sine angle of refraction}}$$

or,     $\mu \times$ sine angle of refraction

           = sine angle of incidence

or,     $\mu \times$ sine 90° = sine critical angle

                  (sine 90° = 1)

Hence     $\mu$ = sine critical angle.

Similarly if we can experimentally determine the critical angle, the refractive index of the medium can be easily determined. This is also a practical method of determination of refractive index.

Total internal reflection is utilised in a number of optical instruments using prisms.

### Refraction through plate of glass

In Fig. 3.4, it is shown that the refraction of light through a plate of glass, whose surfaces are parallel to each other, results in the emergent ray being parallel to the incident ray.

In Fig. 3.4, ABCD is a plate of glass which is a rectangle. An incident ray IN meets the surface AB at N forming the angle of incidence a. This is refracted along the path NN′ meeting the surface CD at N′ and forming the angle of refraction b.

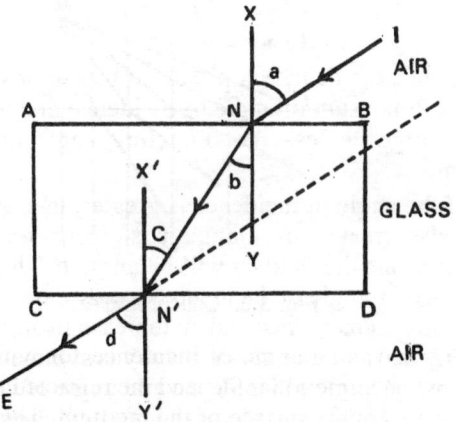

**Fig. 3.4.** Refraction through a plate of glass whose surfaces are parallel to each other.

The refracted ray NN′ acts as the incident ray for the surface CD at N′ forming the second angle of incidence c. It is refracted along NE forming the angle of emergence d.

Now in this figure XY and X′Y′ are parallel to each other being perpendicular to parallel surfaces AB and CD; angle b is equal to angle c.

$$\frac{\text{Sine angle a}}{\text{Sine angle b}} = \mu \qquad \text{(Air/Glass)}$$

and

$$\frac{\text{Sine angle c}}{\text{Sine angle d}} = \mu \qquad \text{(G/A)}$$

or

$$\frac{\text{Sine angle d}}{\text{Sine angle c}} = \mu \qquad \text{(A/G)}$$

or

$$\frac{\text{Sine angle d}}{\text{Sine angle c}} = \frac{\text{Sine angle a}}{\text{Sine angle b}}$$

But        angle b = angle c

Hence     Sine angle a = Sine angle d

or          angle a = angle d

It can be geometrically proved that in such an event emergent ray is parallel to the incident ray.

The emergent ray, though parallel to the incident ray, is displaced; the displacement is dependent upon the refractive index of the media through which it passes, the thickness of the plate and the angle of incidence it makes.

## Refraction through a prism

A prism may be defined as two plane optical surfaces which are not parallel to each other but inclined at a definite angle and with an index of refraction between the surfaces which is different

from that outside them. The angle at which these two refracting surfaces meet is termed the apical or refracting angle and the part of the prism opposite the angle is termed its base.

The prisms have a dual effect on the light rays passing through them. If it is a monochromatic light, the emergent ray bends towards the base. If it is a polychromatic light, it breaks into its coloured components of different wavelengths and each component behaves as a monochromatic beam.

In Fig. 3.5, ABC represents the prism and OP is the incident ray meeting the surface AB of the prism at P. The ray of light is passing from air to glass. OP is, therefore, refracted along PQ the ray bending towards the normal. The refracted ray PQ meets the surface AC at Q. PQ acts as an incident ray for the surface AC and is travelling from glass to air. The ray emerges as QR bending away from the normal and bent towards the base. The emergent ray QR has thus undergone an angular deviation through an angle LKQ.

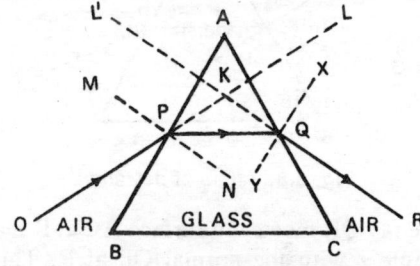

**Fig. 3.5.** Refraction through a glass prism.

In Fig. 3.6, O is a luminous object and ABC is the prism. Let OP and OP′ represent the incident rays which emerge as two divergent rays QR and Q′R′. These emergent rays are received by the observer's eye who projects the image

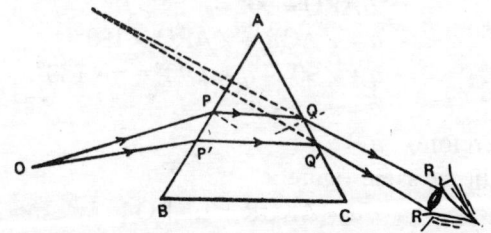

**Fig. 3.6.** Displacement of the image of an object seen through a prism.

towards I. Thus the emergent rays are divergent and deflected towards the base while the image is virtual and deflected towards the apex of the prism (Fig. 3.7).

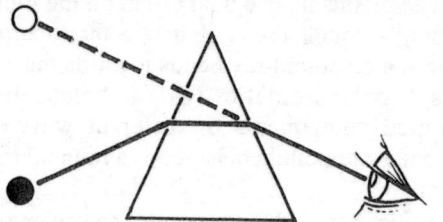

**Fig. 3.7.** Observer views the image through a prism.

In Fig. 3.8, ABC represents the prism. SQ is the incident ray meeting the side AB at Q and making an angle of incidence $i$ with the normal MN at Q. QR is the refracted ray inside the glass prism making an angle $q$ with the normal MN at

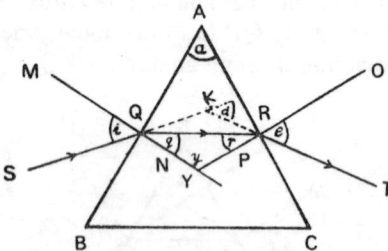

**Fig. 3.8.** Angle of deviation.

Q. The ray QR meets the surface AC at R making the angle $r$ with the normal OP at R. This ray emerges from the prism as an emergent ray RT making an angle of emergence $e$ with normal OP at R. Let $a$ be the apical angle of the prism and $d$ represent the angle of deviation, i.e., the angle between the emergent ray RT and the incident ray SQ.

$$\angle AQR = 90° - q$$
$$\angle ARQ = 90° - r$$
$$a + \angle AQR + \angle ARQ = 180°$$
$$a + \angle 90° - q + \angle 90° - r = 180°$$

or,    $$a - q - r = 0$$
Therefore,    $$a = q + r$$

In the same figure :

$$\angle d = \angle KQR + \angle KRQ$$
$$= (\angle KQY - q) + (\angle KRY - r)$$
$$= i - q + e - r$$

$$= i + e - (q + r)$$
$$= i + e - a$$

Hence the deviation produced by the prism is equal to the sum of angle of incidence and angle of emergence less the refracting angle of the prism.

If the angle of incidence is greater, then angle $q$ is also greater, since angle $y$ is constant, angle $r$ will be smaller and so will be angle $e$. Thus an increase in angle of incidence causes a decrease in angle of emergence and an increase in angle of divergence and vice versa. If a ray is symmetrical (i.e., when angle of incidence and angle of emergence are equal), it undergoes least deviation and may be termed as the ray of minimum deviation.

In minimum deviation

$$i = e$$
and    $$q = r$$
Hence    $$a = q + r = 2r$$
But    $$d = i + e - a$$
Since    $$i = e$$
Hence    $$d = 2i - a$$
$$\text{sine } i = \mu \text{ sine } r$$

When angles are very small, the sines of angles are represented as angles themselves.
Hence    $$i = \mu r$$
or    $$d = 2\mu r - a$$
But    $$2r = a$$
Hence    $$d = \mu a - a = a(\mu - 1)$$

But we usually use glass prism whose refractive index is 1.5.
Hence    $$d = a(1.5 - 1)$$

$$d = \frac{a}{2}$$

The equation shows that the angle of minimum deviation is half of the refracting angle of the prism when glass prisms are used.

In ophthalmology we use glass prisms with small refracting angles and also assume that rays of light strike the prism symmetrically. These conditions are usually produced in crown glass.

Yet another phenomenon that is used is the prentice position of the prisms so that all deviations would result from refraction on the emerging surface. That is achieved by a prism orientation in which the incident ray is perpendicular to

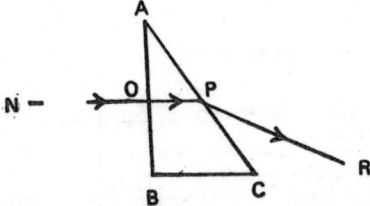

**Fig. 3.9.** Prentice position of prisms.

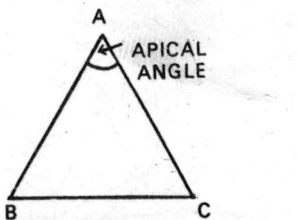

**Fig. 3.11.** Nomenclature of prism—apical angle.

the initial refracting surface of the prism (Fig. 3.9).

### Polychromatic effects

This phenomenon depends upon the fact that the velocity of light in any medium is the function of the wavelength of the light.

The shorter wavelengths have lower velocity. In view of this, the effect of prism on white light is to split the white light after refraction into its coloured components (Fig. 3.10).

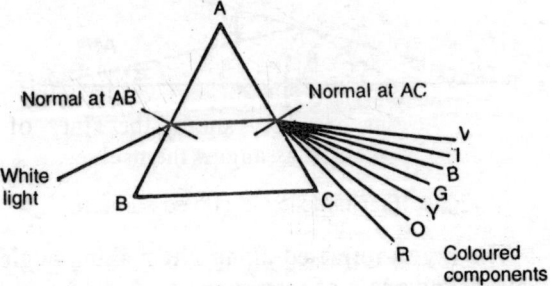

**Fig. 3.10.** Breaking of light into its coloured components.

### Nomenclature of prisms

The prisms may be indicated by one of the following methods :

### Measure in degrees of apical angle (Fig. 3.11)

This method was previously used but is now no more employed as the effectivity of prism does not only depend upon its apical angle but also upon the refractive index of the glass used.

### Measure in degrees of angle of deviation (Fig. 3.12)

This method of denominating a prism is independent of the apical angle and the refractive

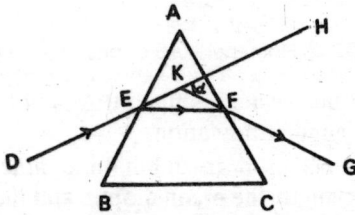

**Fig. 3.12.** Nomenclature of prisms according to angle of deviation.

index of the glass used. It gives an accurate measure of the effectiveness of the prism and can be a good method of nomenclature.

### Centrad (Fig. 3.13)

This measures the angular deviation of the ray by a prism. It denotes the strength of a prism that produces a deviation of 1 cm of arc at a distance of 1 metre. This angular deviation is termed a centrad prism and is equivalent to 34.37747' angle.

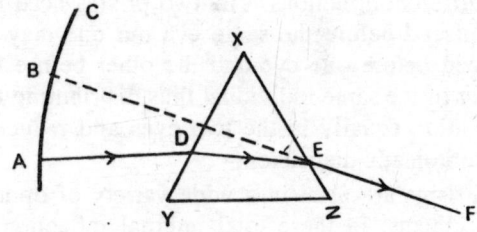

**Fig. 3.13.** Nomenclature of prisms—centrad.

This system has the advantage that 10 centrad deviation is 10 times that of one centrad.

### Prism dioptres (Fig. 3.14)

This method of nomenclature indicates the angular deviation subtended on a vertical line one metre away. It gives an apparent displacement of 1 cm to an object situated one metre away. The

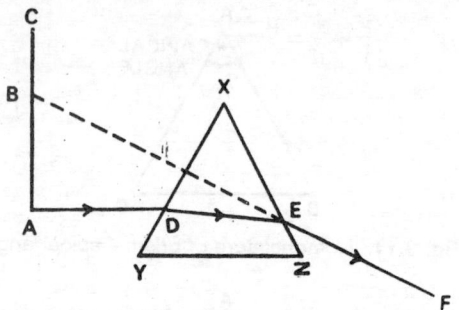

**Fig. 3.14.** Nomenclature of prisms—dioptres.

defect of this system is that 10 Δ is not 10 times one Δ in angular deviation.

In prisms used in ophthalmic practice, the refracting angle, the prism dioptre and the centrad are very nearly equal to each other. The most commonly employed nomenclature is prism dioptres.

## ROTATING PRISMS

If two prisms of equal strength are placed base to base they act as a thick plate of glass. If they are rotated in opposite directions they produce the effect of a single prism of gradually increasing strength which reaches its maximum when they lie apex to apex and the deviation is equal to the sum of the deviating power of the two prisms separately. Such combination of prisms is used to test the power of the eyes to overcome diplopia in different directions. The two prisms need not be placed before the same eye but one may be placed before one eye and the other before the other of the same individual thus distributing the deviation equally in the two eyes and reducing the chromatic dispersion.

Prisms are used in a wide variety of optical instruments. In these total internal reflection is utilised. They permit the designer to bend light rays; since the reflection is total, there is very little loss. The light rays can be made to deviate 180° or 90° as shown in (Fig. 3.15).

### Refraction at curved surfaces

Cornea is a convex curved surface. The refraction at convex surfaces and the formula by which focal distances can be calculated are of practical importance in ophthalmology.

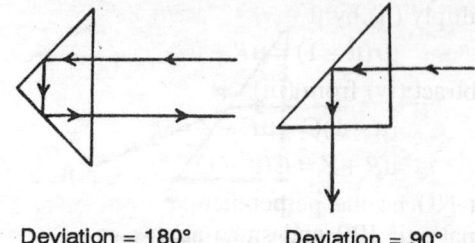

Deviation = 180°          Deviation = 90°

**Fig. 3.15.** Total internal reflection used for deviation of light.

In Fig. 3.16, XPY represents a curved surface which separates air on the incident side with the medium of refractive index on the concave side. C is the centre of curvature and IPC the principal axis. IN is incident ray which meets the convex surface at N making angle INC' ($i$) as angle of incidence. CNC' is the normal at N.

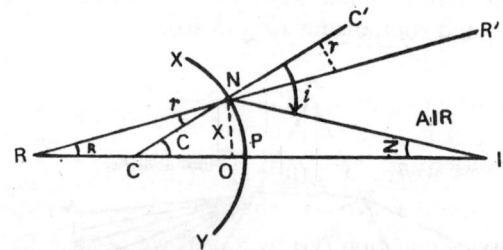

**Fig. 3.16.** Refraction at curved surfaces.

The ray is refracted along NR making angle CNR as the angle of refraction.

$$\angle CNR = \angle C'NR'(r)$$
$$\sin r = \mu$$

or
$$i = \mu r \qquad \text{(for small angles)}$$
$$\angle INR' = \angle INC' - \angle C'NR'$$
$$= i - r$$

But $i = \mu r$

Hence $\angle INR' = \mu r - r = r(\mu - 1)$

and $\angle NIP = Z$

$\angle NCP = C$

$\angle NRP = R$

$\angle INC' = \angle NCP + \angle NIP$

$\mu r = C + Z \qquad \dots(i)$

$\angle INR' = \angle NRP + \angle NIP$

$(\mu - 1)r = R + Z \qquad \dots(ii)$

Multiply (i) by $\mu - 1$

$\mu r(\mu - 1) = C(\mu - 1) + \mu Z - Z \dots(iii)$

Multiply (ii) by $\mu$

$$\mu r(\mu - 1) = \mu R + \mu Z \qquad \ldots\text{(iv)}$$

Subtract (iv) from (iii)

$$(\mu - 1)C - \mu R - Z = 0$$

$$\mu R + Z = C(\mu - 1) \qquad \ldots\text{(v)}$$

Let NO be the perpendicular from N to the principal axis IPR and since angles Z, C, R are small let them be represented by their tangents. O is very near P and, therefore, a great error will not arise if IP is considered equal to IO, OR is considered equal to PR = $-v$ and OC is considered equal to PC = $-r$.

Let NO be equal to $x$ then

$$R = -\frac{x}{v}$$

$$C = -\frac{x}{r}$$

$$Z = \frac{x}{u}$$

Substituting these values in equation (v), we have

$$\frac{ux}{v} + \frac{x}{u} = \frac{(\mu - 1)x}{r} \qquad \ldots\text{(vi)}$$

Divide equation (vi) by $x$, and we have

$$\frac{u}{v} + \frac{1}{u} = \frac{\mu - 1}{r}$$

or

$$\frac{u}{v} = \frac{\mu - 1}{r} - \frac{1}{u} \qquad \ldots\text{(vii)}$$

But

$$\frac{1}{v} + \frac{1}{u} = \frac{1}{f}$$

and if $u$ is infinity, $v = f$, i.e., the focal length. Substituting these values in equation (vii), we have

$$\frac{\mu}{f} = \frac{\mu - 1}{r}$$

or

$$f = \frac{\mu r}{\mu - 1} \qquad \ldots\text{(viii)}$$

If none of the refracting media is one, then

$$\frac{\mu}{1} = \frac{\mu_2}{\mu_1}$$

so that anterior focus will be

$$f_1 = \frac{\mu_1 r}{\mu_2 - \mu_1} \qquad \ldots\text{(ix)}$$

and the posterior focus

$$f_2 = \frac{\mu_2 r}{\mu_2 - \mu_1} \qquad \text{(x)}$$

The formulae (ix) and (x) are actually used for calculating the anterior and posterior focal points of cornea.

# Lenses and Their Combinations

Lenses are portions of transparent medium which are bounded by surfaces which are part of sphere. There are primarily two types of lenses—a convex and a concave.

Convex lenses may be biconvex, plano-convex or concavo-convex, i.e., convex meniscus. Similarly concave lenses may be biconcave, plano-concave or convexo-concave, i.e., concave meniscus (Fig. 4.1).

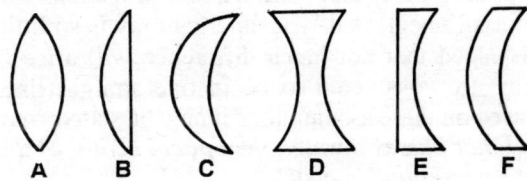

A. Biconvex lens    D. Biconcave lens
B. Plano-convex lens    E. Plano-concave lens
C. Convex meniscus    F. Concave meniscus

**Fig. 4.1.**

A convex lens is usually considered as collection of prisms placed base to base (Fig. 4.2A & B). The line passing through this junction is called the principal axis. A concave lens may be considered as a collection of prisms placed apex

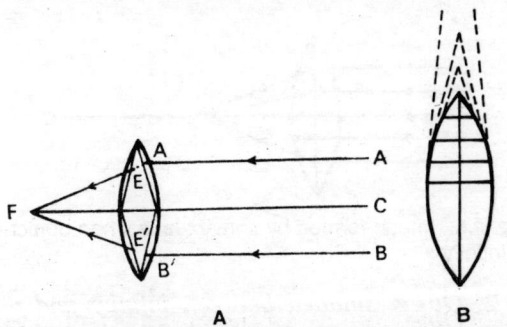

**Fig. 4.2A & B.** Formation of convex lenses.

to apex (Fig. 4.3A & B). The line passing through this junction is called the principal axis.

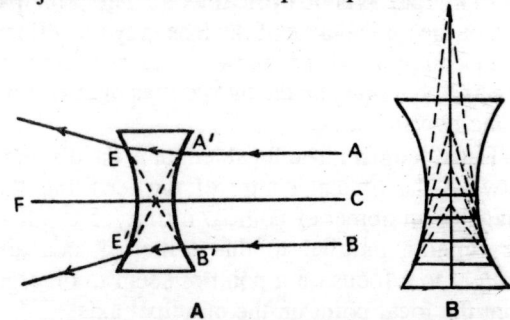

**Fig. 4.3A & B.** Formation of concave lenses.

When the rays of light pass through a convex lens they converge to a point on the principal axis. In Fig. 4.2B, let AA' be a ray of light parallel to the line CF, which is the principal axis. It meets the lens at A'. The ray gets deflected towards the base of the prism and meets the other surface at E. From this point it is further deflected towards the base, similar is the fate of the other ray BB'. These two rays meet at F on the principal axis.

When the rays of light pass through a concave lens they are divergent (Fig. 4.3A & B) and appear to diverge from the principal axis. In Fig. 4.3B, let AA' be a ray of light meeting the lens at A'. It is bent towards the base and meets the other surface at E. From this point it further bends towards the base, i.e., away from the principal axis. Similar is the fate of the ray BB'.

In geometrical construction of images if intersection of any two rays from the object is known, the point of intersection is the image of the object and it is assumed that all rays will intersect at this point. The two rays usually chosen are :

1. One ray emanating from the object running parallel to the principal axis, after refraction

by the lens, must pass through or appear to pass through a point on the principal axis. This point, as in case of mirrors, is the focal point.

2. The second ray passes directly through the centre of the lens and is not deviated by the lens, if the lenses are very thin which we assume for ophthalmic lenses.

Before describing the images formed by various lenses, it would be desirable to define some of the important terms.

**Principal axis or optical axis :** The principal axis or the optical axis of the lens may be defined as the common axis of the two surfaces of revolution and on it must be the two centres of curvature of the two surfaces.

**Focal length :** The focal length is the distance between the optical centre of the lens and the image of an object or point at infinity. Rays that are running parallel to this principal axis are brought to a focus on a point or seem to diverge from the focal point on the principal axis.

**Dioptre :** It is the unit of measurement of the power of the lenses. It is denoted by the abbreviation D. One dioptre corresponds to a lens of the focal length of 1 metre. The dioptric value of the lens is inversely proportional to the focal length of the lens in metres. Thus 1 D means a lens of 1 metre focal length, 2 D means a lens of ½ metre focal length and ½ D means a lens of 2 metre focal length.

## Determination of optical centre of the lens

In Fig. 4.4, let y and v be the two points on the lens at which the two surfaces may be considered to be parallel. Join v and y and let the line cut the axis DD′ at P. Then P is the optical centre of the lens. Draw Cv and C′y as normals from the centres of curvature (C and C′) of the two curved surfaces; C′y and Cv thus become parallel. Triangles CPv and C′Py are similar.

Therefore,

$$\frac{CP}{PC'} = \frac{Cv}{C'y} = \frac{r_1}{r_2}$$

$$\frac{r_1}{r_2} = \frac{CP}{PC'} = \frac{r_1 - CP}{r_2 - PC'} = \frac{D'P}{DP}$$

It, therefore, follows that the point P divides the principal axis DD′ in a definite ratio depend-

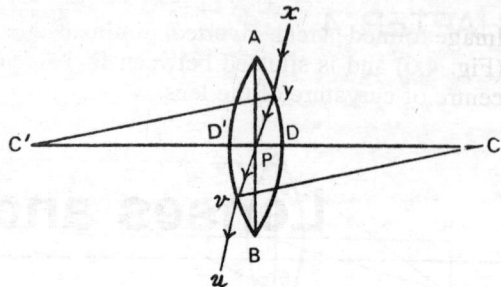

**Fig. 4.4.** Optical centre of lens (P).

ing only upon the radii of the two spherical surfaces. It also proves that the position of the optical centre P lies in between them.

In a biconcave or a biconvex lens it lies within the lens. The lenses with which we deal in ophthalmology are very thin so much so that D and D′ are very near each other and the optical centre P lies in between them. These three points are so near each other that the thickness of the lens can be easily neglected. The emergent ray is so little displaced that not much difference will arise if they are considered to be in one straight line. Based on these assumptions it may be stated *"any ray that passes through the optical centre of the lens passes undeviated."*

### Images formed by various lenses

#### Convex lenses

1. *Object situated at infinity :* If the object is at infinity an image is formed at the focal point (Fig. 4.5). The rays starting from infinity run parallel to the axis of the lens and are, therefore, refracted in a way that they pass through the focus. Thus all the refracted rays meet at the focal point and form its image.

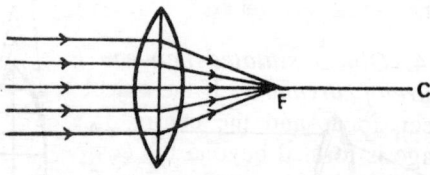

**Fig. 4.5.** Image formed by convex lens when object is at infinity.

2. *Object situated between infinity and the centre of curvature :* If the object is situated between infinity and the centre of curvature the

image formed is real, inverted, diminished in size (Fig. 4.6) and is situated between focus and the centre of curvature of the lens.

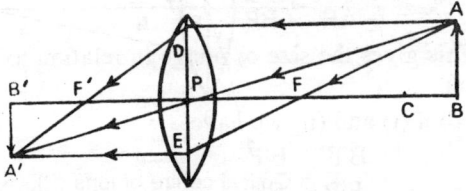

**Fig. 4.6.** Image formed by convex lens when the object is between infinity and centre of curvature.

In Fig. 4.6, let AB be an object and situated beyond the centre of curvature C. The ray AD runs parallel to axis BP and is, therefore, refracted along DF′, i.e., passes through the posterior focal point F′. The ray AP passing through optical centre goes undeviated and the ray AE, passing through F′, i.e., through anterior focal point, is refracted along EA′ which is parallel to the principal axis. All the rays meet at A′ which is, therefore, the image of A. Similarly B′ is the image of B.

3. *Object situated at the centre of curvature :* If the object is situated at the centre of curvature, the image is formed at the centre of curvature on the opposite side. It is real, inverted (Fig. 4.7) and is equal to the size of the object.

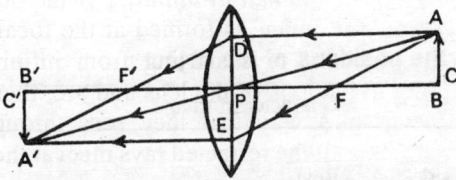

**Fig. 4.7.** Image formed by convex lens when object is at the centre of curvature.

4. *Object situated between focus and the centre of curvature :* If the object is situated between focus and the centre of curvature, the image is formed beyond the centre of curvature (Fig. 4.8); it is inverted, real and enlarged.

5. *Object situated at the focus :* If the object is situated at the focus, the image is formed at infinity (Fig. 4.9).

7. *Object situated between focus and the lens :* If the object is situated between focus and the

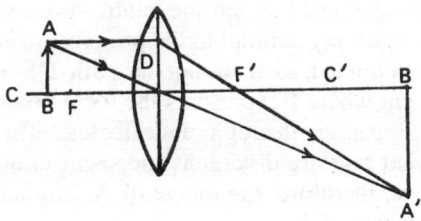

**Fig. 4.8.** Image formed by convex lens when object is between focus and the centre of curvature.

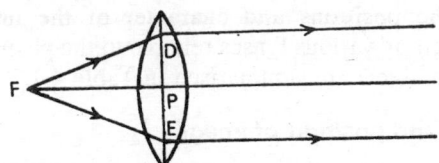

**Fig. 4.9.** Image formed by convex lens when the object is at the focus.

lens, the image is formed on the same side of the lens (Fig. 4.10). It is virtual, enlarged and erect. This is the principle which is utilized in corneal loupes, magnifying glasses and biomicroscopic examination.

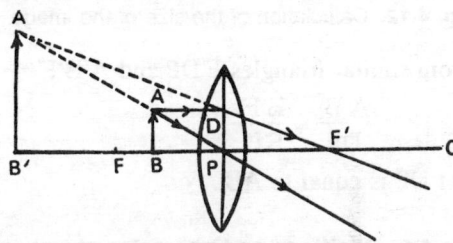

**Fig. 4.10.** Image formed by convex lens when the object is between the focus and the lens.

**Concave lenses**

The image formed by concave lenses is always virtual, erect and diminished in size irrespective of the distance of the object from the lens. It is always situated between the lens and the focus.

In Fig. 4.11, let AB be an object situated in

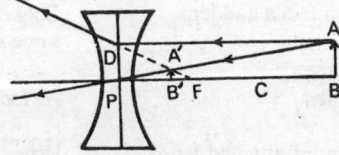

**Fig. 4.11.** Image formed by concave lens.

front of the lens beyond the centre of curvature. Let AD be a ray parallel to the principal axis. The ray is refracted as if along the path DF and is divergent where F represents the focal point. The ray AP passes through undeflected. The two emergent rays are divergent and seem to meet at A'. A' is, therefore, the image of A. Similarly B' is the image of B.

A'B' is situated on the same side as AB. It is erect and diminished is size and is virtual.

The positions and character of the image formed by various lenses relative to the positions of the object are summarised in Table 4.1.

### Size and position of image

In Fig. 4.12, AB is the object and A'B' is the image.

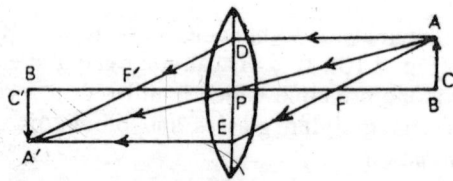

**Fig. 4.12.** Calculation of the size of the image.

From similar triangles F'DP and A'B'F'

$$\frac{A'B'}{DP} = \frac{B'F'}{F'P'}$$

But DP is equal to AB

Hence,

$$\frac{A'B'}{AB} = \frac{B'F'}{F'P'} \tag{i}$$

From similar triangles ABP and A'B'P

$$\frac{A'B'}{AB} = \frac{B'P}{BP} \quad \text{or} \quad \frac{-v}{u} \tag{ii}$$

This gives the size of image in relation to the object.

From (i) and (ii) we have

$$\frac{B'F'}{F'P} = \frac{B'P}{BP} \quad \text{or} \quad \frac{-v}{u} \tag{iii}$$

$$B'F' = -(v-f) = f - v$$

and $\qquad F'P = -f$

Substituting these values in (iii), we have

$$\frac{f-v}{-f} = \frac{-v}{u}$$

or $\qquad uf - uv = vf$

or $\qquad uf - vf = uv$

Dividing by $uvf$, we have

$$\frac{1}{v} - \frac{1}{u} = \frac{1}{f}$$

From (ii) we calculate the size of the image. The size of the object and the image are in the same ratio as their distance from the lens.

It can also be calculated mathematically that the square of the focal length is equal to the product of the distance of image from the focus $(l_1)$ and the distance of the object from the focus $(l_2)$, i.e.,

### Table 4.1. Positions and character of image relative to the positions of the object

| Position of object | Position of image | Character of image |
|---|---|---|
| **Convex lenses** | | |
| 1. At infinity | At focus on the opposite side | Real |
| 2. Between infinity and centre of curvature | Between infinity and centre of curvature on the opposite side | Real, inverted and diminished in size |
| 3. At centre of curvature | At centre of curvature on the opposite side | Real, inverted and of the same size as the object |
| 4. Between centre of curvature and focus | Between centre of curvature and infinity on the opposite side | Real, inverted and enlarged |
| 5. At focus | At infinity | Real |
| 6. Between focus and lens | Between infinity and lens on the same side | Virtual, erect and enlarged |
| **Concave lenses** | | |
| 7. At infinity | At focus on the same side | Virtual, and on the same side as the object |
| 8. Between infinity and lens | Between focus and lens | Virtual, erect and diminished |

$$l_1 \times l_2 = f^2$$

Suppose the image is situated at a distance of $l_1$ and the object is situated at $l_2$ from the focus. Then in Fig. 4.12 from similar triangles A'B'F' and F'DP we have

$$\frac{A'B'}{DP} = \frac{B'F'}{F'P}$$

or

$$\frac{A'B'}{AB} = \frac{l_1}{f} \qquad \text{(iv)}$$

Similarly from similar triangles PEF and ABF, we have

$$\frac{AE}{AB} = \frac{PF}{AB}$$

or

$$\frac{A'B'}{AB} = \frac{f}{l_2} \qquad \text{(v)}$$

From (iv) and (v) we have

$$\frac{l_1}{f} = \frac{f}{l_2}$$

or

$$l_1 \times l_2 = f^2$$

## Cylindrical lenses

These lenses are segments of the cylinder cut parallel to its axis (convex lenses) or segments of the mould cut parallel to its axis (concave lenses). These lenses do not have the same curvature in all meridians. In simple cylinders one meridian is plane and the other has curvature. The axis of the cylindrical lens, which is quite distinct from the optical axis, is parallel to that of the cylinder of which it is a segment. In the simple cylindrical lens, the cylinder acts as a plane lamina with parallel sides in the direction of its axis.

Since these lenses are very thin, the plane lamina does not cause any practical displacement of the rays passing through it. In compound lenses both meridians are curved but to different degrees and produce a complex refractive system. In a direction at right angles to the axis of the cylinder, the lens acts as spherical lens, either as plano-concave or as plano-convex type, leading to divergence or convergence of rays.

Fig. 4.13 describes the path of rays in a single convex cylinder showing that the rays passing along the axis of the lens (AB) go undeviated as it acts as a plane lamina while the rays from O and P which meet the convex surface and which are parallel to the optical axis (XY) are converged

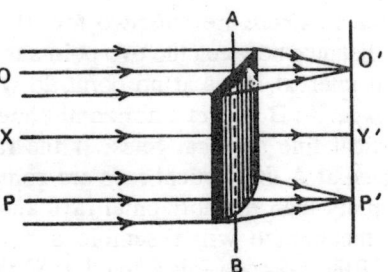

**Fig. 4.13.** Refraction through a convex cylinder.

to a point O' and P'. Thus the focus instead of being a point is a focal line O'P'.

Fig. 4.14 describes the path of light in a similar way in a simple concave cylinder and rays parallel to optical axis (XY) seem to diverge from the focal line O'P'.

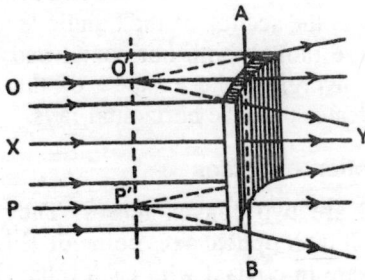

**Fig. 4.14.** Refraction through a concave cylinder.

## Sturm's conoid

In compound cylindrical lenses, the lens has different curvatures in the two meridians, the vertical meridian VV' and the horizontal meridian HH' (Fig. 4.15).

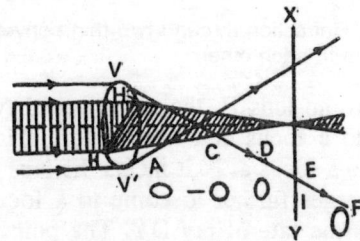

**Fig. 4.15.** Sturm's conoid.

Let us suppose that the vertical meridian has greater curvature than the horizontal meridian so that the rays in the vertical meridian come to a focus at B and rays in horizontal meridian are focused at E. There are thus two foci (B and E) and the distance between the two points is termed the focal interval. Thus at no point do we get a point image. At B we get a horizontal line and at E a vertical line as focal lines. If the rays are intercepted at A the vertical rays are converging more rapidly than the horizontal rays and a section of the bundle will resemble a horizontal ellipse. If the rays are intercepted at C then the divergence of vertical rays is perhaps equal in degree to the convergence of horizontal rays and the section of bundle presents as a circle. This is a point where there is least distortion and such a circle is called the circle of least diffusion. If the rays are intercepted at D the degree of divergence of vertical rays is far greater in expanse than the convergence of horizontal rays and the section of the bundle appears to be an oval ellipse. Beyond E, i.e., at F, the section of the bundle is again an oval ellipse though both horizontal and vertical rays are diverging, the expanse of the vertical rays is greater than the horizontal rays.

## Combination of lenses

A and B are two convex lenses. They are so placed that their optical axes coincide (Fig. 4.16) and they are in contact with each other. Let EX be parallel to F'F''. It meets the lens A at X. If

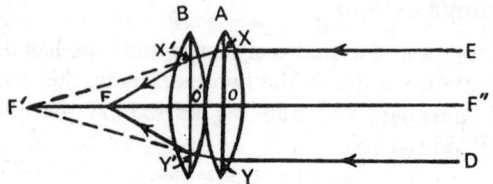

**Fig. 4.16.** Refraction through two thin convex lenses in contact with each other.

there were no lens B, the ray would have been brought to a focus at F' but before this ray is brought to a focus at F' it meets the lens B at X' and converges further to come to a focus at F. Similar is the fate of ray DY. The point F now becomes the focus of the lens combination. Let us suppose that the lenses are very thin and O' and O are very near each other so that not much error will arise if we measure the focal distance from any of these points.

Now if we consider lens A above then

$$\frac{1}{v_1} - \frac{1}{u_1} = \frac{1}{f_1}$$

This $v_1$ will act as $u_2$ for the lens B. Then in lens B,

$$\frac{1}{v_2} - \frac{1}{u_2} = \frac{1}{f_2}$$

But $u_2 = v_1$

Therefore, $\frac{1}{v_2} - \frac{1}{v_1} = \frac{1}{f_2}$

If the object is at infinity then $v_1$ is equal to $f_1$

or $\frac{1}{v_1} = \frac{1}{f_1}$

or $\frac{1}{v_2} - \frac{1}{f_1} = \frac{1}{f_2}$

or $\frac{1}{v_2} = \frac{1}{f_1} + \frac{1}{f_2}$

But the image of the object at infinity by this combination is at the new focus or at F. Therefore, $v_2 = f$

Hence, $\frac{1}{f} = \frac{1}{f_1} + \frac{1}{f_2}$

If there are several lenses then,

$$\frac{1}{f} = \frac{1}{f_1} + \frac{1}{f_2} + \frac{1}{f_3} + \cdots$$

Therefore the power of a combination of thin lenses, as we use in ophthalmology in contact with each other, is the algebraical summation of the power of the lenses.

If the lenses were separated from each other by a distance $d$ (Fig. 4.17), then in this event

$$u_2 = f_1 - d$$

or $\frac{1}{v_2} = \frac{1}{f_1 - d} + \frac{1}{f_2}$

or $\frac{1}{v_2} = \frac{1}{f_2} + \frac{1}{f_1 - d}$

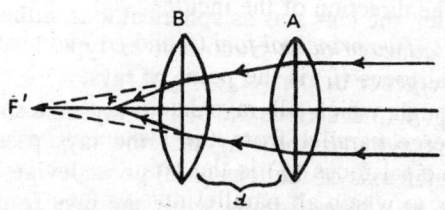

**Fig. 4.17.** Refraction through two thin convex lenses separated by a distance $d$.

or
$$\frac{1}{f} = \frac{1}{f_2} + \frac{1}{f_1 - d}$$

### Gauss' theorem

Now if several lenses were so situated, i.e., they were homocentric and their optical axes coincided with each other, such a mathematical calculation becomes very tedious and in case of thick lenses it will be a task of great difficulty and complexity. Gauss, therefore, devised a simple method and showed that a homocentric system of lenses could be treated as a whole if the object and image distances are measured from two theoretical planes (principal planes). The whole system can be resolved into six cardinal points (Fig. 4.18).

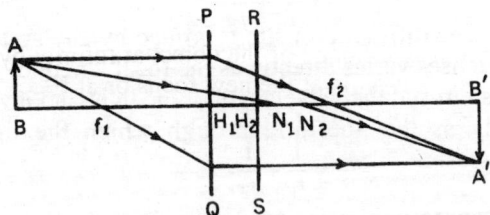

**Fig. 4.18.** Theorem of Gauss (cardinal points).

1. *Two principal points* ($H_1$ and $H_2$) : These are such that an incident ray passing through the first principal point passes, after refraction, through the second principal point also but the incident and emergent rays are not necessarily parallel to each other. These principal points are situated in the principal planes at points where they meet the homocentric optical axis.

2. *Two nodal points* ($N_1$ and $N_2$) : These correspond to a single optical centre of a simple lens. Thus an incident ray directed to the first nodal point will emerge from the system through the second nodal point and take a direction parallel to the direction of the incident ray.

3. *Two principal foci* ($f_1$ and $f_2$) The first principal focus ($f_1$) is the point on the principal axis through which all rays have to pass so as to emerge parallel from the system. The second principal focus ($f_2$) is the point on the principal axis to which all parallel rays to the system are brought to a focus.

In Fig. 4.18, let AB be an object. A ray AP

parallel to the principal axis is brought on to a focus at the second principal focus ($f_2$). AQ is the ray which passes through the first principal focus ($f_1$) and, therefore, emerges parallel to the system. The two emergent rays meet at A'. A ray $AN_1$ meets the first nodal point $N_1$ and emerges from the second nodal point $N_2$ as $N_2A'$. A' is, therefore, the image of A. Similarly B' is the image of B. From this it is clear that the principles of construction of images as laid down in the case of simple lenses are equally applicable to a homocentric system of lenses provided the six cardinal points are known and are taken into account. This has great practicability as will be seen later for the eye is regarded as such a homocentric system of lenses.

### Combination of cylindrical lenses

As in the case of spherical lenses, if two cylindrical lenses are held in contact so that their axes are parallel to each other their combined power will be the algebraic sum of the power of each lens. If these lenses are held with their axes at right angles to each other, they will act as two different cylindrical lenses. In case they are of equal dioptric power and both are convex or both are concave they will resolve themselves into a spherical lens of dioptric strength equal to that of cylinder, e.g., +4 D cyl. axis 90° when added to +4 D cyl. axis 180° the resultant lens is +4 D sphere, or conversely a spherical lens can be broken into its two component cylinders placed at right angles to each other.

If two cylinders (both concave or both convex) are held at right angles to each other but are of different dioptric strength the combination resolves itself into a spherical lens with the common factor as the dioptric strength and the remaining factor as the cylinder in the axis of the cylindrical lens with higher dioptric strength, e.g., if +4 D cyl. axis 180° is added to +2 D cyl. axis 90° then 2 is the common factor and the combination becomes +2 D sphere added to the remaining factor of the higher cylindrical lens in the same axis, i.e., 4 – 2 or +2 D cyl. at 180° axis. The combination, thus, will be +2 D sph. +2 D cyl. axis 180°.

If a spherical lens is combined with a cylindrical lens of the same power but opposite sign, the

## Table 4.2. Optical aberrations

### Aberrations depending upon the nature of light

| Type | Pattern |
| --- | --- |
| 1. Diffraction (Fig. 4.19) | Narrower the aperture, greater the diffraction. |
| 2. Chromatic aberration (Fig. 4.20) | Longitudinal—chromatic difference of focus. Transverse—chromatic difference of magnification. |

### Monochromatic aberrations

| Type | Direction | Type of object with which it occurs |
| --- | --- | --- |
| 1. Spherical (Fig. 4.21) | Longitudinal | Point objects on and off the principal axis |
| 2. Coma or sine (Fig. 4.22) | Transverse | Point objects on and off the principal axis |
| 3. Refraction of eccentric rays | Longitudinal | Point objects off the principal axis |
| 4. (a) Curvature | Longitudinal | Extended objects |
|    (b) Distortion | Transverse | Extended objects |
| 5. Depth of focus | | |

combination will be equal to a cylinder of the power and sign of the sphere whose axis is at right angles to the axis of the given cylinder, i.e., +2 D sph. added to the –2 D cyl. axis 180° will resolve into +2 D cyl. axis 90°.

## Optical defects of image

Some of the aberrations are summarised in Table 4.2.
1. Aberrations depending upon the light :
    (a) Diffraction—which is a monochromatic phenomenon.
    (b) Chromatic aberration—which is a polychromatic phenomenon.
2. Monochromatic aberrations :
    (a) Spherical aberration
    (b) Sine condition
    (c) Refraction of eccentric rays
    (d) Curvature and distortion
    (e) Depth of focus

## Aberrations depending upon the light

### Diffraction of light

The statement that light travels in a straight line is not wholly true. The outer rays tend to spread and form a series of maxima and minima so that they do not travel in straight lines. The edges of the image are, therefore, never sharp. The narrower the waves the greater the diffraction (Fig. 4.19).

The diffraction pattern formed by any system of lenses varies directly as the focal length of the system and the wavelength of the light and inversely as the aperture through which the light passes.

### Chromatic aberration

As rays from the various parts of the spectrum do not travel at the same velocity through a lens, they are unequally refracted; the longer the wavelength the farther it is focused. Thus, in visible light, the long red rays are focused at a longer distance than the short violet rays and the red image is larger in size. In between these two extremes the other intermediate colours of the spectrum are focused in order of their wavelength (Fig. 4.20).

The difference between the focal points is termed the chromatic focal interval and the difference in magnification is called chromatic difference in magnification. This defect in lenses is overcome by the use of a combination of lenses, convex and concave, made of substances of different refractive index. Such a combination of lenses is called an achromatic lens. This lens usually consists of a combination of a convex lens of high refractive power but low dispersive power with a concave lens of low refractive power but high dispersive power so that dispersion is neutralised while much of refractive power remains.

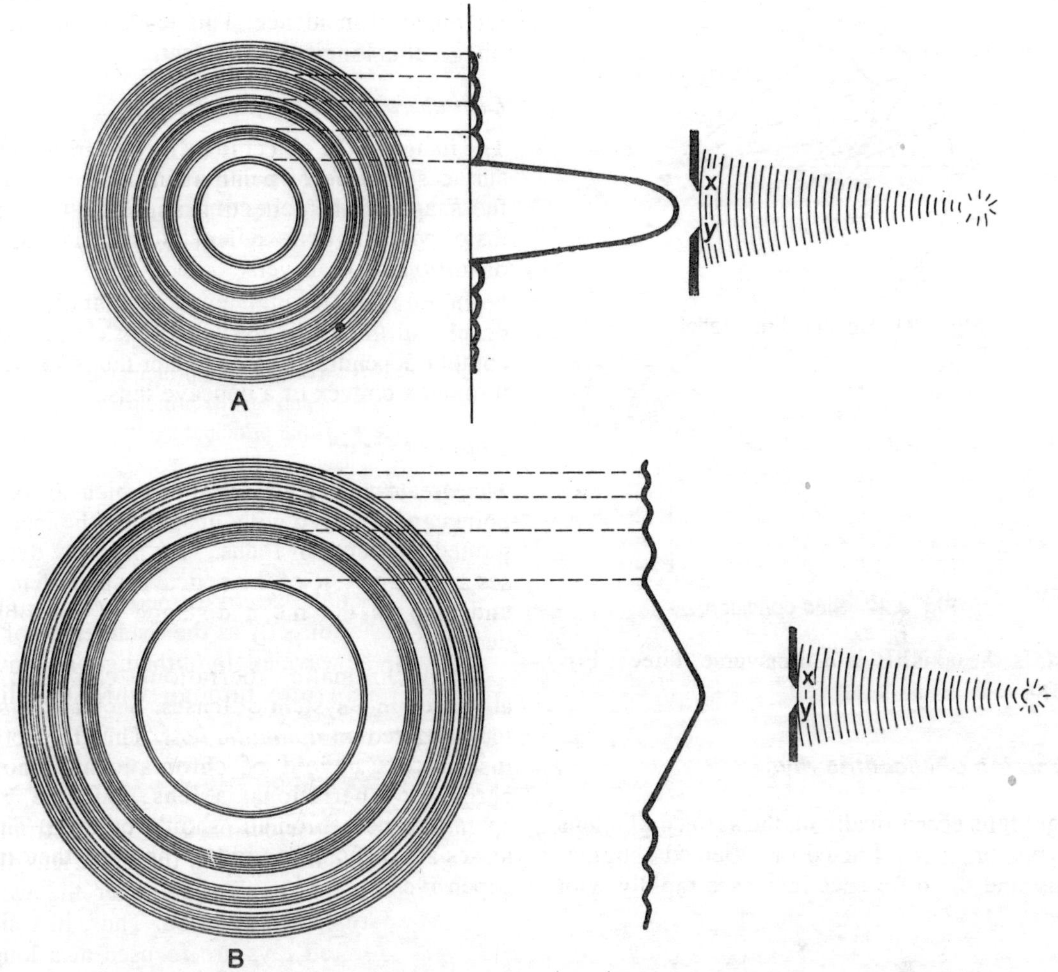

**Fig. 4.19.** Diffraction pattern depending upon aperture. A—Large aperture. B—Small aperture. XY— Size of aperture. Diffraction is inversely proportional to size of aperture.

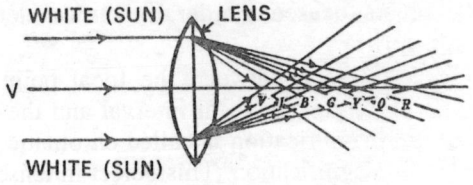

**Fig. 4.20.** Chromatic aberration.

## Monochromatic aberrations

### Spherical aberration

If the pencil of light is large and the aperture of the lens is large, the central rays and the peripheral rays falling on the lens though parallel are not passing through the same principal focus after refraction. The location of images formed by the peripheral and central portions differ and form a caustic curve. The composite image formed is not sharp but blurred and the image has a disc of least confusion. It is a longitudinal defect (Fig. 4.21).

The error can be easily corrected by aplanatic lenses. These lenses are so ground that the curvature decreases from the centre to the periphery.

### Sine condition

Even when the spherical aberration is corrected the different zones of a lens form an image in the shape of a coma, the tail of which is directed

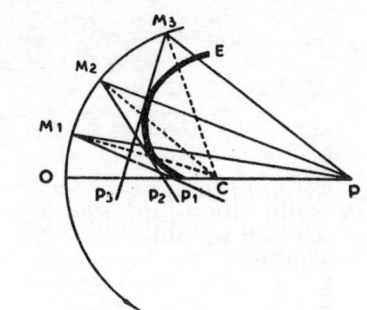

**Fig. 4.21.** Spherical aberration.

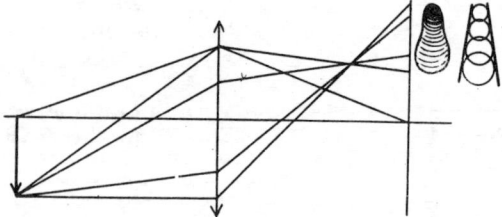

**Fig. 4.22.** Sine condition.

towards the axis. It is a transverse defect (Fig. 4.22).

## Refraction of eccentric rays

If light falls eccentrically on the surface of a lens or a mirror, it is refracted or reflected astigmatically and the difference increases rapidly with the angle of incidence. This leads to blurring of image. It is longitudinal defect.

### Curvature and distortion

The image of the object in reflection from curved surfaces, instead of being a linear one, assumes the shape of the reflecting surface and is thus distorted. Curvature defect is longitudinal and distortion is a transverse defect.

In refraction through lenses similar distortions occur and the shape has a convex or a concave contour depending upon whether the refraction is through a convex or a concave lens.

### Depth of focus

The greatest distance through which an object point can be moved without spoiling the image is termed the depth of focus. This property decreases as the aperture of the optical system increases and also as the mean distance of the object decreases.

Monochromatic aberrations can also be abolished in a system of lenses. Such a lens system is called an *aplanatic lens*. Thus for optical instruments devoid of chromatic and monochromatic aberrations, a lens which is both aplanatic and achromatic should be used. These lenses are difficult to produce and are, therefore, expensive.

# SECTION II

# Physiological Optics

# CHAPTER 5

# General Concepts of Eye as a Refracting Apparatus

The eye is composed of several refracting structures, viz., the cornea, the aqueous humour, the lens and the vitreous. These constitute a homocentric system of lenses which, when combined in action, form a very strong refracting system of a short focal length. The rays are refracted by the anterior surface of the cornea, the posterior surface of the cornea, the aqueous humour, the anterior cortex of the lens, the nucleus of the lens, the posterior cortex of the lens and the vitreous humour.

In an earlier chapter the combination of several lenses has been considered as a coaxial homocentric system of lenses which were resolved by Gauss into six cardinal points. The principles can, by and large, be applied to the eye. The eye, however, is complex because most of the refraction occurs at cornea, yet it must be considered as a thick system of lenses. In eye there are some very important deviations from the assumptions of a co-axial homocentric system of the lenses. The most important being that the refracting surfaces are not isotropic and with accommodation there is a shift in the overall centre of power of the eye when lens assumes a much greater significance. This will result in shifting of the cardinal points. In aphakia again there will be a change in the cardinal points. In view of these, certain optical constants need to be stated for better understanding.

There are at least four groups of optical constants, i.e., the refractive indices, the radii of curvature of major refracting surfaces, the power of optical elements and the cardinal points.

The refractive indices are given in Table 5.1.

From these refractive indices it may be inferred that much inaccuracy would not arise if refractive indices of aqueous and vitreous are

**Table 5.1. Refractive indices of various reflecting surfaces of the eye**

| Refracting medium | Refractive index |
|---|---|
| 1. Cornea | 1.377 |
| 2. Aqueous humour | 1.377 |
| 3. Anterior capsule of lens | 1.359 |
| 4. Anterior cortex of lens | 1.387 |
| 5. Nucleus of lens | 1.406 |
| 6. Posterior cortex of lens | 1.385 |
| 7. Vitreous | 1.336 |

considered equal. 1.336 should be considered as the acceptable refractive index. Refractive indices of the anterior and posterior cortices of the lens have also very slight variation and may be considered as the same. From this point of view the lens may be considered to consist of a central core of lens which is biconvex and which is surrounding by two meniscus lenses (Fig. 5.1). The image formed by A is, therefore, focused by C and this, in turn, is focused by P. The concavo-convex menisci neutralise part of the effect of C but it is less in proportion as their refractive index is lower. However, if A and P had the same refractive index as C, the reduction would have been higher. Thus the lens, as such, has a greater refracting power than it would have if it were a homogeneous medium. The heterogeneous quality of the lens medium not only increases the refractive power of the lens but also diminishes the spherical aberrations thus acting partly as an aplanatic lens.

The principal refracting surfaces have the radii of curvature as given in Table 5.2.

The refracting power in dioptres of the principal optical elements and the eye as a whole are given in Table 5.3.

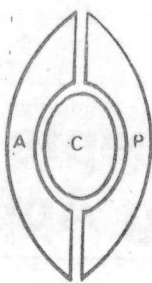

**Fig. 5.1.** Three zones of lenses.

**Table 5.2. Radii of curvature of the principal refracting surfaces**

| Refracting surface | Radius of curvature (in mm) | |
|---|---|---|
| | For distance | For near |
| 1. Anterior cornea | 7.8 | 7.8 |
| 2. Anterior lens | 10.0 | 5.3 |
| 3. Posterior lens | 6.0 | 5.3 |

**Table 5.3. Refracting power of the principal optical elements and the eye as a whole**

| Optical element | Power (in dioptres) | |
|---|---|---|
| | For distance | For near |
| 1. Cornea | 43 | 43 |
| 2. Lens | 20 | 33 |
| 3. Total | 60 | 71 |

The values of the cardinal points from the vertex of the cornea are given in Table 5.4.

**Table 5.4. Values of the cardinal points from the vertex of the cornea**

| Cardinal points | Distance from the vertex of cornea (in mm) | |
|---|---|---|
| | For distance | For near |
| 1. First principal point | 1.5 | 1.8 |
| 2. Second principal point | 1.6 | 2.0 |
| 3. First focal point | 15.2 | 12.3 |
| 4. Second focal point | 22.3 | 18.9 |
| 5. First nodal point | 6.9 | 6.5 |
| 6. Second nodal point | 7.3 | 6.9 |
| 7. First focal length | 16.7 | 14.1 |
| 8. Second focal length | 22.3 | 18.9 |

If a candle is placed in front of and at the same level as the observer and an attempt is made to look into the eye, some images of the candle flame are seen. The images are usually referred to a Purkinje-Sanson images. There are several such images. The formation of these images is dependent upon the principles of catoptric imagery of the eye and these have been utilised to measure the radii of curvature of the refractive media of the eye.

## Catoptric imagery of the eye

If the reflecting surface is regular and smooth, all the reflected light would be thrown back regularly, but such an ideal condition hardly exists. This regularly reflected light is termed *specular reflection*. As is usual, some of the reflected light which forms the catoptric image of source of light, which is actually a part of the regularly reflected light, can be seen by an eye. The light gives rise to the observation of Purkinje-Sanson images. Since some of the surface is irregular, part of the light undergoes *diffuse reflection*.

Besides reflection, some of the light, as stated before, is absorbed and some of it is refracted. In passing through the eye, the light is subjected to all these phenomenon, i.e., some is refracted, some is absorbed and some is reflected, which may be regularly reflected (specular reflection) or irregularly reflected (diffuse reflection). From the six zones of specular reflection (anterior and posterior surfaces of the cornea, anterior and posterior surfaces of lens and anterior and posterior zones of optical discontinuity within the lens) six catoptric images can be seen. Of these four were originally described by Purkinje (Fig. 5.2—only three images are shown).

1. A bright erect image is formed by the anterior surface of the cornea (A) and can be easily recognised.

2. Just to one side of this is a smaller and less distinct image (not shown in the figure) which is formed by the posterior surface of the cornea.

3. Outside these images and nearer to the pupillary area, a diffuse erect and distinct image (B), larger, though less bright, than A is formed by the anterior surface of the lens.

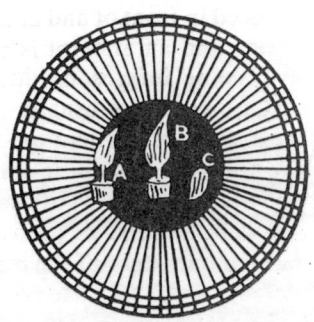

**Fig. 5.2.** Purkinje-Sanson images.

That this image is behind the pupillary plane can be shown by the method of parallax. If pupillary plane is kept as the fixed plane and the head of the observer is moved, B will be found to be moving in the same direction as the head of the observer.

4. A much smaller, inverted, less bright and

real image C towards the other side of the pupillary area is formed by the posterior concave surface of lens. The images formed by the lens are less bright than the first corneal image, because the difference between the refractive indices of the aqueous and the lens, respectively, is slight and consequently, less rays are reflected. The image formed by the posterior part of the lens is smaller because it is reflected by a surface having a radius of curvature less than that of cornea.

To these four images two indistinct images which are reflected by the anterior and posterior surface of the lens nucleus may be added. These images have become less important since the development of the slit lamp as by that apparatus the surfaces themselves can be delineated.

The Purkinje-Sanson images are given in Table 5.5.

### Table 5.5. Purkinje-Sanson images

| Image | Source | Mode | Nature | Brightness | Utility |
|-------|--------|------|--------|------------|---------|
| 1 | Anterior corneal surface | Reflection | Virtual, erect, diminished | Very bright | Keratometry, measurement of thickness of cornea, measurement of angle alpha, diagnosis of strabismus |
| 2 | Posterior corneal surface | Reflection and refraction via the stroma of cornea | Virtual, close to No. 1; erect, diminished, even smaller than No. 1 | Moderately bright | Unimportant and usually not used for clinical purposes |
| 3 | Anterior lens surface | Reflection through aqueous humour and refraction through cornea | Virtual, diminished, but larger than No. 1 | Less bright | Curvature of anterior lens surface, accommodation, measurement of anterior chamber depth |
| 4 | Posterior lens surface | Reflection through lens substance, refraction through cornea | Real, close to No. 1, inverted and diminished | Less bright but almost as bright as No. 3 | Curvature of posterior lens surface, accommodation |

# The Corneal and Lenticular System

## CORNEAL SYSTEM

The refractive power of the corneal system is dependent upon the following :

1. The bathing fluid on the anterior surface, i.e., the lacrimal fluid.
2. The refractive index.
3. The curvature of the surfaces.
4. The thickness of the cornea.
5. Bathing fluid on the posterior surface, i.e., the aqueous humour.

### Lacrimal fluid

It covers the cornea as a thin film in the form of a parallel lamina. In view of a thin parallel lamina, the effect of this fluid on the optical system of the eye is negligible. It is, therefore, ignored.

### Refractive index of the cornea

As stated in the previous chapter, the refractive index of the cornea is 1.377. This can be determined by Abbe's refractometer.

### Curvature of the anterior surface

The radius of curvature of the anterior surface of the cornea is 7.8 mm. It is not possible to measure directly the form of the anterior surface of the cornea in the living and the conditions are grossly altered in the dead.

The cornea also acts as a convex mirror.

In an earlier chapter, it has been stated that the convex mirror forms an erect image, diminished in size and placed apparently behind the cornea, i.e., towards the side of the concavity. The size of image varies with the curvature; the greater the curvature the smaller the size. It is possible to deduce the radius of curvature of the mirror by measuring the size of the image of a given object formed by a convex mirror.

### Calculations of radius of curvature of convex mirror

In Fig. 6.1, AB is the object and A′B′ is the image formed. In this figure, from the law of proportions, we have

$$\frac{A'B'}{AB} = \frac{PB'}{BP}$$

or

$$PB' = PB \times \frac{A'B'}{AB}$$

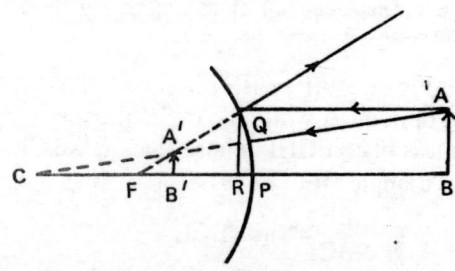

Fig. 6.1. Calculation of radius of curvature of convex mirror.

Now if AB is at infinity then A′B′ is very small and is situated at the focus F in which case BP is the focal distance or ½ of the radius of curvature.

If AB = $O$, A′B′ = $I$, BP = $u$ and CP = $R$,

then

$$\frac{R}{2} = u \times \frac{I}{O} \qquad \ldots(1)$$

or

$$R = \frac{2uI}{O} \qquad \ldots(2)$$

Therefore, if the size of the image of a known object at a given distance is measured, the radius of curvature can be calculated.

The accurate measurement of such an image

presents difficulty in the living eye due to inability to immobilise the living eye while under observation. To measure the size of the image of a given distance the principle that in a parallel plate of glass each point of the image undergoes displacement is utilized. The size of the image, therefore, can be calculated by the total displacement undergone by the rays in a plane lamina (Fig. 6.2).

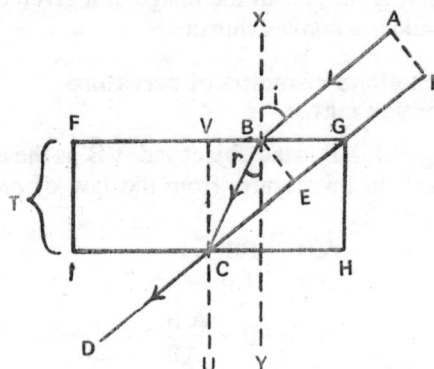

**Fig. 6.2.** Displacement of emergent ray by a plane lamina.

In Fig. 6.2, AP or BE represents the displacement of point A while the ray is passing through the glass plate FGHI, whose thickness is T.

In triangle BEC,

$$\frac{BE}{BC} = \sin \angle BCE$$

$$= \sin (\angle VCE - \angle VCB)$$

$$= \sin (i - r)$$

$$\frac{VC}{BC} = \cos \angle VCB$$

$$= \cos r$$

$$BC = \frac{VC}{\cos r} = \frac{T}{\cos r}$$

Therefore, $BE = \dfrac{T}{\cos r} (\sin i - \sin r)$

$$2BE = 2T \frac{(\sin i - \sin r)}{\cos r} \qquad ...(3)$$

These calculations have been utilized for measuring the image in the eye by Helmholtz ophthalmometer where there is double displacement of images.

Helmholtz ophthalmometer consists of two plates. Each plate displaces the image through

half its length and the total displacement gives the size of the images. The doubling of image dispenses with the necessity of immobilizing the living eye. If the eye moves during the process, both the images move together and, therefore, difficulties in adjustment are avoided.

The Helmholtz ophthalmometer consists of two plates of glass of known thickness and index of refraction, placed side by side, so that each covers half of the object of a short distance telescope. The axis of telescope coincides with the plane of separation of the glass plates. These plates can be inclined one to the other at known angles and the angle of incidence of light falling on them from a point in front can be varied and measured (Fig. 6.3).

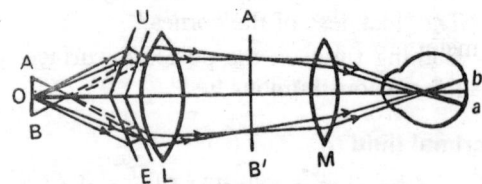

**Fig. 6.3.** Principle of Helmholtz ophthalmometer.

In Fig. 6.3, rays from point O meet the plates U and E and undergo lateral displacement after refraction. As viewed through L, the two objects appear at A and B. The eyepiece M is so arranged that its principal focus coincides with the images A′ and B′ and receives parallel rays which come to the focus without accommodation on the retina at a and b. If the position of the plates is such that the two images A and B just touch at O then each plate has displaced the image through half its length and the total displacement gives the size of the image (Fig. 6.4).

We have already seen from equation (1) that

$$R = \frac{2uI}{O}$$

and from equation (2)

$$I = \frac{2T \sin (i - r)}{\cos r}$$

In this instrument, $u$ and $O$ are known and $I$ has been calculated as above, hence $R$ can be easily calculated. This is one of the most accurate instruments from the scientific point of view. The instrument has undergone several modifications and now-a-days several keratometers are in use.

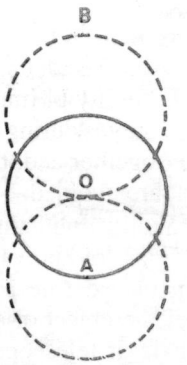

**Fig. 6.4.** Measurement of the size of image.

### Keratometers in clinical use

Some keratometers are based on constant object size and variable image size.

Among the most important uses of keratometer are :

- Helps in measurement of corneal astigmatic error.
- Helps to estimate the radius of curvature of the anterior surface of cornea (useful in contact lens fitting).
- Can monitor the shape of the cornea as in keratoconus.

Among the less frequent uses are :

- Assess the axis and value of the corneal cylindrical refractive error.
- May be able to assess the refractive error in cases with media haze (rough estimate on the presumption that the normal measurement is 43.5 D—comparison of the two eyes in these cases is useful).
- Useful to take K readings along with corneal thickness and axial length of eyeball (with other means) to find out the IOL power required.

Ideally keratometers are essentially based on one of the two principles :

- Where object size is kept constant (commonly employed) as in Javal & Schiötz keratometer and Bausch & Lomb keratometer.
- Where image size is constant (not in common use).

An ideal keratometer must be able to measure the radii in various meridians about the axis of the cornea. Thus the instruments are designed to rotate them with respect to a particular axis.

The objects are called mires. In order to avoid inaccuracies due to constant motion of the eyes, a doubling device was introduced in Helmholtz ophthalmometer already described above.

Two commonly used keratometers in this country are :

1. Bausch & Lomb keratometer
2. Javal and Schiötz keratometer

There are other keratometers which work on the principle of constant image size and are hardly ever used in this country.

### Bausch & Lomb keratometer

This instrument works on the principle of constant object size and variable image size for its operation. Fig. 6.5 shows the optical system of the instrument in its simplified form. A lamp illuminates the mires by means of a diagonal mirror. Light from the mires strikes the patient's cornea and produces an image behind it. Since the dimensions of the mire are fixed, the size of the image formed is dependent on the radius of the cornea. The image thus produced acts as an object for the rest of the optical system. Light from this object is gathered by an objective lens and is focused to a plane farther along the central axis. A four-aperture diaphragm is situated near the objective lens. Beyond this diaphragm are two doubling prisms, one with its base up and other with its base out. The prisms can be moved independently parallel to the central axis of the instrument. Light passing through the left aperture (A) of the diaphragm is made to deviate above the central optical axis by a base up prism. Light passing through the right aperture (O) is deviated by the base out prism, placing the second image to the right of the central axis. Light passing through the upper (B) and lower (C) apertures of the diaphragm does not pass through either prism and an image is produced in the axis. The total collective area of the upper and lower apertures is equal to the area of each of the other two apertures. Thus, the brightness of all the three images is equal. The upper and lower apertures also act as a Scheiner's disc, doubling the central image, whenever the instrument is not focused precisely

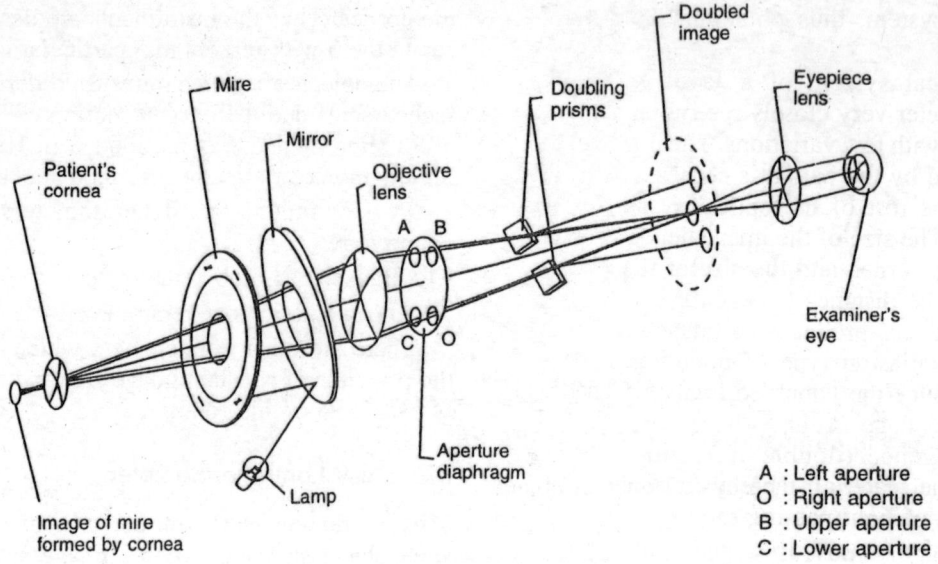

**Fig. 6.5.** Optical system of keratometer.

Labels in figure:
- Patient's cornea
- Mire
- Mirror
- Objective lens
- Doubling prisms
- Doubled image
- Eyepiece lens
- Examiner's eye
- Aperture diaphragm
- Lamp
- Image of mire formed by cornea

A : Left aperture
O : Right aperture
B : Upper aperture
C : Lower aperture

**Table 6.1.** Comparison of Bausch & Lomb keratometer and Javal & Schiötz ophthalmometer

|  | Bausch & Lomb | Javal & Schiötz |
|---|---|---|
| Principle | Constant object; variable doubling | Variable object; fixed doubling |
| Prism | Doubling prism (base out and base up) | Wollaston type prism (birefringent) |
| Position of image | Side to side | 90° to each other |
| Mirror position for checking both the axes | Required; one position | Not required; two positions |

on the central mire image. Thus a continuous monitoring of correct focus can be done by the examiner. The function of the eyepiece is to provide a magnified view of the doubled image.

The cornea acts as a convex mirror. A virtual erect image of the mires is formed 4 mm behind the cornea. The size of the mires on a Bausch & Lomb keratometer is 64 mm and the image size is 3.0 mm. The distance between the cornea and the mires is 75 mm. The mires have a variable separation on the same instrument depending on the radius of curvature of the cornea being tested. Mires of different instruments have a variable separation for the same corneal curvature. On a cornea of 7.94 mm radius, the separation of mires for a Bausch & Lomb keratometer is 3.1 mm. The image is magnified 1.304 times by the objective lens and magnified finally to 6.197 times by the eyepiece.

**Javal & Schiötz ophthalmometer**

The working of a Javal & Schiötz keratometer is based on variable object size and constant image size. It employs a fixed image doubling device. In this system, the object consists of two mires (one stepped and the other a square mire), illuminated by lamps enclosed in a housing behind them. The stepped mire has a green filter and the square mire is covered by a red filter. Any area of superimposition due to overlapping of the two mires appears yellow. The two mires move synchronously along a curved track which is situated below the housings. When the central knob is rotated in one direction, each of the mires moves closer together towards the central axis of the instrument. Rotation of the controls in the opposite direction causes both mires to move away from the central axis. Thus both the two mires collectively act as an object for the rest of the optical system, thus obtaining the variable object size.

The optical system of a Javal & Schiötz ophthalmometer very closely resembles that of a keratometer with few variations. The image of the mires formed by the patient's cornea acts as the object for the rest of the optical system of the instrument. The size of the image depends on the radius of the cornea and the size of the original object, i.e., the distance between the two mires. An objective lens produces an image of the new object. A Wallaston type of doubling prism is used to produce the "doubled image". The doubling of the image in this prism is attributed to the birefringence (double refracting) characteristic of the material, thereby implying that a single beam of light passing through it emerges as two beams. An eyepiece lens helps in magnification of the viewed double image, the two images are separated from each other. By changing the separation of the mires, the patterns in the image can be made to overlap. When the two central images just meet, the scales associated with a mire separation indicate the correct corneal radius of curvature and the dioptric power of the cornea. The relationship between the dioptric power and the radius of curvature is as follows :

$$D = \frac{n-1}{r}$$

where $D$ = dioptric power of the cornea,

$n$ = index of refraction of the cornea,

$r$ = radius of curvature (in metres).

Index of refraction of cornea for calibrating a keratometer is 1.3375.

Therefore,   $r$ (in metres) $= \dfrac{0.3375}{D}$

$r$ (in millimetres) $= \dfrac{337.5}{D}$

Radius of curvature of the cornea is first found in one meridian. Then the entire optical system is rotated by 90° about its central axis for the measurement of the radius of curvature in the second meridian which is perpendicular to the first one.

## Procedure of keratometry

### Step 1

*Instrument adjustment :* A white paper is held before the objective. Focus a black line or hair on the paper. This is followed by calibration of the keratometer with steel balls (as previously discussed). The range of the instrument may be extended in very steep or very flat corneas by adding +1.25 D or –1.00 D respectively to the objective.

### Step 2

*Patient adjustment :* The patient puts his chin on the chin rest and head against the head rest. The chin is raised or lowered to bring the line in apposition with the black line on Bausch & Lomb keratometer. The eye which is not being examined is covered till the patient's pupil and the projecting knob are at the same level. The instrument is moved forwards and backwards till the mires are accurately focused. The dial is then rotated till the mires are approximated. The plus mires should be aligned so that they overlap with each other. This may be done by adjustment of mire size and separation by the knob or adjustment of the axis by tilting the instrument along axis to overlap the mires. The value of the horizontal meridian is read. The mires are then realigned in the vertical meridian and mires are overlapped.

Mires in Bausch & Lomb keratometer may be spherical which will be seen in majority of corneas. Horizontally oval and vertically oval mires indicate the presence of 'with the rule' and 'against the rule' astigmatism respectively. Pulsating mires are suggestive of keratoconus.

## One and two position keratometers

The axes of a toric surface are always at 90° to each other. Therefore, in a 'one position' keratometer (i.e., Bausch & Lomb keratometer), two separate doubling systems operating in perpendicular meridians are used. These instruments have to be rotated about the anteroposterior axis in order to determine one of the principle meridians of the cornea; having achieved this, no further rotation is required to obtain the measurement along the second principle meridian. This type of keratometer is called as one position instrument. The keratometer requiring rotation through 90° in order to measure the curvature of the second principle meridian is known as two position instrument (i.e., Javal & Schiötz keratometer).

**Table 6.2. Conversion from radius of curvature in mm to dioptres**

$$D = \frac{n-1}{r} \qquad n = 1.3375$$

| mm | Dioptres | mm | Dioptres | mm | Dioptres | mm | Dioptres |
|------|----------|------|----------|------|----------|-------|----------|
| 5.00 | 67.50 | 6.30 | 53.57 | 7.60 | 44.41 | 8.90 | 37.92 |
| 5.05 | 66.83 | 6.35 | 53.15 | 7.65 | 44.12 | 8.95 | 37.71 |
| 5.10 | 66.18 | 6.40 | 52.73 | 7.70 | 43.83 | 9.00 | 37.50 |
| 5.15 | 66.53 | 6.45 | 52.43 | 7.75 | 43.55 | 9.05 | 37.29 |
| 5.20 | 64.90 | 6.50 | 51.92 | 7.80 | 43.27 | 9.10 | 37.09 |
| 5.25 | 64.29 | 6.55 | 51.53 | 7.85 | 42.99 | 9.15 | 36.88 |
| 5.30 | 63.68 | 6.60 | 51.14 | 7.90 | 42.72 | 9.20 | 36.68 |
| 5.35 | 63.08 | 6.65 | 50.75 | 7.95 | 42.45 | 9.25 | 36.49 |
| 5.40 | 62.50 | 6.70 | 50.37 | 8.00 | 42.19 | 9.30 | 36.29 |
| 5.45 | 61.93 | 6.75 | 50.00 | 8.05 | 41.93 | 9.35 | 36.10 |
| 5.50 | 61.36 | 6.80 | 49.63 | 8.10 | 41.67 | 9.40 | 35.90 |
| 5.55 | 60.81 | 6.85 | 49.27 | 8.15 | 41.41 | 9.45 | 35.71 |
| 5.60 | 60.27 | 6.90 | 48.91 | 8.20 | 41.16 | 9.50 | 35.53 |
| 5.65 | 59.73 | 6.95 | 48.56 | 8.25 | 40.91 | 9.55 | 35.34 |
| 5.70 | 59.21 | 7.00 | 48.21 | 8.30 | 40.66 | 9.60 | 35.17 |
| 5.75 | 58.70 | 7.05 | 47.87 | 8.35 | 40.42 | 9.65 | 34.98 |
| 5.80 | 58.19 | 7.10 | 47.53 | 8.40 | 40.18 | 9.70 | 34.79 |
| 5.85 | 57.69 | 7.15 | 47.30 | 8.45 | 39.94 | 9.75 | 34.62 |
| 5.90 | 57.20 | 7.20 | 46.87 | 8.50 | 39.70 | 9.80 | 34.42 |
| 5.95 | 56.72 | 7.25 | 46.56 | 8.55 | 39.47 | 9.85 | 34.25 |
| 6.00 | 56.25 | 7.30 | 46.23 | 8.60 | 39.24 | 9.90 | 34.08 |
| 6.05 | 55.78 | 7.35 | 45.92 | 8.65 | 39.10 | 9.95 | 33.90 |
| 6.10 | 55.33 | 7.40 | 45.61 | 8.70 | 38.79 | 10.00 | 33.75 |
| 6.15 | 54.88 | 7.45 | 45.30 | 8.75 | 38.42 | | |
| 6.20 | 54.44 | 7.50 | 45.00 | 8.80 | 38.35 | | |
| 6.25 | 54.00 | 7.55 | 44.70 | 8.85 | 38.14 | | |

In place of flames as objects diffuse light reflected from white surfaces disposed on a circular arc is employed. This arc can be rotated round the axis of the instrument. The instrument measures only the central area of the cornea. The peripheral radii measured by Helmholtz ophthalmometer were greater. The curvature of cornea was, therefore, considered as an ellipsoid but this contention has not been accepted. The keratoscopic disc and keratographic procedures have shown the presence of certain degree of physiological astigmatism.

This instrument is calibrated both for radius of curvature and corresponding dioptres. The conversion can also be obtained by the following equation.

$$D = \frac{n-1}{r}$$

where $D$ is dioptre, $n$ is a constant (1.3375) and $r$ is the radius of curvature. The conversion is given in Table 6.2.

On the calibrated arc are mounted two linear objects A and B (Figs. 6.6 and 6.7) which can be adjusted by a knob. In the centre of the arc is a telescope T through which the images of A and B can be seen as mires a and b (Fig. 6.8). These mires can be considered as the ends of the linear object AB. The arc is adjusted in a position and the length of the object AB is adjusted by moving A and B on the arc so that the images a and b touch each other (Fig. 6.8). The mire has steps and each step corresponds to a dioptre. On rotat-

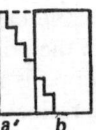

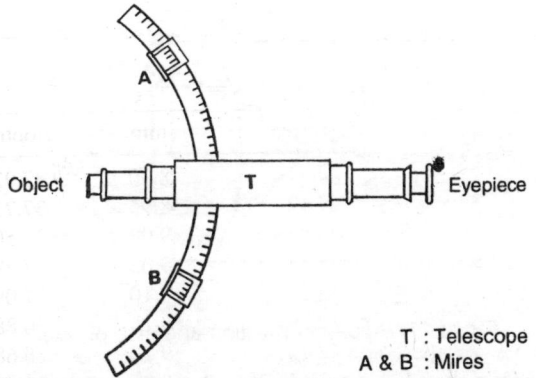

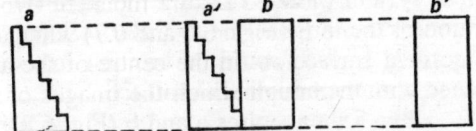 

**Fig. 6.6.** Arc of telescope of Javal & Schiötz ophthalmometer (diagrammatic).

T : Telescope
A & B : Mires

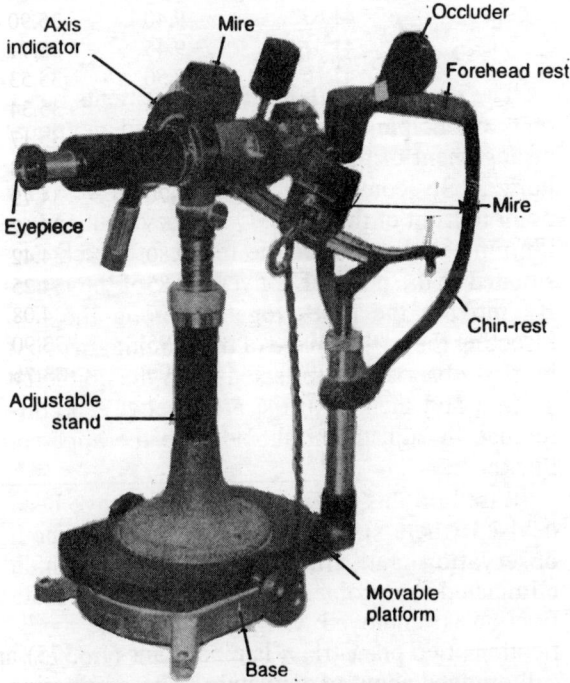

**Fig. 6.7.** Javal & Schiötz ophthalmometer.

**Fig. 6.8.** Images of two targets in coincidence.

ing through 90° there may be an overlapping (Fig. 6.9).

The number of steps overlapped will give the approximate difference in the dioptric strength of

**Fig. 6.9.** Images of two targets overlapping.

the two meridia. The objects are moved so that once again the position given in Fig. 6.8 is achieved. The readings in the two axes are recorded and the difference between the two gives the astigmatic error.

**Measurement of thickness of transparent media**

If in ophthalmometry Nernst lamp is used, a ratio between the reflex images of the anterior and posterior surfaces can be found which will correspond to the ratio between the two radii of the curvature. Assuming that the radius of curvature of the anterior surface of the cornea is 7.8 mm and the radius of curvature of the posterior surface of the cornea is 6.7 mm, the thickness of the cornea can be measured by the observation of images reflected from the two surfaces by applying the principles of an ophthalmophakometer (Fig. 6.10).

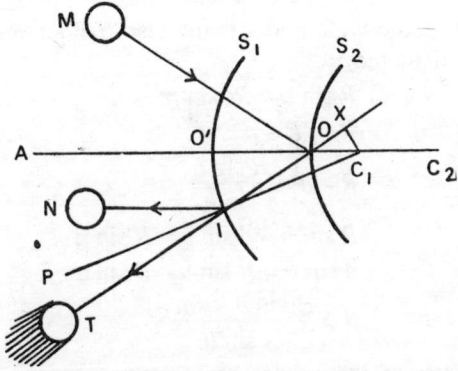

**Fig. 6.10.** Measurement of the thickness of cornea by ophthalmophakometer.

In Fig. 6.10, let $S_1$ and $S_2$ be the anterior and posterior surfaces of the cornea having their centre of curvature at $C_1$ and $C_2$. OO' represents the distance $d$ between them. $O'C_1$ is the radius of curvature ($R$) of the anterior surface of the cornea. OO'A is the visual axis of the eye which fixes the object A on a graduated arc. Two sources of light M and N and a telescope T are mounted on the movable carriages of the arc. A ray MO is directed to the posterior surface of the cornea and the telescope is moved about the arc until it receives the reflected ray from O. The angle MOT ($2b$) is measured on the arc.

With another source of light N the image is formed at the anterior surface of the cornea and carriage of this light is displaced until the image of N is superimposed upon that of M and the angle NIT ($2a$) is measured.

In the same figure produce TIO to X and drop a perpendicular $C_1X$ on it from $C_1$ at X. Then in the triangle $C_1XI$,

$$\frac{C_1X}{C_1I} = \sin a$$

or

$$\frac{C_1X}{R} = \sin a$$

or

$$C_1X = R \sin a$$

In the triangle $C_1OX$,

$$\frac{C_1X}{OC_1} = \sin b$$

or

$$\frac{C_1X}{R_2} = \sin b$$

or

$$C_1X = R_2 \sin b$$

or

$$R_2 \sin b = R \sin a$$

We know $\angle a$ and $\angle b$ and also $R_1$ then $R_2$ can be calculated.

$$R \sin a = R_2 \sin b \qquad \ldots(3)$$

But

$$R_2 = R - d \qquad \ldots(4)$$

$$R - d = \frac{R \sin a}{\sin b}$$

$$R \sin b - d \sin b = R \sin a$$

$$d \sin b = R \sin b - R \sin d$$

$$d = \frac{R(\sin b - \sin a)}{\sin b}$$

Sine of the angles are known and so is $R$, hence $d$ can be calculated.

In Fig. 6.11, we have $R - R_2 = d$ and from equation (4) we know $R$ and $R_2$, hence $d$ can be calculated.

The method, however, gives an apparent position of the surface. The object is situated within the focal distance of the concave surface of the media and, therefore, gives a virtual, erect and magnified image displaced towards the anterior surface of the cornea (Fig. 6.11). In this figure,

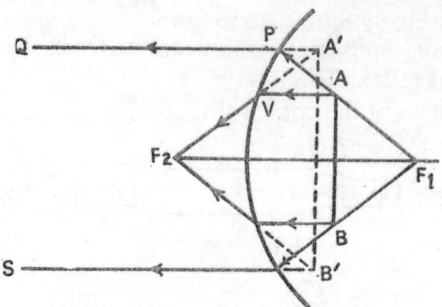

Fig. 6.11. Apparent position and size of pupil.

AB is the object and A'B' is the image. Knowing the apparent position, the real position can be calculated from

$$\frac{F_1}{u} - \frac{F_2}{v} = l$$

The practical method of measurements based on the principle of Blix who employed an optical arrangement of two identical microscopic tubes, horizontally converging at an angle of 40° to a point in front of the tubes. One tube contained an illuminated diaphragm, the image of which was situated at the point of convergence of the tubes. By moving the tubes together along the line bisecting them, the image of the diaphragm could be first observed as reflected from the epithelial surface and then from the endothelial. The difference in adjustment should give the apparent thickness.

Based on this system, instruments have been devised where simultaneous adjustment of both observation and illumination system which eliminated the problem of maintaining accurate fixation is employed. Originally in these modifications two plane glass lamina were symmetrically moved about vertical axis before both optical systems. The rays of the lower half of the optical system passed through the laminae. By rotation of the laminae the specular reflection of the corneal surface could be brought into coincidence with the endothelial surface.

### Maurice and Giardini's instrument

This can be attached to Haag-Streit slit-lamp. A plastic plate is used between the lens and the slit-lamp. It achieves the same purpose as two glass laminae. The plastic plate contains a 1 mm wide slit covered by coloured celluloid and rotated by an arm over a fixed scale to align the coloured epithelial reflex with the white endothelial reflex. The rotation of the arm gives the thickness of the cornea (Fig. 6.12).

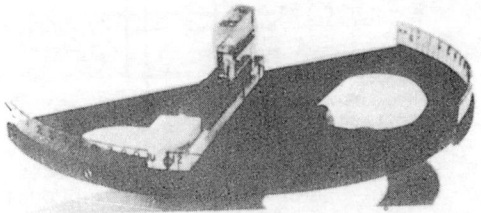

Fig. 6.12. The pachometer of Maurice.

### Donaldson's instrument

The principle employed in this instrument is the same as of splitting of images by plane glass lamina or some other device. In Donaldson's apparatus a split ocular eyepiece is employed instead of the standard eyepiece on the slit-lamp. This divides the images by producing a horizontal prismatic effect when one of the eye lenses is moved in relation to the other (Fig. 6.13).

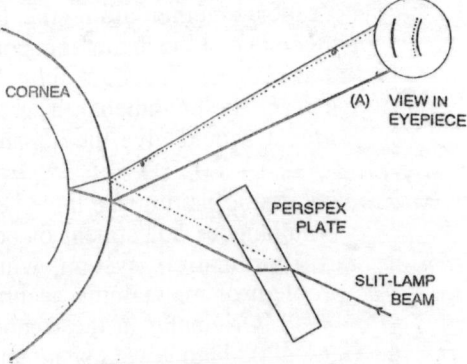

Fig. 6.13. The corneal thickness.

Similarly the relative position of surface of lens can be determined (Fig. 6.14).

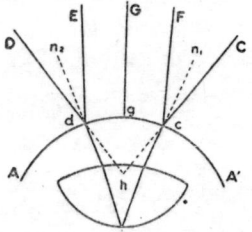

Fig. 6.14. Relative position of surfaces of lens.

In addition to the optical pachometer, the ultrasonic pachometer (Fig. 6.15) is gaining more widespread use for the measurement of corneal thickness. Its ease of use and its portability make

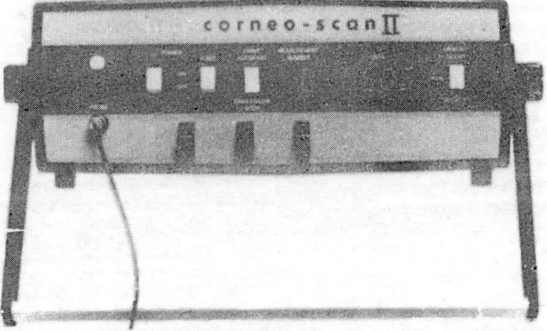

Fig. 6.15. Ultrasound pachometer used to measure the corneal thickness.

it much simpler and more convenient to handle and use. Ultrasonic waves are passed through the cornea to provide a digital read-out of the corneal thickness. The head of the pachometer is either of solid type or fluid-filled. The probe is directly applied to the cornea. The read-outs are given in microns of thickness of the cornea.

# CHAPTER 7

# Optical Resolution of the Eye

According to Gauss' concept, a coaxial homo-centric system of lenses can be resolved into six cardinal points, i.e., two principal foci, two nodal points and two principal planes.

The refractive indices of the aqueous and the vitreous are almost identical while cornea has an insignificantly higher refractive index than this. In view of these facts Listing expressed that the optical system of the eye may be considered to consist of two elements :

1. The corneal surface separating air from the common medium.
2. The lens in the common medium.

### Schematic eye of Gullstrand

On this presumption, Gullstrand considered the eye to consist of coaxial homocentric system of lenses and, therefore, can also be resolved into six cardinal points.

In Fig. 7.1 such a system is represented. There are two principal points ($H_1$ and $H_2$) with their planes situated somewhere in the anterior chamber and they are very near to each other; two nodal points ($N_1$ and $N_2$) which are situated on either side of the posterior pole of the lens and the two principal foci ($F_1$ and $F_2$). The anterior focal point is situated, roughly speaking, about 15

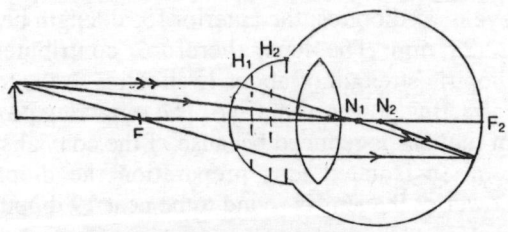

**Fig. 7.1.** Cardinal points.

mm in front of the cornea and the posterior focal point lies on the retina in an emmetropic eye.

### Listing's reduced eye (Fig. 7.2)

Listing felt that the data and the geometrical optics of the eye looked rather complex and he, therefore, simplified the data and laid steps towards the ultimate concepts of the reduced eye.

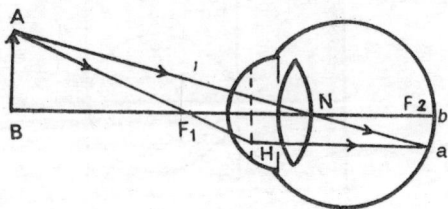

**Fig. 7.2.** Listing's reduced eye.

The two principal points are very near to each other, and, therefore, no significant error will arise if an intermediate point is taken as the principal point which might be considered to be situated about 1.5 mm behind the anterior surface of the cornea. Similarly the two nodal points are situated very near to each other and no significant error will arise if they are resolved into a single nodal point situated in between the two, i.e., about 7.8 mm behind the anterior surface for the cornea. This distance corresponds to just behind the posterior pole of the lens. The final optical system (Fig. 7.2) of the eye, therefore, can be resolved into a principal point H, a nodal point N and two foci, anterior and posterior ($F_1$ and $F_2$).

According to Listing, the anterior focal point is 15.2 mm in front and the posterior focal point is 22.3 mm behind the anterior surface of the cornea. The anterior focal length is 16.7 mm and the posterior focal length is 22.32 mm and the dioptric power of the eye is 60 dioptres.

### Donders' reduced eye (Fig. 7.3)

Donders in the interest of simplicity treated the eye as a single refracting surface, the plane being situated 2 mm behind the cornea with a radius of 5 mm and the anterior and posterior focal length of 15 and 20 mm respectively, whose relative index of refraction is 1.33. This carries simplification much too far but it makes the remembering of figures quite easy. This over-simplification introduces several errors and inaccuracies.

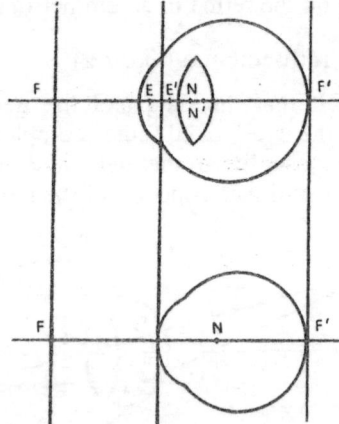

**Fig. 7.3.** Donders' reduced eye.

Thus according to this concept the following assumptions have been made :
1. There is a single refracting surface of 60 D power.
2. The intraocular index of refraction for all refractive media is uniform and is 1.33.
3. The first principal plane is superimposed on the second principal plane and are located at an imaginary 'cornea' situated 2 mm behind the anatomical cornea.
4. The first nodal point is superimposed on the second nodal point and is 5 mm posterior to the principal plane.
5. The second focal point is 20 mm posteriorly from the surface of the principal plane.

This concept, however, is useful and practical for locating images employing the two ray trace procedure.

### Construction of image on this concept

With reduced eye of Donders it is neither difficult to construct a retinal image nor to calculate its size.

In Fig. 7.4, let AD be a ray passing through the anterior focus meeting the principal plane at D, it is refracted as Da which is parallel to the axis Bb. AN is a ray passing through the nodal point N and, therefore, goes undeviated meeting the ray Da at a. a, therefore, is the image of the A, and similarly b is the image of B. Thus ab is the image of AB.

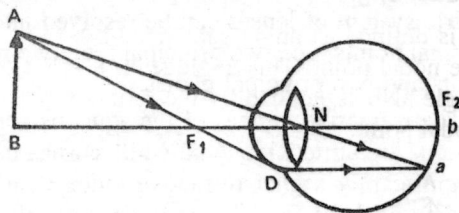

**Fig. 7.4.** Construction of image on reduced eye concept.

In similar triangles ANB and aNb,

$$\frac{ab}{AB} = \frac{bN}{NB}$$

If NB = d and, from Donders' reduced eye bN = 15 mm then the ratio between the size of the image and the size of the object is equal to the ratio between 15 mm and the distance of the object from the eye. If d is 30 mm then the size of the retinal image is 15/30 = 1/2.

When the lens is removed, i.e., the eye becomes aphakic, the position of these cardinal points is altered. According to Gullstrand the principal points remain unaltered. The ideal surface has now a radius of curvature of 7.8 mm as against 5.73 mm. The anterior focal length changes to 22.23 mm from 16.7 mm and the posterior focal length to 31.03 mm from 22.78 mm.

The refracting power of a normal eye is about 60 dioptres and the dioptric power of the aphakic eye is 45 dioptres, the anterior focal length being 22.23 mm. The lens, therefore, contributes a dioptric strength of about 15 dioptres to the total refracting power of the eye. The refracting power of the lens is reduced because of the coaxial system. In isolated lens preparation the dioptric power of the lens is found to be near 19 dioptres.

In aphakia the nodal point also shifts forwards and almost coincides with the principal point.

# CHAPTER 8

# Visual Angles, Visual Acuity, Visual Axes and Axial Length of Eye

## Visual angle

It is defined as angle subtended by an object at the nodal point. This angle (Fig. 8.1) is equal to angle aNb subtended by the retinal image at the nodal point.

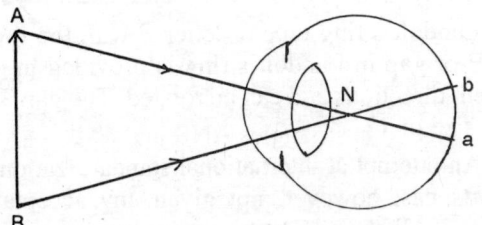

**Fig. 8.1.** Visual angle.

The macular area has a large number of cones herded together. These cones are the visual end organs. If two luminous points are to be distinguished separately, two cones must be stimulated while the intermediate cone should remain unstimulated. The distance is termed the minimum resolvable distance, which is about 0.002 mm. The minimum resolvable distance is the tangent of the angle that the retinal image makes at the nodal point, i.e.,

$$\tan aNb = \frac{ab}{bN} = \frac{0.002}{17.054}$$
$$= \tan 24'14''$$

**Line acuity**: The problem of visibility of a line is a function, to some degree, of the length of line. In addition, the thickness of the line, the general illumination level and contrast are important variables. Most persons can distinguish these images with a minimum visible angle of 1′ and this is considered to be a practical limit.

**Vernier acuity :** Vernier acuity or aligning power refers to the ability to determine when two parallel straight lines are exactly in line. The vernier acuity is defined as the minimum detectable displacement from perfect alignment. The threshold is lower for longer lines, and adaptation and illumination are important variables.

**Fig. 8.2.** Vernier acuity.

**Visual acuity :** Visual acuity is defined as the power to distinguish one object from the other and to appreciate the details of the visible objects. It consists of a form sense, a colour sense and a light sense.

To measure the visual acuity it is necessary to find the minimum angle at which two points are seen as separate points. The visual angle can be increased or decreased by either increasing or decreasing the size of the object; decreasing or increasing the distance of the object from the eye.

The knowledge of a minimum practical visual angle of 1′ has been utilized for devising tests for visual acuity. The most commonly employed test is the Snellen's test. Snellen found that an object such as a letter is required to subtend an angle five times greater than the lines or the dots of which it is composed (Fig. 8.3). He so constructed his letters that they formed visual angle of 5′ from varying distances, i.e., 60, 36, 24, 18, 12, 6 and 5 metres (Figs. 8.4 and 8.5). These letters are made on a chart which is placed at a distance of 6 metres from the patient and is illuminated in such a way that illumination does not fall below 3 foot candles. An illumination of

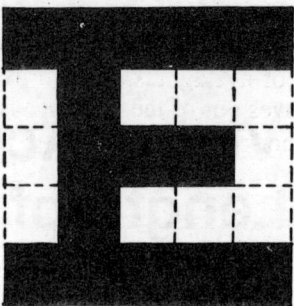

**Fig. 8.3.** A letter on Snellen's principles.

20-40 foot candles is ideal for the purpose. The visual acuity is described as *d/D* where *d* is the distance of the chart from the patient (usually 6 metres) and *D* is the distance at which the letter would subtend an angle of 5′, i.e., 6/60, 6/36, 6/24, 6/18, 6/12, 6/9, 6/6, 6/5, etc. The normal vision at the time Snellen constructed his chart was thought by him to be of the order of 6/6 but in practice we find that the normal vision is 6/5.

6 metre distance of the patient from the chart has been chosen on the assumption that for all practical purposes the rays of light coming from this distance meet the eye parallel to its axis.

If at 6 metres the letter which subtends an angle of 5′ from 60 metres cannot be comprehended, the distance should be reduced by moving the patient forwards gradually so that the vision can be recorded as 5/60, 4/60, 3/60, 2/60, 1/60 etc. If the letter cannot be seen even from one metre distance then, with the light behind the patient, he is asked to count the fingers of the outstretched hand which are brought gradually nearer to the eye. The vision is then recorded as F.C. (finger counting) from 1 metre, 1/2 metre, etc. If he cannot appreciate this then the outstretched hand is moved just near the eye and the vision is recorded as H.M. (hand movements). Failing this he may be able to perceive the light only and the vision is recorded as P.L.

A large variety of test types have been introduced from time to time as Snellen's charts were not considered to be ideal. Since most people are familiar with alphabets it was thought that it interferes with the exactitude of the test. A letter of somewhat blurred outline may be correctly interpreted by an experienced observer.

Landolt's ring type or letter E with the limbs of E or gap in Landolt's ring is provided in different directions and can be rotated. The gap is of the size of 1′.

An attempt at international standardization of charts has, however, not given any acceptable norms. All the test types devised are tests of a subjective nature. Among these types even today most widely used charts are the Snellen's types.

Charts used in this country are in different languages and present many difficulties in adoption. The author, however, standardized the Hindi and Urdu charts based on Snellen's principles. These are now usually commercially utilised in this country.

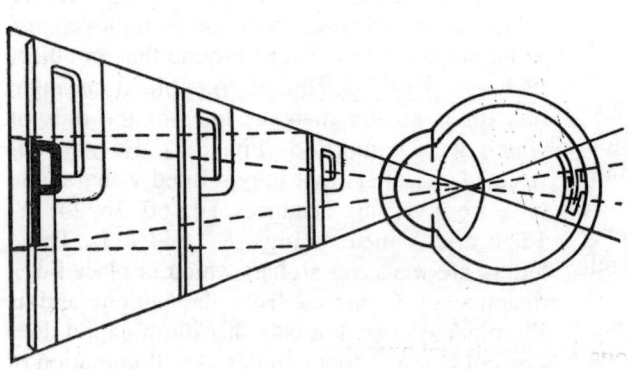

**Fig. 8.4.** Principle of Snellen's chart.

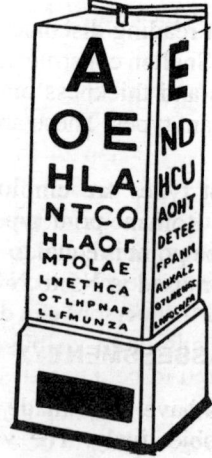

**Fig. 8.5.** Snellen's chart.

An international visual acuity transcription as approved by the International Council of Ophthalmology (1994) and adopted as notation by many ophthalmologists is in vogue. The same is summarised in Table 8.1.

**Table 8.1. Visual acuity transcription tables**

| Decimal visual acuity notation | 6 metre equivalent | 20 foot equivalent | Visual angle in minutes |
|---|---|---|---|
| 1.0 | 6/6 | 20/20 | 1.0 |
| 0.9 | — | — | 1.1 |
| 0.8 | 5/6 | 20/25 | 1.3 |
| 0.7 | 6/9 | 20/30 | 1.4 |
| 0.6 | 5/9 | 15/25 | 1.6 |
| 0.5 | 6/12 | 20/40 | 2.0 |
| 0.4 | 5/12 | 20/50 | 2.5 |
| 0.3 | 6/18 | 20/70 | 3.3 |
| 0.2 | — | — | 5.0 |
| 0.1 | 6/60 | 20/200 | 10.0 |

The amount of illumination has a considerable effect on the visual acuity. It is essential that the test types are well and uniformly illuminated. In the normal eye, below 2 lumens per square foot the efficiency falls very rapidly and above this value it rises slowly by a small amount until illumination of 50 lumens/sq. ft. is attained. In practice, however, an illumination of 100 lumens/sq. ft. is provided which is easy to attain with tube or strip lighting.

### Testing of near vision

Visual acuity at reading distance is measured on near test types. Snellen constructed a set of letters of graded sizes and thickness on the same principle as his distant types. These are, however, not used now.

Jaeger's test types are employed which are now in 'Times Roman' print types from point 5 to 48 in size (one point is equal to 1/72 of an inch) and the notation used is N5 to N48.

### OBJECTIVE ASSESSMENT OF VISION

Many attempts have been made to measure the visual acuity objectively. The various methods are grouped as under :

### Optokinetic nystagmus

The instruments in this group aim at producing a jerking type of nystagmus as soon as the object of regard moves out of the field of vision.

The method cannot be used if an existing larger nystagmus exists, if disturbances in central nervous system are present, or if the patient shows inability to observe correctly.

### Oscillatory motion

The tests aim at eliciting oscillating eye movements when the test is presented at varying distances from the eye. The objections against these techniques are several including the difficulty of observation of small eye movements.

### Arresting nystagmus

Nystagmus is induced by targets and then arrested by the introduction of target which permits steady fixation when the target site becomes large enough for resolution.

For the objective methods it is necessary that the cooperation of the patient required should be minimum; it should be possible to examine patients of all ages; the IQ should not be the altering factor in assessing the visual acuity and that the correlation between subjective and objective methods should be present over a wide range of visual acuities.

From these criteria the optokinetic methods seem to be the most satisfactory. In actual practice, however, Snellen's method still seems to be the best method of measuring visual acuity.

The diminution in vision may be due to a diminution in dioptric power of the eye. The record of visual acuity with an uncorrected refractive error is relative visual acuity and is expressed as naked eye vision. If the refractive error of the eye is corrected and the vision is recorded with glasses it is termed as an absolute visual acuity. The visual acuity of each eye separately is slightly less than the visual acuity recorded when both eyes are uncovered.

### Axes of the eye

The eye has three principal axes :
1. Optical axis
2. Visual axis
3. Fixation axis

The *optical axis* of the eye (OCD) passes through the centre of the cornea. The various refracting surfaces of the eye centre round the axis. It does not cut the fundus at the macula but cuts it somewhat towards the inner side. On this line are situated the two foci, the nodal points and the principal axis. On this axis is also situated the centre of rotation of the eye which is about 13.5 mm behind the anterior surface of the cornea. This axis cannot be precisely defined because there is uncertainty on the exact location of optical centres of each optical element, through which this line is supposed to pass. For practical purposes this axis is taken to coincide with the pupillary line which is a line drawn through the apparent centre of the pupil perpendicular to the surface of the cornea. This line is not entirely symmetrically passing through the remainder of the optical system because the pupil is slightly nasally located.

The *visual axis* (FNM) does not coincide with the assumed optical axis. It is along a line joining the nodal point, the macula and the fixation point. It crosses the cornea 4° down and 5° to the nasal side of the cornea.

The *fixation axis* (FC) is the line joining the fixation points and the centre of rotation of the eye. The three axes are shown in Fig. 8.6.

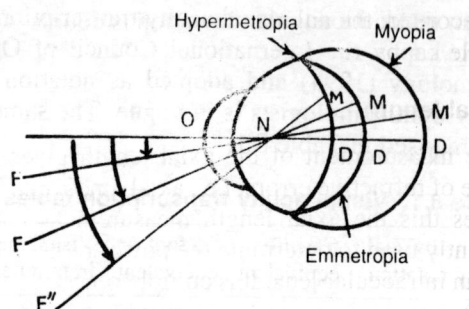

**Fig. 8.7.** Variations of angle alpha with refractive errors.

angle is then negative. It happens in high degree of myopia. This gives rise to an apparent convergent squint. In high hypermetropia the angle alpha is high and positive and it gives a deceptive appearance of a divergent squint.

The angle between the assumed optical axis and the fixation axis is angle gamma. Angle gamma is slightly larger than angle alpha.

As stated above the size of angle alpha is of some importance in the diagnosis of strabismus associated with refractive errors. It is not possible to measure angle alpha clinically. Another angle kappa, which is nearly of the same size as angle alpha and angle gamma, is measured clinically. Angle kappa is an angle formed between the central pupillary line and the visual axis at the centre of the pupil. Angle kappa is smaller than angle alpha and angle gamma (Fig. 8.8).

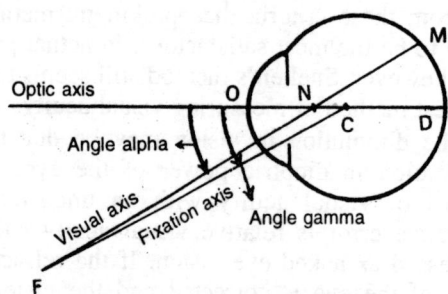

**Fig. 8.6.** Angle alpha and gamma.

### Visual angles

The angle between the visual axis and the assumed optic axis is angle alpha (Fig. 8.6) which is about 5° in a normal emmetropic eye. As long as the visual axis cuts to the nasal side of the assumed optical axis, it is positive. In some instances it may be that the visual axis cuts to the temporal side of the optical axis (Fig. 8.7) the

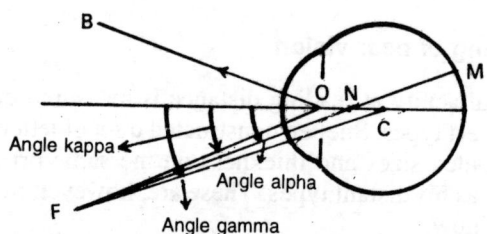

**Fig. 8.8.** Angles alpha, gamma and kappa.

The practical angle kappa is measured on the arc of a perimeter. At the summit of the perimeter at mark zero is placed a lighted candle and the visual axis of the observer is directed to the candle. Now the observer moves his eye on the arc of the perimeter from the temporal side till the shadow of the candle appears in the centre of the pupil of the observed eye. The reading on the arc is recorded; the angular deviation is double of the angle kappa.

## Axial length

The measurement of the axial length gives one type of refractive errors, i.e., axial ametropia. Besides this the axial length measurement is frequently used to determine the power requirement of an intraocular lens. It is entirely objective (Fig. 8.9).

Ultrasound consists of high frequency sound waves in the range of 8 to 10 MHz. Electric impulses are converted to sound by a vibrating quartz crystal (transducer). These sound waves are made to travel through tissues at varying speed and are reflected from interfaces between tissues of different acoustic densities. After emitting a pulse the transducer 'waits' for the reflected waves to return, strokes the quartz crystal and initiates the reverse process. The impulses are then electronically modified and recorded. The A scan is the recording of the behaviour of A wave. It is a single beam, linear wave which is directed through a probe to detect interference

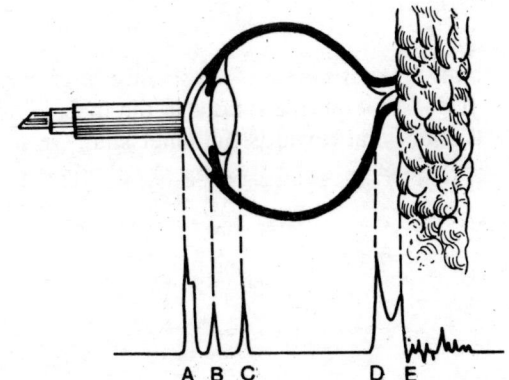

**Fig. 8.9.** Schematic representation of A scan.

along its pathway which are seen as peaks in the echogram. The distance between various peaks are used to determine the position and distances between these surfaces and the axial length of the eyeball.

In Fig. 8.9, A represents the corneal surface, B the anterior surface of lens, and C the posterior surface of lens. D and E represent the posterior bulbar wall. AD is the axial length of the eyeball.

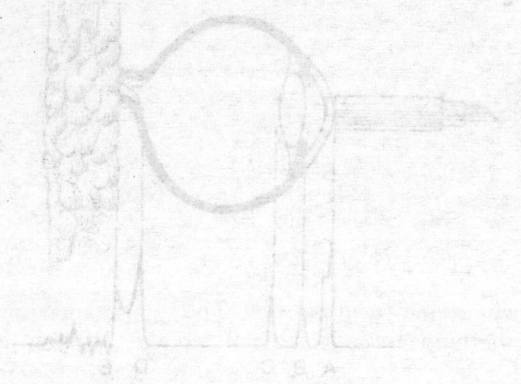

Fig. 8.5. Schematic representation of A-scan

# CHAPTER 9

# Optical Aberrations of the Eye

As in the case of lenses, so in the eye, the optical system produces many aberrations. As pointed out earlier, for the purposes of geometrical optics the eye is considered to be a co-axial system of small aperture lenses made up of homogeneous media bounded by perfectly spherical surfaces and as if only monochromatic light meets the dioptric surface almost at right angles. It is only on these assumptions that the theory of Gauss can essentially be applied to any system of lenses. In spite of the assumption, the eye does not constitute such a system but special adaptations by the eye nearly make it so.

The first condition to be fulfilled is the co-axial nature of the refracting surfaces, but, as has been pointed out in the previous chapter, the ray enters the eye rather obliquely forming an angle alpha with the optical axis. Since the determining ray is an eccentric ray, the eye suffers from astigmatism.

The size of aperture in this co-axial system should not exceed 10°, but the size of the pupil ordinarily is not less than 4 mm in diameter which corresponds to a size of 20°. This produces circles of diffusion at the retina.

As explained in an earlier chapter, the wave of light suffers from a phenomenon called diffraction, i.e., the peripheral part of the wave tends to deviate because it has no support. This is particularly true of a pencil of rays passing through the pupillary aperture which is small. As a result of this phenomenon, the rays do not converge to a point but make a series of concentric rings of light with a bright spot at their centre.

## Chromatic aberration

As in the lenticular system, the differential refraction of the different wavelengths of a composite light causes a chromatic aberration. There is a chromatic focal interval. The total dispersion of the human eye is subject to some variation. It is usually between 1.5 to 2 D from the red to the blue ends of the spectrum. The chromatic aberration is also responsible for certain degree of myopia in night vision. In night vision the sensitivity is probably shifted from 555 nm to 510 nm, changing from photopic to scotopic vision. The eye accommodates itself to the yellow-green rays, i.e., the rays of maximum luminosity so that the rays towards the violet end of the spectrum come to a focus in front of the retina and those towards the red behind the retina (Fig. 9.1).

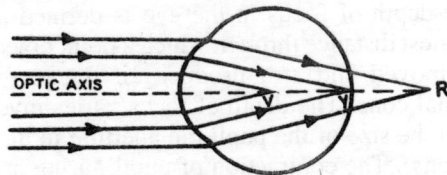

**Fig. 9.1.** Chromatic interval (V to R).

In lenses, as has already been referred to, this can be compensated by an achromatic combination, but no such correction is affected in the eye.

If a screen is kept at the focus of the violet rays, it will give a violet dot surrounded by a red ring. If the screen is kept at the red focus it will give a red dot surrounded by a violet ring.

Besides the difference in focus and the chromatic focal interval, there also exists a chromatic difference in magnification which is responsible for colour stereoscopy. When the eye is focused for green-yellow light the error introduced is very small and insignificant.

## Monochromatic aberrations

The eye suffers from monochromatic aberrations

like any other optical instrument but to a considerably smaller degree.

## Spherical aberration

Spherical aberration in the eye is typical and important but not to the same extent as might be anticipated. The eye is not essentially an aplanatic apparatus. The effects of spherical aberration are decreased because of the following reasons :

The cornea is flatter in the periphery than in the centre which results in less refraction by the peripheral cornea.

The lens core has a higher refractive index and is more refractile. The lens, therefore, refracts the central rays to a greater degree than the peripheral rays.

There is a lesser contribution to the brightness sensation in cone vision by the light rays entering the eye through the peripheral cornea. If the pupil is widely dilated, the peripheral flattening of cornea may cause negative aberration.

## Depth of focus

The depth of focus in the eye is defined as the greatest distance through which a point object can be moved and still produce an image on the retinal cone. The depth of focus varies inversely with the size of the pupil (an aperture in the case of lens). The contraction of pupil during accommodation serves a useful purpose of increasing the depth of focus. Though optically this is an aberration in the system yet it is of practical usefulness in the eye as a visual apparatus.

## Sine condition

The eye obeys the sine condition in a way identical to any other optical instrument. This is, however, partly compensated by the displacement of fovea to the side of the optical axis.

## Curvature and distortion

The eye has a curved image plane which helps to compensate for the curvature and distortion produced in an ordinary spherical optical system.

As a recording apparatus the eye shows several defects, e.g., scattering of light, halation and flare.

When the rays of light are focused onto the retina, considerable light is reflected back. No doubt, very little confusion is caused in the appreciation of image. The phenomenon is utilized in darkroom examinations of the eye, particularly in funduscopy and retinoscopy, as the emergent light is allowed to pass out of the pupil. Some of the light, however, falls on the peripheral part of the retina which is relatively insensitive.

Some of the reflected light may fall back upon the sensitive part of the retina from the surface above it and may cause confusion. This phenomenon is termed *halation*. In the eye it appears to be negligible.

When the light passes through several media, some of it is reflected back from each interface while passing from one medium to another and this process causes confusion. The phenomenon is called *flare* and is of negligible amount in the eye as the refractive indices of the media of the eye show insignificant difference. The lens is immersed in a medium of approximately the same refractive index as itself so that the reflected light is minimal and causes hardly any confusion.

The eye may suffer from the anomalies of the dioptric system itself (Fig. 9.2). The rays of light focused by the dioptric system may not fall upon the retina. If they fall in front, it is termed

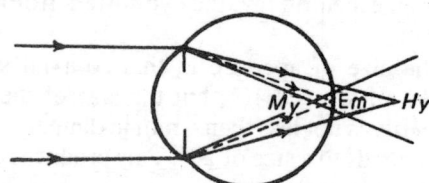

**Fig. 9.2.** Defect of eye as a dioptric apparatus.

myopia; and if they fall behind, it is called hypermetropia. It may be that the rays may be brought to different foci in different axis. Such a condition is termed astigmatism (Fig. 9.3).

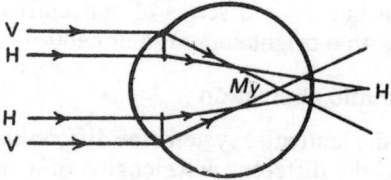

**Fig. 9.3.** Astigmatism.

# Principles of Ophthalmic Procedures

# CHAPTER 10

# Darkroom Procedures

For the examination of the internal eye and for detailed examination of the anterior and posterior segments of the eyeball, the patient is examined in a darkroom.

## OBLIQUE ILLUMINATION

### Anterior segment of the eye

The basic principle of the method is the concentration of light upon a spot in the eye by a convex lens (condensing lens) which is usually of a focal length of 7.5 cm (+13 D). A more complex system of condensation of light is utilised in examination by slit-lamp. The condensing lens can be utilised to concentrate even the daylight as a cone on the structure to be examined and make it stand out as a brilliantly illuminated part against comparatively dark background. The daylight is not always satisfactory. Most commonly artificial light is employed in the darkroom. Once the light is concentrated on the part, it is examined with the help of a magnifying device to get an accurate information. The magnification is obtained either by a corneal loupe (binocular 3 to 5 times or uniocular 6 to 20 times) or a corneal microscope which is a part of slit-lamp apparatus (10 to 72 times).

### Examination by oblique illumination

A source of light is placed at the level of the eye to be examined. It is placed 2 to 3 ft. in front and on the same side. The light is then concentrated upon the part of the eye to be examined by a +13 D condensing lens (Fig. 10.1) held with one hand. A lens with a handle is more convenient than the one without a handle. The handle is held between the thumb and the index finger. The little and ring fingers rest on the face of the patient in a way that the surface of the lens is at right angles to the

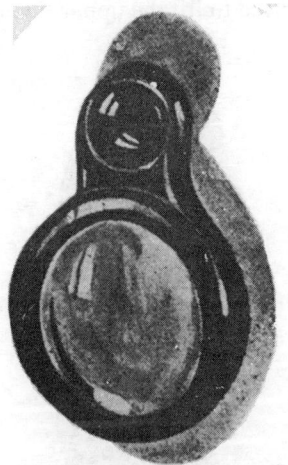

**Fig. 10.1.** Condensing lens.

direction of the path of light. The support of the fingers allows to and fro movement of the lens without much difficulty.

The examiner who is wearing a binocular loupe (Fig. 10.2) now moves his head towards the

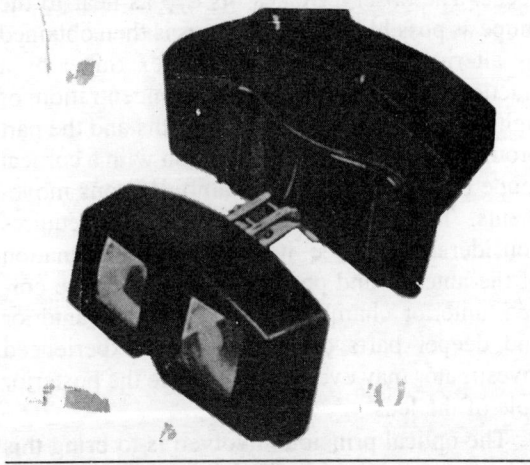

**Fig. 10.2.** Binocular loupe.

patient's eye till the illuminated spot comes in focus. If the head is now moved a little nearer, the details of the part to be examined can be made out under low magnification. Though the magnification is low the examination provides stereoscopic effect.

In examination by the uniocular loupe (Fig. 10.3) the shoulder of the loupe is held between the thumb and the forefinger and the middle finger is utilised to lift the upper lid. The ring and

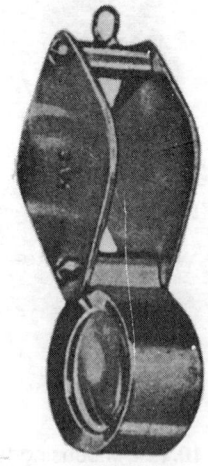

**Fig. 10.3.** Uniocular loupes.

little fingers rest on the forehead near the eye to be examined. The examiner looks through the loupe, standing a little to the side of the eye to be examined. The illuminated spot is brought to a focus. The observer takes his eye as near to the loupe as possible. Accurate focus is then obtained by altering the flexion of the index finger by a fraction of a millimetre. The concentration of light can be altered to various depths and the part brought into focus for examination with a corneal loupe by carefully adjusted ambidextrous movements. The procedure is difficult and requires considerable practice. It enables the examination of the anterior and posterior surfaces of the cornea, anterior chamber, the iris and the anterior and deeper parts of the lens. An experienced investigator may even be able to see the posterior pole of the lens.

The optical principle involved is to bring this illuminated spot within focal distance of a convex lens of high dioptric power forming a virtual,

magnified and erect image on the same side of the lens as the object (Fig. 10.4).

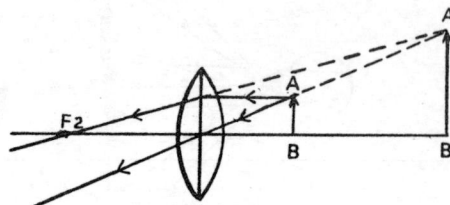

**Fig. 10.4.** Optical principle of corneal loupe.

Electrically operated torches are now available which can focus a spot or a slit-like light on the ocular structures cutting their sections. The uniocular loupe can then be utilised for examination as in slit-lamp.

### Slit-lamp examination

To obtain higher magnification and to make precise observations, but essentially based on the same principles, slit-lamp examination is undertaken.

The slit-lamp essentially consists of a strong illuminating system which can focus a slit, a spot, or a circular area of light on the part to be examined. Two systems of illumination in general use are the Gullstrand system and the Kohler-Vogt system.

The differences between these two systems are of basic nature. In the Gullstrand technique a luminous ellipse is formed (Fig. 10.5) many times the size of the illuminating lens. The light suffers considerable chromatic aberration so that the borders of the image show a variety of colours. This scattering of light is annoying both to the observer and the subject. Another disadvantage of the system is that spirals of the filament are discernible in the focal part of the light and edges are not well-defined. In Kohler-Vogt's method (Fig. 10.6) light is concentrated on the surface of the illuminated lens where the image of the filament is sharply outlined avoiding the luminous ellipse. The part of the beam of light is more homogeneous and contains no image of filament. This gives greater intensity of illumination and reduces the chromatic aberration to a negligible minimum. In the Gullstrand system the image of

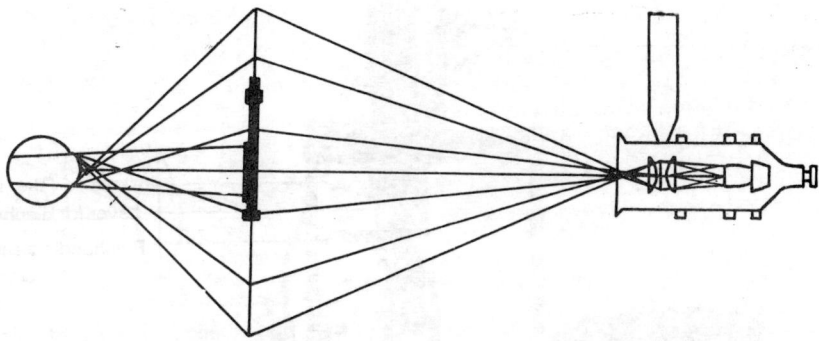

**Fig. 10.5.** Gullstrand's illuminating system.

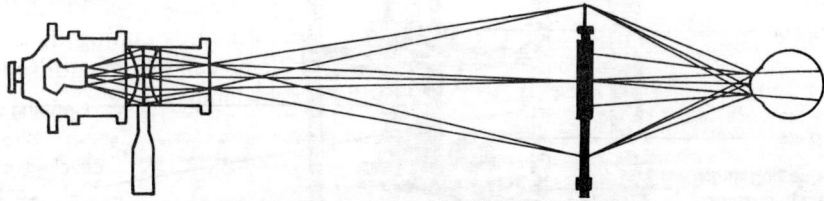

**Fig. 10.6.** Kohler-Vogt's illuminating system.

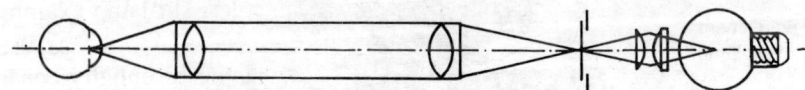

**Fig. 10.7.** Modified Gullstrand's illuminating system.

filament can be avoided by placing a fine ground glass disc in front of the condensing lens which thus produces an even illumination of great intensity (Fig. 10.7).

The illuminated spot is observed by a binocular microscope mounted on a stand. The optical principles involved are similar to any other binocular microscope (Fig. 10.8).

Thus slit-lamp examination is essentially an oblique illumination. The illumination system replaces the condensing lens and the microscope replaces the loupe. The microscope and the beam can be moved from side to side and up and down besides to and fro movements. These movements help in accurate and stereoscopic examination of the eye.

The mechanical mounting of the illumination system allows it to be rotated about nominal focal point. Variable angles of illumination are possible without continuous adjustment of the arm and focusing of the illuminating beam.

The viewing system is essentially a low power,

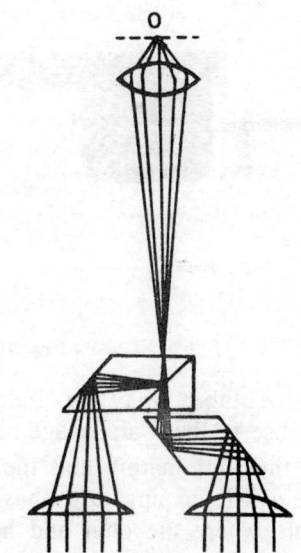

**Fig. 10.8.** Optical principle of binocular microscope.

stereoscopic microscope. This is an important contribution in depth perception and localization both in the anterior segment and in the fundus.

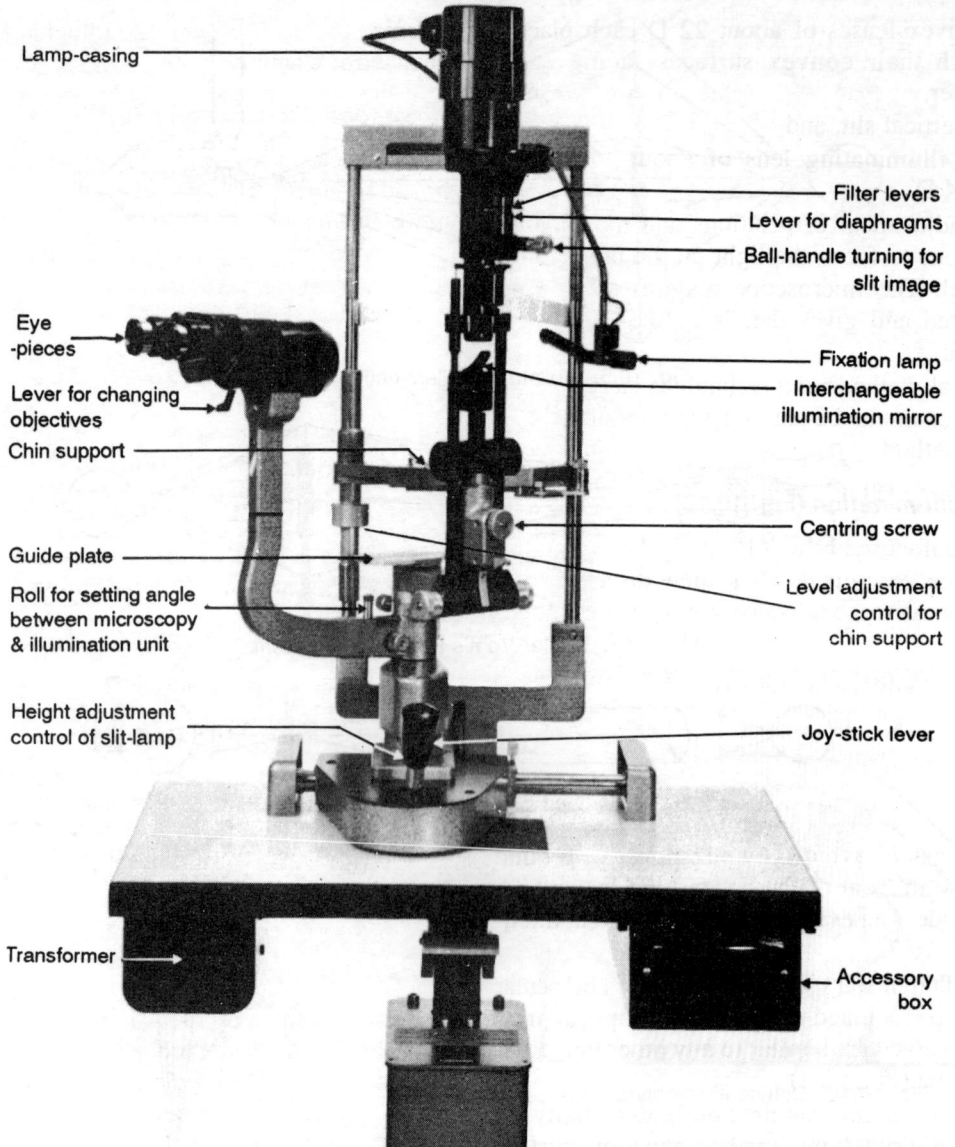

**Fig. 10.9.** The Haag-Streit slit-lamp 900.

The eyepiece tubes may be independently focused to observe the sharp image of the slit.

Besides the illuminating and the observing system, the slit-lamp apparatus has accessory arrangements where the chin and head of the patient can rest (Fig. 10.9) and can be moved up and down.

With special attachments to the slit-lamp the apparatus can be utilised for funduscopy, gonio-scopy (observation of angle of anterior chamber) and applanation tonometry. There are several other examinations for which slit-lamp can be used.

The instrument consists (as described) of an illuminating system and a corneal microscope. The illuminating system comprises

- lamp,
- collecting system consisting of two plano-

convex lenses of about 22 D each placed with their convex surfaces facing each other,

- a vertical slit, and
- an illuminating lens of about +10 D to +14 D.

The adjustment of positions and movements enables one to focus the light on the point to be examined. The microscope magnifies the area illuminated and gives details of the part to be examined.

Several methods and techniques can be employed to examine the anterior segment of the eye by this method.

### Diffuse illumination (Fig. 10.10)

A large unfocused beam of light is thrown on the part to be examined. It is then directly seen through a microscope which gives a stereoscopic

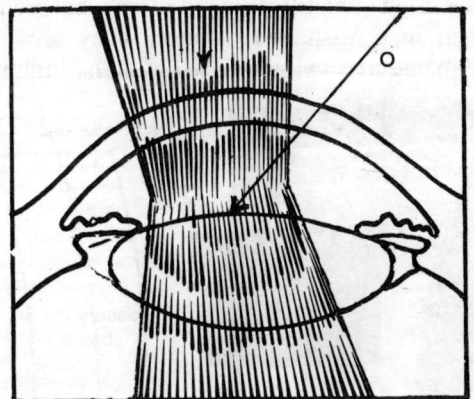

**Fig. 10.10.** Diffuse illumination.

magnification. By this method entire surface of the cornea, iris and lens may be examined. A cobalt filter and fluorescein may be used to inspect position, bearing and movements of a corneal contact lens over the anterior surface of the cornea. It gives an idea of its fitting. Similarly with this method by using a monochromatic light precise viewing of conjunctival and/or episcleral vessels is made possible.

The method is also useful in getting an idea about the entire scar or opacity of the cornea, the folds in Descemet's membrane, invading abnormal blood vessels of the cornea and the iris,

oedema of the cornea and the epithelialization of the anterior chamber.

### Direct focal illumination (Fig. 10.11)

In this method a beam of light is obliquely directed into the eye and focused. The beam is viewed from the side. The focal point of the beam is regulated until it coincides with the exact focus of the microscope. The optically homogeneous media appear dark.

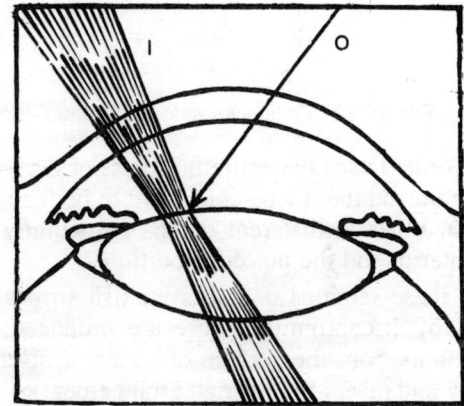

**Fig. 10.11.** Direct focal illumination.

The beam may be classified as an optical section, parallelepiped or a conical beam.

The optical section of the cornea or the lens is obtained by focusing a very narrow slit of the light from an angle of about 45° for the cornea and from an angle of about 15° for the lens. The illuminated part can be brought into a sharp focus from directly in front, with the microscope.

The beam can be moved across the surface of the part to be examined from side to side and, with the simultaneous movement of the microscope, can be kept in focus for detailed examination of the optical section of the various areas of the focused part. With the change in angle of the beam deeper areas of the focused part can be seen.

In the cornea the optical section consists of a segment of an arc with a tear layer as a bright first zone, the epithelium as a dark line immediately behind it, a brighter light of Bowman's membrane, a wider granular and grayer zone of stroma showing structures of various types under higher magnification, and a final brighter and inner endothelial zone (Fig. 10.12).

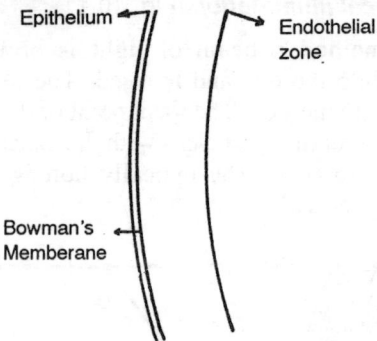

**Fig. 10.12.** Optical section of cornea.

In order to see the entire thickness of the lens, the beam and the microscope have to be focused several times at different depths particularly at the anterior and the posterior portions.

In these sections one sees whitish stripes or zones of discontinuity. These are produced by reflections from the surface of zones of discontinuity and reveal the internal arrangement of the lens material in an optical section. There are six clear-cut stripes and two faint ones (Fig. 10.13) from the anterior to the posterior surface. They are :

1. Anterior capsule
2. Anterior surface of the adult nucleus
3. Anterior surface of foetal nucleus

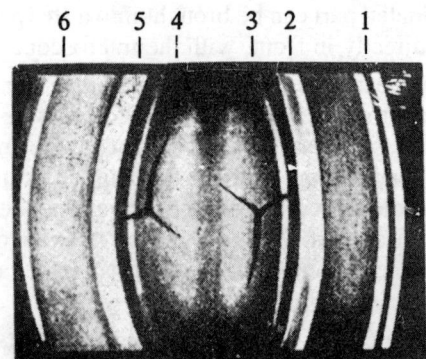

**Fig. 10.13.** Optical section of lens. 1, anterior capsule; 2, anterior surface of adult nucleus; 3, anterior surface of foetal nucleus; 4, posterior surface of foetal nucleus; 5, posterior surface of adult nucleus; 6, posterior capsule.

4. Posterior surface of foetal nucleus
5. Posterior surface of the adult nucleus
6. The posterior capsule

Between these stripes are the darker areas which represent the lens substance. Sometimes fainter stripes of adolescent nucleus between the adult and the foetal nuclei are seen.

The apparent depth of the corneal or lenticular opacities is much less than actual depth. In cornea the apparent depth of opacities is 2/3 of the real depth.

*Parallelepiped :* In this the slit used is much wider than the optical section. It is usually 2 mm wide. The parallelepiped is similar to the optic section.

The cornea is a divergent meniscus. The vertical edges, although curved, are not exactly parallel (Fig. 10.14). In this the opaque area of the cornea appears whiter than the surrounding and corneal nerves can be seen as white threads. Under high magnification they can be seen to branch in a Y-shaped manner. They are non-myelinated axis cylinders except at the limbus.

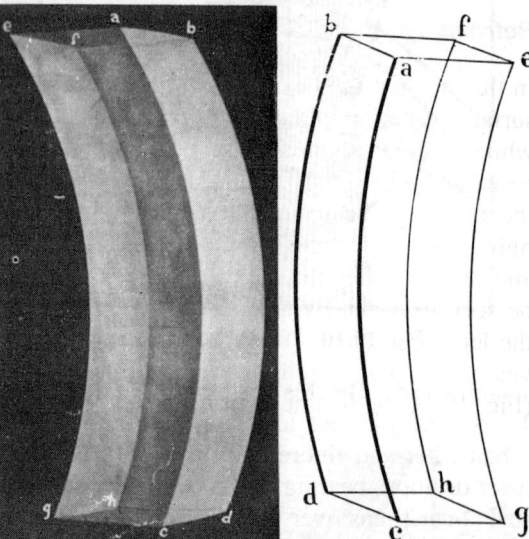

**Fig. 10.14.** Parallelepiped of cornea. abdc—anterior epithelial surface; efhg—posterior endothelial surface.

In parallelepiped it is easy to examine anterior and posterior surfaces for any irregularities, though endothelium of cornea is better studied by the technique of observing the zone of specular reflection.

*The conical beam* (Fig. 10.15) : It is a small circular beam preferably used to test the aqueous flare. A marked flare indicates a pathology in the aqueous humour. It can be quantitatively and qualitatively studied.

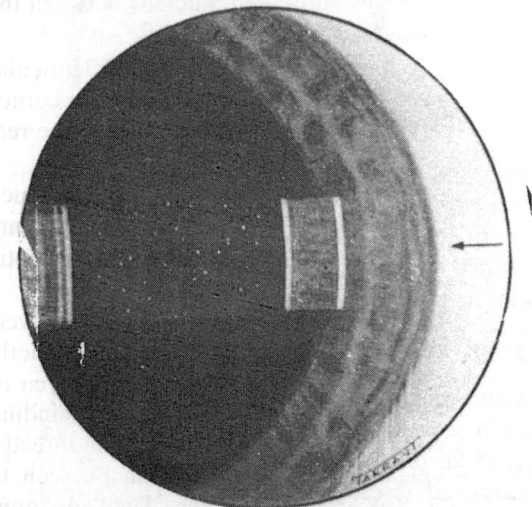

**Fig. 10.15.** Aqueous flare.

### Retroillumination

In this method the beam of light is focused on a surface posterior to the object under observation while the microscope is focused on the object to be examined (Fig. 10.16). This method enables the object to be examined under the reflected light. For application of this method the cornea and the lens offer the best field. The cornea can be seen from the light reflected from the iris or the lens. Descemet's membrane, invading blood vessels, epithelial oedema, keratitic precipitates (Fig. 10.16) and some faint opacities of the cor-

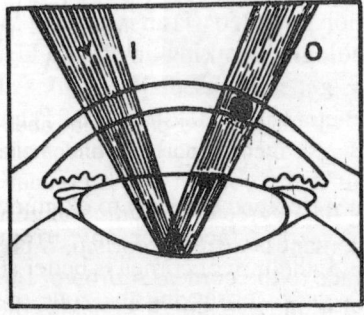

**Fig. 10.16.** Retroillumination.

nea are best seen by this method. The posterior surface of the iris can also be seen by the reflected light from the lens. Vascularization, atrophy and vacuoles of iris can be seen by this method. In the lens, capsular and subcapsular vacuoles and many types of lenticular opacities can be observed.

### Zones of specular reflection

When a beam of light passes from one medium to another, part of the light is transmitted and part of it is reflected back. In living tissues, due to the surface being not highly polished and not as regular as in mirrors, part of the light is regularly reflected (i.e., the angle of incidence is equal to the angle of reflection) and part of it is reflected in a diffuse irregular manner. Both types of reflection (regular and irregular) are observed at each zone of discontinuity of the eye (Fig. 10.17).

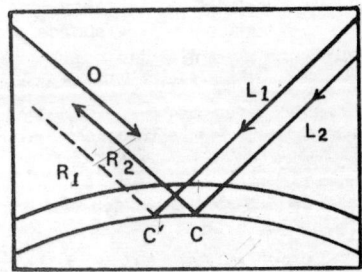

**Fig. 10.17.** Zones of specular reflection.

In this method of examination, the microscope and the light beam are so aligned to the surface that the angle of incidence and the angle of reflection become equal. Surface elevations and depressions appear as dark defects in brilliant zone of reflected light owing to the fact that the light reflected from them is irregular or diffuse. In the cornea this method reveals :

- Elevations and depressions in the anterior surface.
- Folds and tears in the Descemet's membrane and its reduplication.
- Details of precorneal fluid.
- Most important of all is the endothelial mosaic and defects in them in the posterior part of the corneal parallelepiped.

This principle is employed in specular endothelial microscopy.

In the lens this method reveals :

- Folds and thickenings of the anterior capsule.
- To a certain extent the internal architecture of the lens especially the senile nuclear sclerosis.

In Fig. 10.17, the beam $L_2$ impinges on C. Regular reflection occurs at point C on the posterior corneal surface and is observed along the direction O when the angle of observation is equal to the angle of incidence. Beam $L_1$ impinges on an area where there is a defect (C′). Consequently no light will be reflected at this point (C′) and it will appear dark in the surrounding specular areas. This would correspond to the imperfections in the polish of a mirror.

The method is used to study the normal corneal surfaces and abnormalities therein (Fig. 10.18).

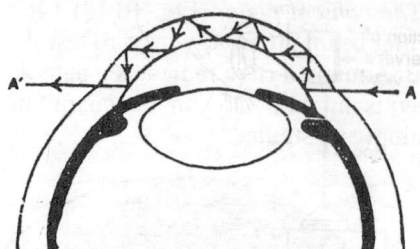

**Fig. 10.19.** Sclerotic scatter.

scars and lines in the cornea which appear white against a dark background. This method can also be utilised for observing haemorrhages in the iris stroma, presence of chromatophores in the iris and the structure of the iris sphincter.

### Oscillating illumination

In this method the microscope is focused on a given area in the field and the focused beam is given an oscillatory movement. The area so illuminated is closely observed. This affords an opportunity to observe the area alternately by direct and indirect illumination. This method is useful to see the flare and small opacities which can be seen against a dark background.

### Tangential surface grazing or sunset illumination

This method is useful in observing changes in the iris. A wide beam is focused on the iris at a tangent to the iris surface while the microscope is focused in front. It is only an alternate of sclerotic scatter. By this method one can see iris strands, freckles, nodules, tumours and pupillary border nodules.

### Applanation tonometry

Applanation tonometry is an important tool for an ophthalmologist working in the field of glaucoma. It is generally used along with a slit-lamp. The tonometer (Figs. 10.20 and 10.21) consists of two parts : a mechanical device which exerts force against the cornea; and a contact element indicating the degree of flattening of cornea. The contact element is a small biprism. It presents as a flat surface to the cornea. A drop of fluorescein is instilled in the eye and this enables the area of flattening to be delineated visually by the menis-

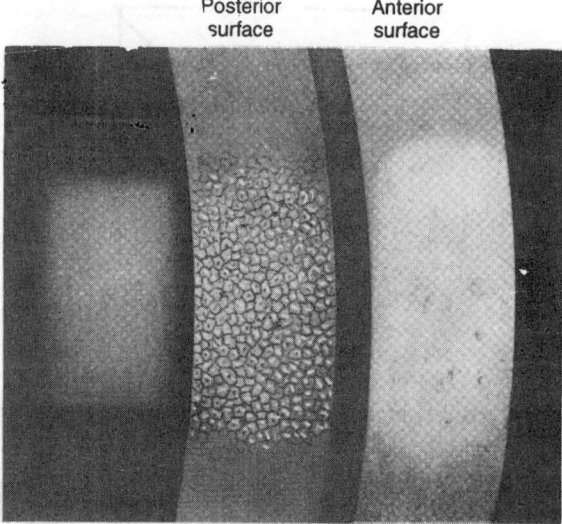

Posterior surface   Anterior surface

**Fig. 10.18.**

### Sclerotic scatter

If the focused broad beam of light is directed on the corneoscleral limbus, there occurs a scattering of light in the region of perilimbal sclera producing a crescentic halo of light around the cornea and is more noticeable at the opposite limbus of the same eye. There should be a large angle between the line of incidence of the beam and direction of observation with the microscope (Fig. 10.19). The method is useful for the detection of fine nebulae, maculae, interstitial deposits,

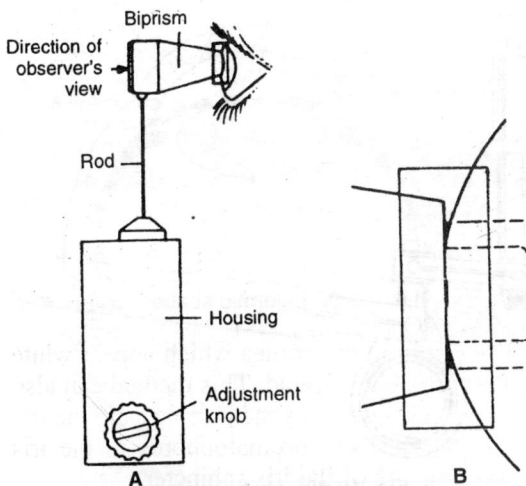

**Fig. 10.20.** Applanation tonometer.

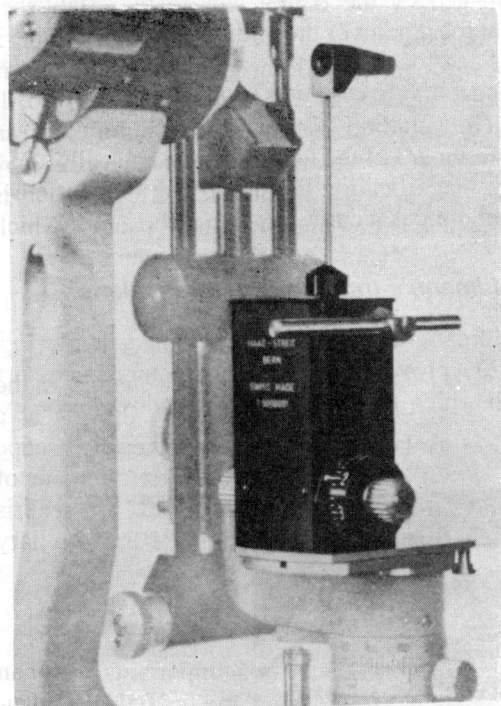

**Fig. 10.21.**

cus of the fluorescein-stained tear film. The biprism performs two functions : (1) splits the field in half; and (2) the angle of the prism is adjusted to displace the two half images. The end point is measured by applying the principle of vernier acuity. The optics is represented in Fig. 10.22.

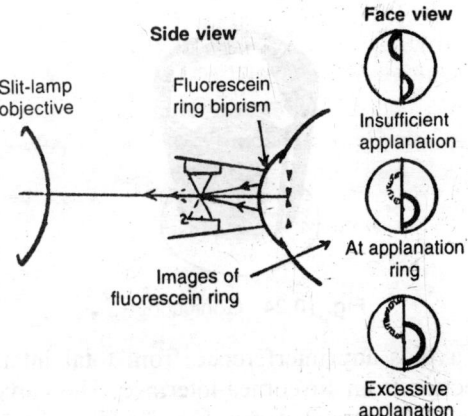

**Fig. 10.22.** Optics of applanation tonometer.

### Gonioscopy

The angle of the anterior chamber has been made accessible to the slit-lamp by diverting the beam of light at an angle with the help of a gonioprism. The commonly used contact lens for the purpose is the one devised by Goldmann. The contact lens not only acts as a prism which transmits the emergent rays from the angle region to the observer but magnifies the area significantly. Goldmann's lens is a flat surfaced lens (Figs. 10.23 and 10.24) which contains a mirror placed at an angle of 64° with the flat surface. The lens is rotated to observe the different meridia of the circumference

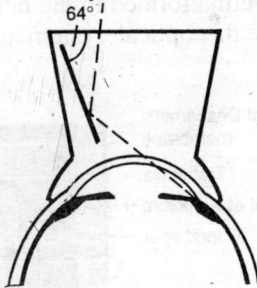

**Fig. 10.23.** Goldmann's gonio-contact lenses (line drawing).

of the angle. A special prism attached to slit-lamp permits the observation illumination angle to be reduced to 5°. Four-mirror gonioscopes are also available which almost enable one to observe all segments of the angle at one time.

The contact lens is virtually indispensable for gonioscopy. The optical continuity between the lens and the eye eliminates corneal reflections,

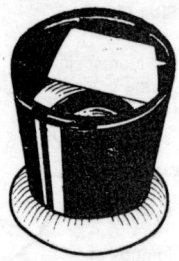

**Fig. 10.24.** Gonioscope.

and avoids any interference from total internal reflection from air-cornea interface. The parts of angle visible are shown in Fig. 10.25.

### Slit-lamp funduscopy

Two most commonly employed accessories for this purpose are (1) Hruby's lens, and (2) Goldmann's three-mirror contact lens.

### Hruby lens (Fig. 10.26)

This is a useful lens and has a –55 D dioptric strength. The lens is used to compensate for the refractive power of the eye, i.e., the convergent action of the anterior media is counteracted in such a way that an image of the retina is presented for examination by the microscope and the posterior parts of the eye are brought within the field of observation. It may be stated that an image of the retina formed in the neighbourhood of infinity by the optical system of the eye is

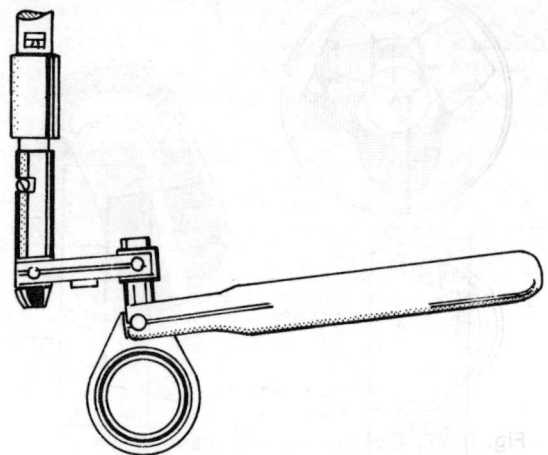

**Fig. 10.26.** Hruby's lens.

reimaged by the Hruby lens to the established front focal point of the microscope. With Hruby's lens and focal beam the examination has become comparatively easy and simple.

The method allows the examination of posterior 2/3 of the fundus stereoscopically under high magnification besides giving the advantage of an optical section.

### Goldmann's three-mirror contact lens

Goldmann's three-mirror contact lens (Fig. 10.27) provides a very satisfactory accessory with which the whole of the fundus can be ex-

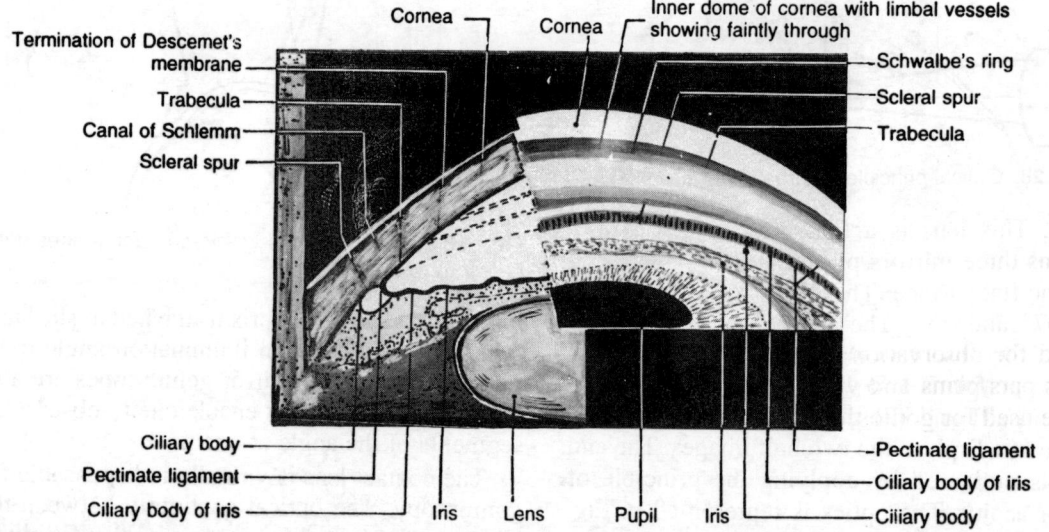

**Fig. 10.25.** Parts of angle of anterior chamber.

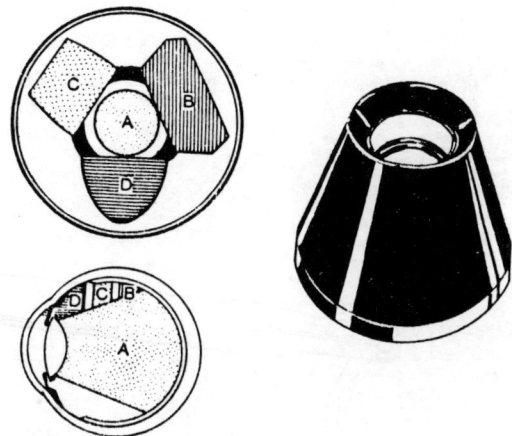

**Fig. 10.27.** Goldmann's three-mirror contact lens.

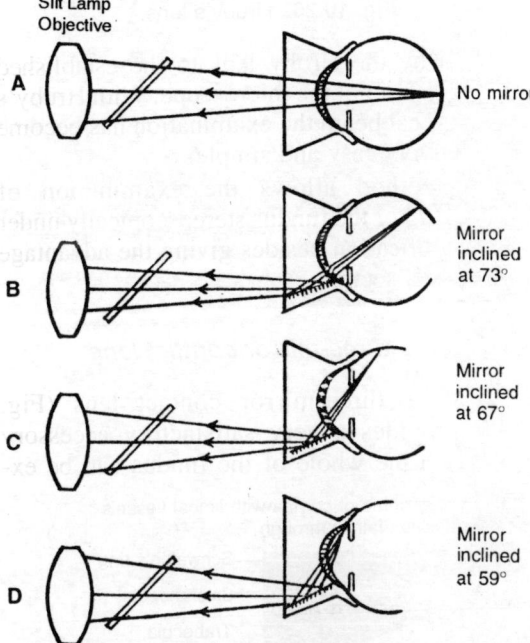

Slit Lamp
Objective

A — No mirror

B — Mirror inclined at 73°

C — Mirror inclined at 67°

D — Mirror inclined at 59°

**Fig. 10.28.** Optical principle of three-mirror contact lens.

plored. This lens is a flat-surfaced lens which contains three mirrors placed at different angles with the flat surface. The mirrors are inclined at 59°, 67° and 73°. The mirror at 59° angle is utilised for observation of the periphery of the fundus pars plana and vitreous at the ora. It can also be used for gonioscopy.

The posterior pole of the eye may be observed in similar manner as with fundus contact lens by using the central part of the contact lens without the mirror (Fig. 10.28A). With 73° inclination the zone from macula to 30° is observed (Fig. 10.28B). With mirror inclined at 67° the peripheral parts of the fundus can be seen (Fig 10.28C). Considerable overlapping of the field: is provided by different mirrors. This may be increased by the movements of the eye and the lens. Recently the contact lens has been provided with an indentor for ease in examination of the extreme periphery and better view of fovea. The optical principles of the three-mirror Goldmann contact lens are shown in Fig. 10.28.

### Posterior fundus contact lens

This is a modified Koeppe's lens. The image produced is virtual and erect, situated in the anterior vitreous cavity and is most helpful in exploring the posterior fundus (Figs. 10.29 and 10.30).

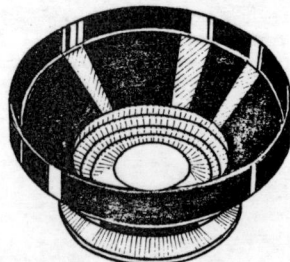

**Fig. 10.29.** Posterior fundus contact lens (modified Koeppe's lens).

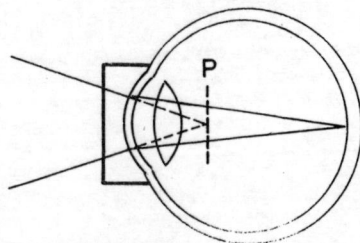

**Fig. 10.30.** Posterior fundus with the image appearing at P.

# CHAPTER 11

# Ophthalmoscopy

Ophthalmoscopy is an objective method of examining the posterior segment of the eye. The main objective of the examination is to determine the presence or absence of abnormalities in the posterior segment—structural or pathological. This also affords an opportunity to exclusively view the vascular and neurological structures of a living organ in situ. This may well result in gathering information of the state of central nervous system and the general vasculature.

In order to properly examine the posterior segment some conditions need to be fulfilled as under :

- The room should be dark.
- The pupil should be under effect of a mydriatic and preferably a cycloplegic if retinoscopy has to be done in younger patients.
- The light should be so adjusted that the face remains in darkness.
- A proper choice of a mirror should be made, i.e., a plane mirror for distant direct and a concave mirror for direct and indirect ophthalmoscopy.
- The examination should be conducted from an appropriate distance, i.e., 25 centimetres for distant direct, 50 centimetres for indirect and as near the eye as possible for direct ophthalmoscopy.

## Historical

Ophthalmoscope was first invented by Helmholtz in 1851 in which he used a small concave mirror for reflecting the light inside the eye. Since then the ophthalmoscope has undergone many changes. The modern ophthalmoscope (Fig. 11.1A & B) is a self-illuminated instrument which has made the examination comparatively easy and precise. The electrical energy in this ophthalmoscope is derived from dry battery cells or directly from the mains. A micro-lamp serves as the source of illumination. The light is collected by a condensing system and is reflected into the patient's pupil by either a silvered mirror or by a silvered back surface of a glass prism. The lens disc is placed behind the reflecting mirror or the reflecting prism with a series of lenses which appear in the peep hole in a regular order. Any lens can be placed behind the hole in the reflecting system which is utilized for observation. Most of the ophthalmoscopes have a rheostat for regulating the amount of light required for examination.

### Principles of ophthalmoscopy

Ophthalmoscopy is based on the principle that very little light can enter the eye through the pupil and that some of it is reflected back through the pupil in the same direction by which it entered and so could only be appreciated by an observer if his own pupil happens to coincide with the path of this narrow bundle of rays of light. The earliest experiments performed enabled Bruck to see the glow in the human eye.

In a darkroom a light L is held in front of the observed eye and the person is instructed not to accommodate for the light. The observer moves his eyes behind the light into the path of rays from the source of light illuminating the interior of the eye. Thus the reflected light from the illuminated spot on the retina could be received and seen (Fig. 11.2). Helmholtz used to illuminate the fundus by virtual image of the source of light formed in a glass plate and was thus able to place the observer's eye behind the glass plate so as to inter-

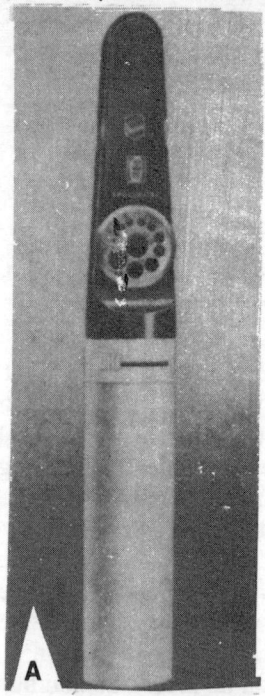

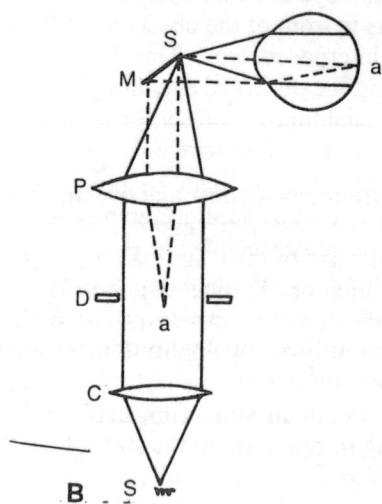

**Fig. 11.1. A.** A modern electric ophthalmoscope (Keeler). **B.** The optical system ⸍ an electric ophthalmoscope. Light from a source, S, is collimated by a condenser, C. The lens, P, then images ⸍e source at S′, at the top of a half-mirror, M. Any point a, in the plane of aperture, D, is also in the front focal ⸍ane of lens P. The broken lines show that a is imaged on the emmetropic retina at a′, and hence the circular ⸍ ⸍erture, D, may be imaged on the fundus as a sharply defined disc of light.

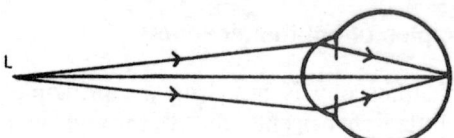

**Fig. 11.2.** Focus of retinal spot at anterior focal plane.

cept some of the rays which were reflected by the fundus of the observed eye (Fig. 11.3).

Let L be the light source striking a glass plate CD. A large part of the light passes through glass plate in the direction of I and is lost (Fig. 11.3).

Some of the rays are reflected along i and enter the observed eye S. These rays are reflected back along their own path and will form an image P. If the observer's eye O be placed behind the plate CD he will be able to see the image of the fundus. The image will be faint as some more light will be lost due to reflection in the direction of L. If both eyes are emmetropic it will be possible to see the details of the retina of the observed eye. If a plano-concave lens is placed before the observer's eye a magnified erect image

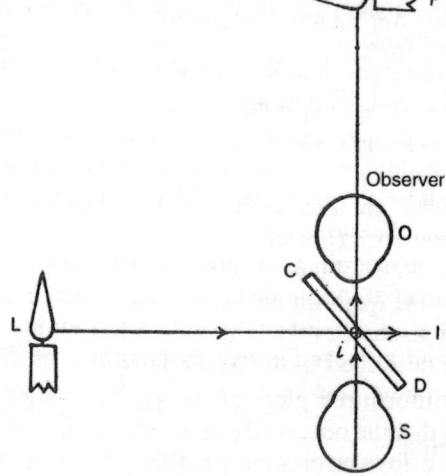

**Fig. 11.3.** Principle of Helmholtz ophthalmoscopy.

of the fundus can be seen. In this system the reflecting surface used can be a silvered mirror. This method gives a direct method of ophthalmoscopy, i.e., the examination of the erect image of the retina.

If a high convex lens is introduced near the observed eye the method is termed indirect ophthalmoscopy. In this method the rays are reflected into the eye by a concave silvered mirror and after leaving the eye are made to converge and come to a focus in front of the observed eye by the high convex interposed lens. This has the effect of converting the observed eye into a highly myopic eye and enabling the observer to see a real, inverted and magnified image.

The examinations can be placed under four groups and they should preferably be performed in the order given below :

1. Preliminary examination at one metre distance.
2. Distant direct ophthalmoscopy (at 25 cm to 28 cm distance).
3. Indirect ophthalmoscopy (50 cm distance).
4. Direct ophthalmoscopy (as near the eye as possible).

**Preliminary examination**

This gives a rough idea of the nature of the refraction of the eye. The patient is seated on a stool and the observer sits almost a metre away from the patient. The observer reflects the light from the plane mirror into the eye to be observed and looks through the sight hole. A red reflex from the pupil is seen which is uniformly illuminated and shows no dark spots in the field if no opacities are present. Sometimes a hazy image of the fundus can be seen. By slight movements of the mirror an idea with regard to the type of refractive error (myopia or hypermetropia) of the patient can be obtained. A more elaborate procedure for the quantitative estimation of the error of refraction objectively is termed retinoscopy and will be described in the next chapter.

A uniform red glow of the pupillary area indicates that the observed eye is either emmetropic or has a low error of refraction. If some hazy image of the fundus is seen it gives an indication of a high degree of refractive error of the observed eye. If the movement of the shadow is in the direction of the movement of the mirror, it may be hypermetropia, or myopia less than ID or emmetropia and if the movement is in the opposite direction it is myopia of more than ID.

**Distant direct ophthalmoscopy**

After conducting the preliminary examination, the observer now stands up and approaches the patient till he is about 25 centimetres from the eye under observation. The examination reveals

- opacities in the refractive media and their relative position;
- a detached retina, a tumour, vitreous haemorrhage, a foreign body or other matter just behind or in the neighbourhood of the lens.

Any opaque or translucent object in the course of the light presents as a dark or semi-dark spot. If there is no red reflex seen and the whole field is black or grey it may be that the lens is totally opaque or that there is haemorrhage inside the eye or that there is a total retinal detachment.

In Fig. 11.4, if 4 is the centre of rotation of the eye and if there are opacities at 1, 2, 3, 4 and 5 then when the eye is rotated a small amount, all the opacities except 4 will move, the amount being greater the further the opacity is from the centre of rotation. Since all the movements can be judged only from the edge of the pupil or the anterior capsule of the lens, the relative positions of the opacities is determined by parallax. The patient is now asked to move the eye. The parallax is determined with the pupillary plane as the fixed point (anterior capsule of the lens). The following information can be obtained (Fig 11.4).

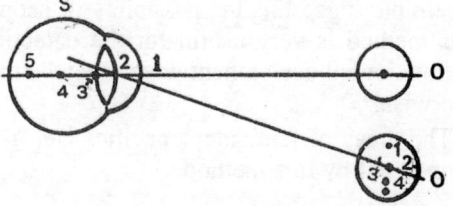

**Fig. 11.4.** Principle of distant direct ophthalmoscopy.

- If the opacity moves in the direction of the movement of the eyeball it is either situated in the cornea or in the aqueous humour. In the case of the latter the opacity will float and continue to move after the eye is brought to rest.
- If the opacity moves in the direction opposite to the movement of the eyeball it is

either in the lens or in the vitreous. The degree of parallax gives a rough idea with regard to the position of the opacity in relation to the pupillary plane.

- If the opacity is situated behind the pupillary plane and continues to move after the eye has been brought to rest, it is situated in the vitreous and this vitreous is fluid.
- If the opacity does not change its position it is in the anterior surface of the lens.
- The opacity at 5 will seem to be lost behind the iris.
- In the subluxated lens with one of its edges in the pupillary area or in ectopia lentis the edge is easily detected by this method as it presents as a black crescentic ring in the pupillary area.

Normally the pupillary area is uniformly illuminated and gives a uniform red glow. Sometimes, this red glow is not uniformly seen. The sites of the greyish patches in the pupillary area correspond to the place of retinal changes, e.g., a retinal detachment, new growth or chorioretinal degenerations. By examining the pupillary glow in various directions of ocular gaze these areas can be roughly marked out. If the blood vessels of the retina are seen in this area then it is due either to a retinal detachment, or due to a tumour, otherwise the grey areas are patches of chorioretinal atrophy. Sometimes the folds of retina may be clearly visible indicating a retinal detachment while at times neo-vascularization may be discernible suggesting the possibility of neoplasm. This method is very useful for the detection of shallow retinal detachment which may be missed otherwise.

The areas of lenticular opacities can also be mapped out by this method.

### Indirect ophthalmoscopy

The examination is based on the principle that the observed eye is converted into a highly myopic eye by placing a high convex lens in front of it which enables the observer to get an inverted, real and magnified image of the fundus of the eye to be examined. The image is formed between the high convex lens and the observer. When the eye is either myopic or is made myopic and is

illuminated, the rays of light will emerge from the eye to form an inverted and real image in front of the eye and if this image be in a suitable position the observer will be able to focus the image on his retina by an effort of accommodation. This effect can be relaxed by placing a weaker convex lens (usually +2 D lens) in the peep hole. In myopia the image is formed in front of the focal point, in emmetropia at the focal point and in hypermetropia it is formed beyond the focal point (Fig. 11.5).

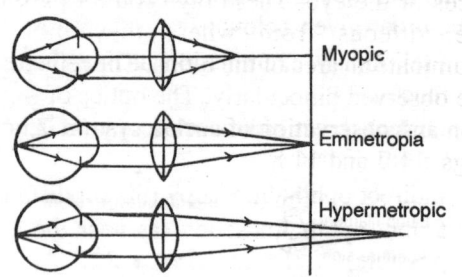

**Fig. 11.5.** Position of image in indirect ophthalmoscopy in various refractive states of the eye.

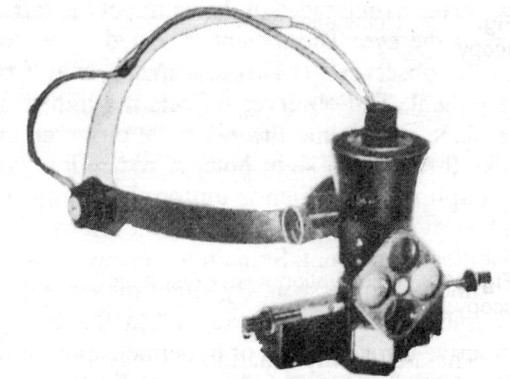

**Fig. 11.6.** Fison's indirect ophthalmoscope.

In this method the light is placed near the eye to be examined. The observer stands at about half a metre away from the patient. With a concave mirror the light is reflected onto the observed eye and the patient's pupil is immediately filled with a glow. A strong condensing lens (about +13 D) is introduced in the path of the reflected light so that anterior principal focus of the lens coincides with the nodal point of the eye. The inverted image of the fundus is formed between the observer and the lens. This conventional method, however, is gradually becoming obsolete and, in fact, has already become so in most parts of the world because of the development of self-luminous indirect ophthalmoscopes (Fig. 11.6). While doing indirect ophthalmoscopy with self-luminous ophthalmoscopes the light is thrown onto the observed eye and a condensing lens is interposed in between the observed eye and the examiner. The lens renders these rays convergent. These convergent rays meet the cornea and are converged further by the various refracting surfaces of the eye. These rays come to a focus in the vitreous from where they diverge to illuminate an area of the retina. The reflected rays are observed binocularly. The optics of illumination and observation of such a system is given in Figs. 11.7 and 11.8.

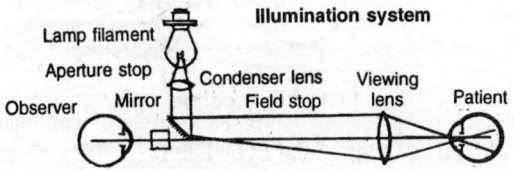

**Fig. 11.7.** Illumination system in indirect ophthalmoscopy.

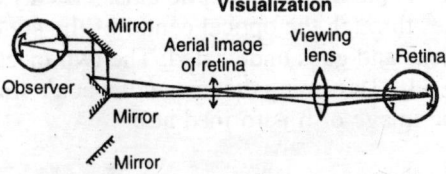

**Fig. 11.8.** Observation system in indirect ophthalmoscopy.

The area of illumination is biggest in myopia and smallest in hypermetropia (Fig. 11.9).

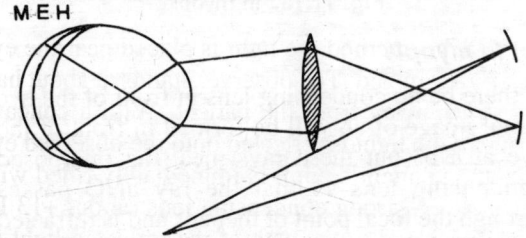

**Fig. 11.9.** Field of illumination in various refractive errors.

The examination must be carried out in a perfect darkroom in which the only source of light

is that to be used in the examination. This helps in getting a better contrast and it also makes the examination easier by greater dilatation of the pupil.

The patient lies comfortably on the examination couch. The light is thrown on the patient's eye by the mirror and the patient's pupil is immediately filled with a glow. A strong condensing lens varying from about +13 D to +30 D is now introduced into the path of the reflected light so that the anterior principal focus of the lens coincides with the nodal point of the eye. The inverted image of the fundus is formed between the observer and the condensing lens. The interposition of the condensing lens is likely to introduce the factor of spherical aberration until and unless the size of the lens introduced is small. A lens of more than 2½ inches in diameter should not be used.

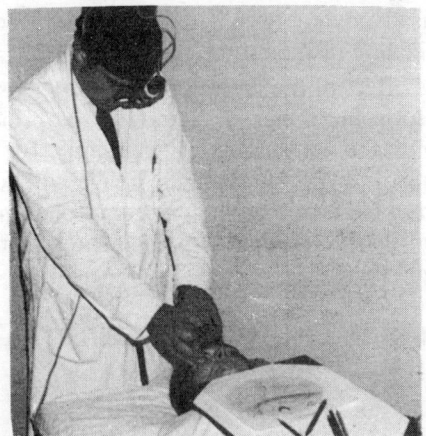

**Fig. 11.10.** Method of indirect ophthalmoscopy by binocular indirect ophthalmoscope.

Three very bright reflexes disturb the examination : images of the mirror one each from the anterior and posterior surfaces of the lens and an image formed by the reflection at the anterior surface of the cornea. To avoid the two formed by the lens, the condensing lens is slightly tilted. One image, i.e., formed by the posterior surface being inverted and real and the other, i.e., formed by the anterior surface of lens being erect and virtual, move in opposite directions clearing sufficient space between the two. The condensing lens forms a real inverted image of the fundus near its principal focus between the lens and the observer. If the lens be moved slightly upwards the image of the fundus moves in the same direction. The corneal image remains fixed and thus the annoying corneal reflex is avoided.

In order to examine the disc the patient is asked to look slightly inward towards the nose and the disc comes in focus. When the patient looks straight in the light and the lens is moved slightly upwards the macula can be examined easily. By various ocular movements the various parts of the fundus can be seen. The guiding principle is that the movements of the eye are such that area to be examined comes opposite to the observer's pupil thus falling in line with the visual axis of the observer.

A monocular indirect ophthalmoscope is also available. It has the advantage of permitting visualization through an undilated pupil. The image formed is erect rather than inverted. It has the disadvantage of not allowing stereoscopic visualization of the retina.

The effect of the convex condensing lens will be to form the image of fundus at the principal focus of the lens. This is true only for emmetropia. In hypermetropia the image will be farther from the lens than the principal focus and in myopia it is formed at a point nearer than the principal focus.

## FORMATION OF IMAGES IN INDIRECT OPHTHALMOSCOPY

### 1. When the principal focus of the lens coincides with the nodal point of the eye

#### (a) In emmetropia (Fig. 11.11)

Let ab be a part of fundus of an emmetropic eye whose nodal point N coincides with the anterior focus of the condensing lens the emergent rays PQ and $aQ_2$ starting from retina would emerge parallel to each other forming the image of ab at infinity which would act as an object for the con-

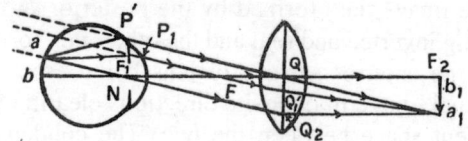

**Fig. 11.11.** In emmetropia.

densing lens which in turn forms the images at a'b' the posterior focus. $F_2PQ$ is the ray passing through the optical centre of the lens hence goes undeviated and the ray $aNQ_2$ passing through the principal focus of the condensing lens is refracted in a direction parallel to the optic axis. The two meet at a' to give the image of a, similarly b' is the image of b.

#### (b) In hypermetropia (Fig. 11.12)

If there be no condensing lens in front of the observed eye then the image of ab will be a"b". This will act as an object for the condensing lens

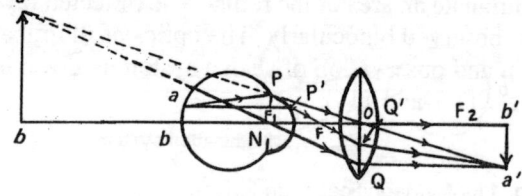

**Fig. 11.12.** In hypermetropia.

if placed in front of the eye. The ray a"NQ passes through the anterior focal point meeting the condensing lens at Q and is refracted along Qa' which is parallel to the optic axis. The ray a"PO passes through the optical centre of the condensing lens and goes undeviated. The two meet at a' (Fig. 11.13) forming the image of a at a'. Similarly the image of b is formed at b'.

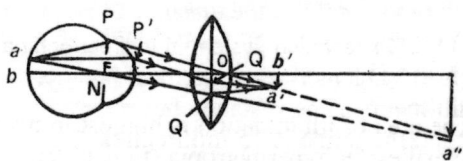

**Fig. 11.13.** In myopia.

#### (c) In myopia

If there be no condensing lens in front of the eye a real image of ab will be formed in front of the eye at a"b" but these rays meet the interposed condensing lens so that the ray aNQ passes through the focal point of the lens and is refracted along Qa'. The ray aP is reflected by the eye along PO which passes through the optical centre of the lens and meets Qa' at a' thus forming the image of a at a' (Fig. 11.13). Similarly b' is the image of b.

## (d) Magnification of images

The image is real, inverted and magnified (Fig. 11.14). The magnification is expressed as

$$\frac{I}{O} = M$$

In Fig. 11.14,

$$\frac{a'b'}{ab} = M$$

In parallelogram $Ob'a'Q$, $a'b' = OQ$
Hence

$$M = \frac{OQ}{ab}$$

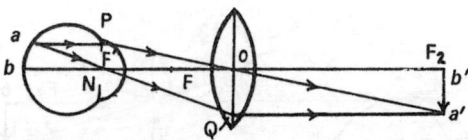

**Fig. 11.14.** Magnification in indirect ophthalmoscopy.

The $\Delta$s $abF'$ and $F'OQ$ are equiangular, because $\angle aF'b = \angle OF'q$ and $\angle F'ab$ and $\angle QOF'$ are right angles.

Hence

$$\frac{OQ}{ab} = \frac{OF}{bF'}$$

or

$$\frac{a'b'}{ab} = \frac{f}{n}$$

where $f$ is the focal length of the condensing lens in millimetres and $n$ is the distance of nodal point from the retina.

If a +13 D lens is used, its focal length is near 75 millimetres. The distance between the nodal point and the retina is 15 millimetres.

Thus $\quad \dfrac{a'b'}{ab} = \dfrac{f}{n} = \dfrac{75}{15} = 5$

i.e., the magnification is about 5 times.

The magnification is dependent upon the focal length of the condensing lens used provided it is so placed that its anterior focal point coincides with the nodal point of the eye.

## 2. When principal focus of the lens coincides with the anterior focus of the observed eye

In such an event the rays parallel to the optic axis of the eye are converged to the anterior principal focus of the eye. These rays then meet the condensing lens passing through its anterior focus and are refracted along a line parallel to the axis of the condensing lens (Fig. 11.15). The image of the part of the fundus will be along this refracted ray. The size of the image will, therefore, remain unaltered irrespective of the distance at which it is formed from the lens.

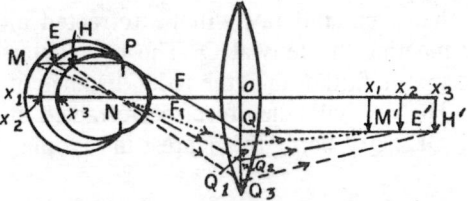

**Fig. 11.15.** Images in indirect ophthalmoscopy when principal focus of the lens coincides with the anterior focus of the observed eye.

In Fig. 11.15, let MP or EP or HP represent a ray parallel to the optic axis of the eye. This ray is converged to the focus F of the eye which coincides with the anterior focus $F_1$ of the condensing lens. The emergent ray $PF_1Q$ meets the lens at Q and is refracted along $QM'$, $QE'$, and $QH'$ parallel to the axis of the lens. In myopia, the ray $MNQ_1$ passes through the nodal point of the eye, leaves the eye convergent in relation to $PFQ$ and is further converged along $Q_1M'$ meeting $QM'E'H'$ earlier at $M'$. In emmetropia the ray $ENQ_2$ passes through the nodal point and emerges parallel to $PFQ$. It is converged along $Q_2E'$ meeting $QM'E'H'$ at $E'$. In hypermetropia, the ray $HNQ_3$ passes through the nodal point N and is divergent in relation to the ray $PEQ$. It is converged along $Q_3H'$ meeting $QM'E'H'$ at $H'$ farther from the emmetropic ray $Q_2E'$.

Since $M'$, $H'$ and $E'$ are all lying on a line parallel to the optical axis of the lens and $x_1$, $x_2$ and $x_3$ are the images of $X_1$, $X_2$ and $X_3$, and image $X_1M'$, $X_2E'$ and $X_3H'$ are equal to the size of each other.

The hypothesis needs a little clarification in as much as the anterior principal focal point in three conditions described varies in position so that the distance of condensing lens from the anterior surface of the cornea of the observed eye will also vary accordingly. The image will be equal only when in each case the principal focus of the condensing lens coincides with the anterior principal focus of the observed eye.

### 3. When the principal focus of the condensing lens is farther from the observed eye than its anterior principal focus (Fig. 11.16)

Applying the same principles as above we will find that a parallel ray will be refracted along PFQ meeting the lens at Q. The ray is starting from a point farther than the focal distance of the lens. The ray will, therefore, be refracted along QM', QE', QH' being the nearest in myopia.

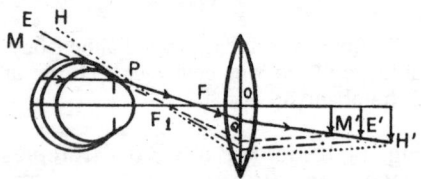

**Fig. 11.16.** Formation of images in indirect ophthalmoscopy when the principal focus of the lens is farther from the eye than its anterior principal focus.

Thus the image in hypermetropia will diminish in size and in myopia it will increase while in emmetropia it will remain unaltered. The image in myopia increases and in hypermetropia it diminishes in size, if the lens is moved away from the eye.

### 4. When the principal focus of the condensing lens is nearer the eye than its anterior principal focus (Fig. 11.17)

Applying similar principles as above it will be found that emergent ray PFQ will be refracted as a divergent ray along QM', QE' or QH' being nearest in myopia. Thus the image in hypermetropia will be largest and in myopia smallest

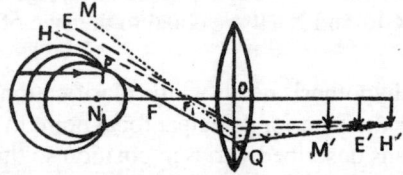

**Fig. 11.17.** Formation of images in indirect ophthalmoscopy when the principal focus of the lens is nearer the eye than its anterior principal focus.

while in emmetropia it is unaltered in size. The image in myopia decreases and in hypermetropia it increases in size if the condensing lens is moved towards the eye.

To simplify we may represent the optics of refractive errors vis-à-vis indirect ophthalmoscopy in Figs 11.18, 11.19 and 11.20.

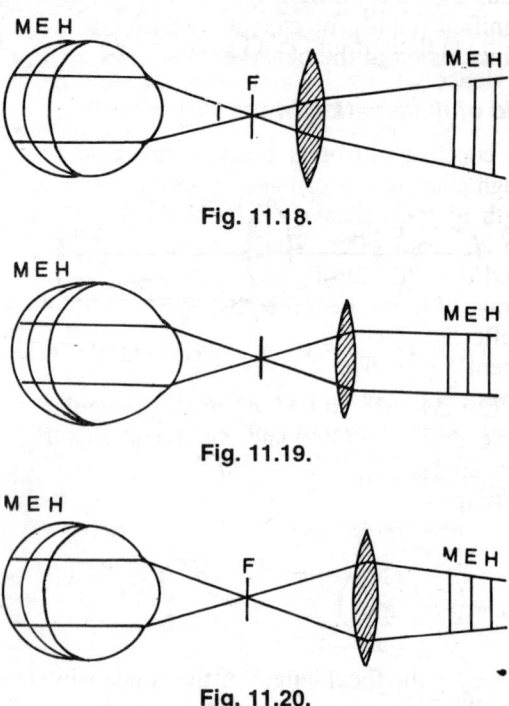

**Fig. 11.18.**

**Fig. 11.19.**

**Fig. 11.20.**

### *Field of illumination and observation*

The ophthalmoscopic field of vision is always larger than the field of illumination in indirect method of ophthalmoscopy. The size of pupil does not affect the size of ophthalmoscopic field provided it is larger than the image of the observer's pupil formed by condensing lens in the observed pupil.

In Fig. 11.21, if OP represents the size of the pupil of the observer's eye, it is focused as O'P'

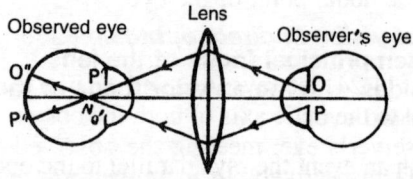

**Fig. 11.21.** Field of vision in indirect ophthalmoscopy.

on the pupil of the observed eye as the focus of the condensing lens coincides with the pupillary plane of the observed eye. The limits of field of vision are O″P″.

## Direct ophthalmoscopy

The method aims at observing the image of the fundus as an erect image. The image is virtual and magnified and is projected at the least distance of distinct vision of the observer.

### Field of illumination in the direct method

The concave mirror is chosen for examination though plane mirror can also be utilized. The focal length of the concave mirror used is not more than 20 centimetres. The light is usually so adjusted that it is farther than its focal length and the rays of lights meet the observed eye. The light is reflected flooding the observed eye as a convergent beam. The convergent beam is further converged by the dioptric system of the observed eye so that the rays come to a focus in the vitreous (Fig. 11.22). The field of illumination is largest in myopia and smallest in hypermetropia. If the light

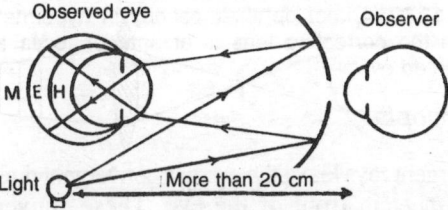

**Fig. 11.22.** Field of illumination in direct ophthalmoscopy when light is more than 20 cm from the mirror.

was at a distance less than 20 cm, the reflected rays from the mirror would be divergent when meeting the eye and the rays will be brought to a focus behind the eye and thus the field of illumination will be smallest in myopia (Fig. 11.23).

Similar result will follow if the observer stands at a much greater distance so that the rays meet in the air and meet the eye as divergent rays.

### Field of vision in direct ophthalmoscopy

In Fig. 11.24, let rays AC and BD be the rays parallel to the optic axis of both the observed and the observer's eye, meeting the observed eye at C and D, respectively. In an emmetropic eye they are focused to F and continue in the direction of

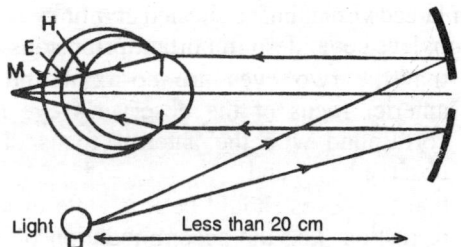

**Fig. 11.23.** Field of illumination in direct ophthalmoscopy when light is less than 20 cm from the mirror.

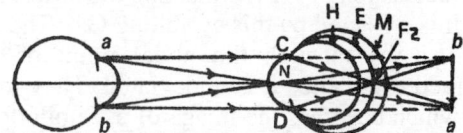

**Fig. 11.24.** Field of vision in direct ophthalmoscopy.

$CF_2a'$ and $DF_2b'$. The rays $aNa'$ and $bNb'$ pass through the nodal point of the eye and, therefore, go undeviated. They form $a'$ and $b'$ as images of a and b. The field of vision is greatest in hypermetropia, intermediate in emmetropia and smallest in myopia. The ophthalmoscopic field of vision, however, differs with

- the size of pupil of the observed eye (the greater the size, the greater the field of vision);
- the size of the pupil of the observer's eye or the sight hole of the ophthalmoscope whichever is smaller (the smaller the hole, the better the field of vision);
- the axial length of the observed eye;
- the distance between the observed and the observer's eye (the lesser the distance, the greater the field of vision).

In the direct method, the field of vision is always smaller than the field of illumination because at the distance of examination the reflected rays from the mirror are convergent and give a large field of illumination.

## Observation of fundus in various refractive states of eye

### In emmetropia

The emergent rays from an emmetropic eye are parallel in direction and when they are received by an emmetropic eye by suitable lenses, they are focused onto the retina of the observed eye. To the observer the rays will appear to have come from an enlarged virtual image situated at infinity behind the observed eye. Two important provisions are :

1. that the two eyes are co-axial and the anterior focus of the observer's eye must correspond with the anterior focus of the observed eye; and

2. that both eyes should be in a state of static refraction, i.e., the accommodation of each eye is completely eliminated.

In Fig. 11.25, a ray aP parallel to the optic axis is refracted along PF($F_1$)Q meeting the observer's eye. It is refracted by this eye along Qa'. The ray RNa' passes through the nodal point of the observed eye; hence it is undeviated. They meet at a' which becomes the image of a. Similarly b' is the the image of b. The size of image a'b' is equal to the part of the observed fundus ab.

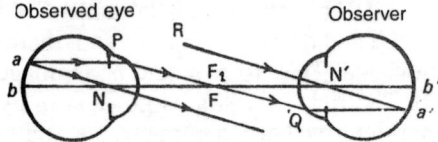

**Fig. 11.25.** Direct ophthalmoscopy of emmetropic eye.

### In hypermetropia

In hypermetropia, the emergent rays are divergent and they seem to diverge from the virtual image of the fundus. The image acts as an object for the observer's eye. Without accommodation the image of this will be formed behind the observer's retina. If now the image has to be formed at the retina the observer must accommodate.

In Fig. 11.26, the ray aP is parallel to the optic axis and, therefore, after refraction passes as PFQ. This ray meets the observer's eye at Q and is refracted along Qa'. The ray aN passes through the nodal point and, therefore, is not deviated. aN and PFQ are divergent and therefore form a virtual image as a' behind the observed eye. The ray a'N' passes through the nodal point of the observer's eye and therefore passes undeviated. It meets Qa" at a". Similarly ray b'N' meets at b" forming the image a"b" of ab behind the observer's retina. The image a"b" is equal in size to the object ab. Now if the observer's eye accommodates the ray a'PQ instead of being refracted parallel to the optic axis as Qa" will be converged along the direction Qa"' meeting the ray a'N' at the observer's retina at a"' forming the image of

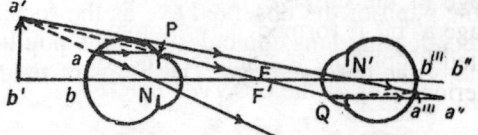

**Fig. 11.26.** Direct ophthalmoscopy in uncorrected hypermetropic eye.

a at a"'. Similarly the image of b will be formed at b"'. Thus the image of ab will be a"'b"'. This image is smaller than the image in emmetropia.

To correct this anomaly a suitable convergent lens is placed at the anterior focus of the eye and the divergent rays are made parallel creating the conditions of emmetropia. The power of convex lens so placed will be equal to the power of the correcting lens worn at the anterior focus of the observed eye. Thus it can help one to approximately estimate the degree of hypermetropia by the direct method (Fig. 11.27).

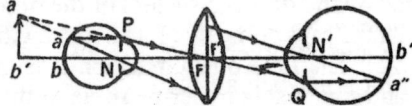

**Fig. 11.27.** Direct ophthalmoscopy in hypermetropia when the correcting lens is at anterior focus of the observed eye.

### In myopia

Emergent rays leave the eye in a convergent direction and meet in front of the eye. These convergent rays meet the observer's eye and after refraction form an image in front of the retina (Fig. 11.28).

In Fig. 11.28, the ray aP which is parallel to the optic axis is refracted along PFa'. The ray aN passing through the nodal point N passes undeviated. The two rays PF and aN meet at a' to form the image a'b'. This acts as object for the observer's eye. The ray PFa" meets the observer's eye at Q and is refracted along Qa". The ray RN' meets the refracted ray Qa" thus forming the image a"b". The observer's eye cannot form a focused

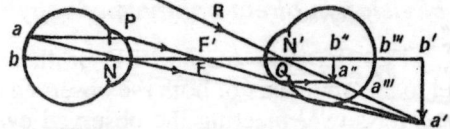

**Fig. 11.28.** Direct ophthalmoscopy in uncorrected myopia eye.

image of the observed eye. A blurred enlarged image a‴b‴ is formed. The anomaly can be corrected by placing a suitable concave lens at the anterior focus of the observed eye (Fig. 11.29).

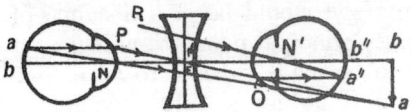

**Fig. 11.29.** Direct ophthalmoscopy in myopia when correcting lens is at anterior focus of the observed eye.

The convergent ray is thus made parallel to the refracted ray PFQ.

Thus, besides a detailed funduscopy, the examination by direct ophthalmoscopy can be used for a rough estimation of the refractive error of the observed eye, but is seldom employed.

### Magnification in direct ophthalmoscopy

The portion of retina observed sends rays which emerge as parallel rays and pass through the focus of the observer's eye. These parallel rays intercepted by the observer's eye are projected backwards to a point behind the observed eye as a″. Similarly b″ is the projected image of b. The points are situated at the observer's minimal distance of distinct vision which is about 25 cm from the observer's eye (Fig. 11.30). Admittedly this distance is arbitrary but we usually hold the objects for near work at this distance. The image (a′b′) of the observed fundus in emmetropia is equal to the size of the part of fundus observed (ab).

In Fig. 11.30, $\Delta$s a″b″N′ and a′b′N′ are equiangular. Therefore,

$$\frac{a''b''}{a'b'} = \frac{b''N'}{b'N'}$$

But $\qquad$ a′b′ = ab

Hence $\qquad \dfrac{a''b''}{ab} = \dfrac{b''N'}{b'N'} = \dfrac{250}{15}$ mm = 16.5 times

Hence the image is magnified about 16.5 times in emmetropia. In hypermetropia the size is smaller and in myopia it is larger.

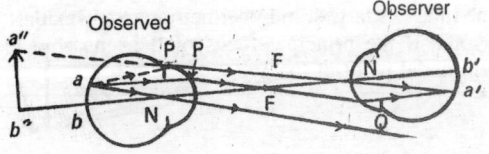

**Fig. 11.30.** Magnification in direct ophthalmoscopy.

### Method of examination (Fig. 11.31)

Before the examination is commenced the pupil of the observed eye should be fully dilated and the room should be a perfect darkroom, the only source of illumination being the one used for ophthalmoscopy. The source of light must give illumination throughout. With the modern battery or mains ophthalmoscopes the problems of illumination and reflection of light have been greatly simplified. The ophthalmoscope used must have a magazine of lenses, as is usually provided for, with an arrangement that the desired lens can be rotated in the sight hole. The right eye is used to examine the right eye of the patient and the left for the left.

To start the examination, a +12 D lens is brought opposite the sight hole by rotating the magazine of lenses. The ophthalmoscope is held vertically and as near the eye as possible. The patient's head is kept erect and fixed in position. The light is reflected on the patient's eye, the observer's eye being at a slightly higher level. The lens is immediately brought into focus and studied. The media between the lens and the retina can be easily explored by gradually rotating lenses of lesser dioptric strength in the sight hole till with no lens in the sight hole an emmetropic retina can be easily examined.

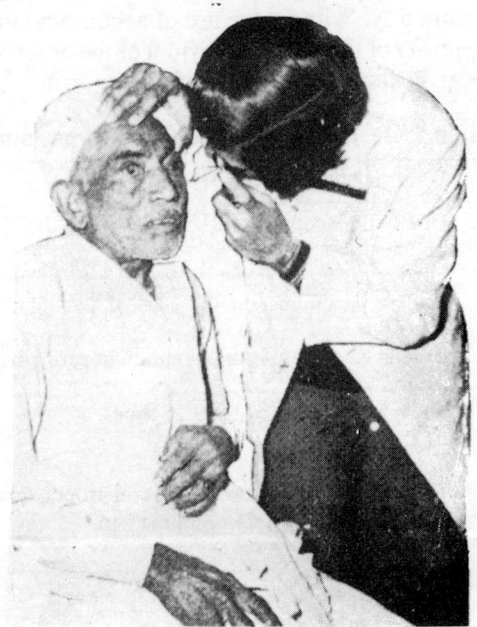

**Fig. 11.31.** Method of direct ophthalmoscopy.

A regular order of examination should be followed and practised to avoid confusion. The patient should be asked to look straight ahead and the disc and large vessels which come in view should be seen. The patient is then asked to look upwards, downwards to the nasal side and to the temporal side to explore the various parts of the periphery of the fundus. Last of all, the patient should be asked to look into the sight hole of the ophthalmoscope and the macula thoroughly examined. The focusing of light on the macula dazzles the patient and intensity of light reflected should be reduced by a rheostatic control, if one is present. The macula should be examined last of all as otherwise the dazzling may reduce the cooperation of the patient and ophthalmoscopy may become difficult.

A rough estimate of the refractive error of the eye can be made by the direct method. The basic principle involved in this method is that the punctum remotum of the observer should coincide with the punctum remotum of the patient's eye to get a clearly defined image. If the patient's eye is myopic with its punctum remotum some distance in front of the eye and the observer's eye is made hypermetropic by putting minus lenses in front of his eye so that its punctum remotum coincides with that of patient's eye then the observer's eye can receive a sharp and clear image of the details of the examined eye without the use of accommodation. The power of the lens used in front of the observer's eye gives the approximate refractive error of the observed eye. This is not the exact measurement. This may be elucidated by two examples.

Let us suppose that the observed eye is +5 D hypermetropic. The image formed by the hypermetropic eye would be at a distance of 20 cm behind its principal point. Now if the observer's eye is to be made myopic to an extent that its punctum remotum should coincide with the punctum remotum of the observed eye it should be at a distance equal to the sum of the anterior focal distance of the two eyes, i.e., 20 + 3 cm (23 cm), or the punctum remotum of the observer's eye should be at 23 cm. The lens required to produce the desired effect would be about +4.5 D. Thus the refractive error of the observed eye would be estimated as +4.5 D instead of +5 D. In myopia the punctum remotum will be at 20 cm minus the sum of anterior focal lengths of the observed and the observer's eye, i.e., 20 − 3 = 17 cm. This refractive error will be estimated at about −6 D instead of −5 D. The formulae for calculation of refractive powers can be expressed as under :

$$H = \frac{100}{PR + 3}$$

where H is the estimated hypermetropia of the observed eye

$$M = \frac{100}{PR - 3}$$

where M is the estimated myopia of observed eye.

The comparison between the direct and indirect ophthalmoscopy is summarised in Table 11.1.

### Table 11.1. Comparison between direct and indirect ophthalmoscopy

| | Direct ophthalmoscopy | Indirect ophthalmoscopy |
|---|---|---|
| 1. | Ophthalmoscopic field is less than the field of illumination. | Field of illumination is less than the field of vision. |
| 2. | Field of vision is largest in hypermetropia, smallest in myopia depending on the size of the pupil of the patient. | Field of vision is largest in myopia and smallest in hypermetropia. It is independent of the size of the pupil of the patient. |
| 3. | Brightness of field is maximum in hypermetropia and least in myopia. | The brightness of field does not depend upon the error of refraction. |
| 4. | The magnification is 14 to 16 times. | Magnification is 5 times with +13 D sph. and is dependent upon the dioptric power of the condensing lens. The higher the dioptric power, the lower the magnification. |
| 5. | The image is smaller in hypermetropia, bigger in myopia and distorted in astigmatism. | The image is largest in hypermetropia and smallest in myopia if the principal focus of the lens coincides with nodal point of the eye. |

# CHAPTER 12

# Retinoscopy

The principle of retinoscopy is to convert the observed eye into a degree of myopia that the image formed by the fundus in front of the observed eye coincides with the pupillary plane of the observer. Principally a spot of the fundus of the patient's eye is illuminated by reflecting light into the eye with a plane or concave mirror and the image of this illuminated spot formed by the patient's eye, when the light is reflected back, is observed. In the use of the plane mirror to obtain results the opening in the mirror should be 4 mm in size. The advantage is, however, counterbalanced by the appearance of a circular dark patch. To get over this difficulty a concave mirror of about 150 cm focal length should be employed. It acts as a plane mirror for all practical purposes and gives a bright light to play with.

Nowadays self-illuminating retinoscopes (Fig. 12.1) are being used based on the above principles. They are alternative more easily manipulated systems with the advantage that the intensity and size of the beam can be readily controlled. Both types of mirror effect can be provided by moving a strong converging lens to and from the bulb to vary the angularity of the light leaving the mirror, so that at one extreme the rays converge

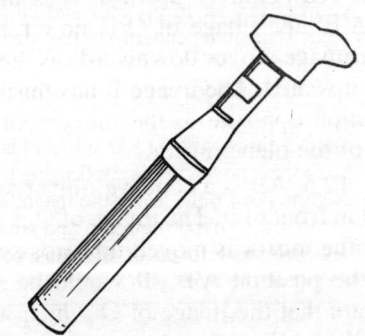

**Fig. 12.1.** Self-illuminating retinoscope.

at a point close to the instrument (concave type mirror) and at the other the rays are parallel (plane type mirror) (Fig. 12.2). As long as this image is not coinciding with the pupillary plane of the observer there remains some parallax and

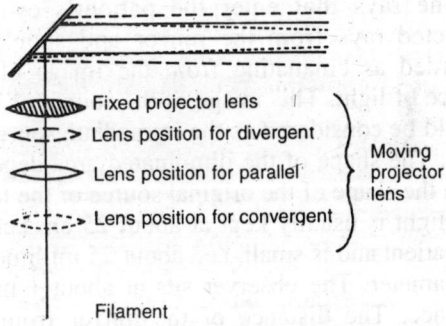

**Fig. 12.2.** Optical construction of the electric retinoscope.

by placing suitable lenses in front of the observed eye this parallax is eliminated. Retinoscopy is carried out preferably by some from a distance of one metre purely as a matter of convenience both for the manipulations required during the procedures and subsequent mathematical calculations. Many ophthalmologists prefer to do retinoscopy at about 2/3 metre distance, i.e., at about an arm's length away from the patient which they regard as a working distance. The choice of distance should be left to the observer as long as it is understood that the mathematical correction is to be accurately applied according to the formula $100/d$; where $d$ is the distance in centimetres at which retinoscopy is done.

It should also be borne in mind that lesser the distance used for retinoscopy, the greater are the errors in this objective assessment of the refractive error. A distance of more than one metre hampers the manipulations. The movement of the image (or shadow as it is called) is estimated in relation to the movement of the mirror performed by the observer. If a distance of *one metre* is used with the plane mirror and if the image moves in the same direction as the movement of the mirror the refractive state of the eye is (a) emmetropia, (b) hypermetropia, or (c) myopia of less than one dioptre. If the image moves in the direction opposite to the movement of the mirror the refractive state of the eye is myopia of more than one dioptre. With a concave mirror the findings opposite to those obtained with the plane mirror are recorded. With either mirror if there is no parallax in the movement of the image the refractive state of the eye is myopia of one dioptre.

The rays that enter the patient's eye are reflected rays from the mirror and should be regarded as emanating from the image of the source of light. This image of the source of light should be considered as the immediate source of light. The shape of the illuminated area depends upon the shape of the original source of the light. The light is usually kept at about 25 cm behind the patient and is small, i.e., about 25 millimetres in diameter. The observer sits at about 1 metre distance. The distance of the mirror from the source of the light is, therefore, 1.25 metres. In a plane mirror the image will form as far behind as the object is in front and will be equal in size. The eye of the patient will, therefore, be 2.25 metres from the immediate source of light. The diameter of the retinal image I (Fig. 12.3) is :

$$I = \frac{dv}{u}$$

But $\qquad v = N$

and $\qquad u = D$

Hence $\qquad I = \frac{dN}{D}$

where $d$ is the diameter of the source of light, $N$ is the distance of the nodal point from the retina,

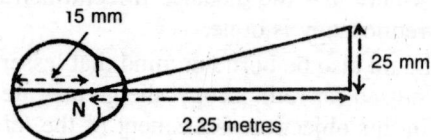

**Fig. 12.3.** Size of retinal image in retinoscopy.

and $D$ is the distance of the nodal point from the immediate source of light.

or $\qquad \dfrac{25 \times 15}{2250} = 0.16$ mm

which is rather very small. In streak retinoscopy we use a linear source of light and a linear image upon the fundus is formed. The intensity of illumination of the fundus will depend upon (1) clarity of the media, (2) refraction of the patient's eye, (3) type of mirror—plane or concave, (4) distance of original source of light from the mirror, and (5) the intensity of the original source of light.

The portion of the illuminated fundus that can be seen at any one time depends upon the size of the pupil and the distance at which the observer sits, i.e.,

$$\frac{4 \times 15}{1000} = 0.06 \text{ mm}$$

We know that the illuminated area of the fundus is 0.16 mm, i.e., only a small area of the illuminated fundus is seen at one time and the surrounding fundus is invisible. If the immediate source of light be moved, i.e., the movement of the mirror, the illuminated area of the fundus will be succeeded by a dark area, usually termed as the shadow. It is on the junction of the illuminated area that one's attention is concentrated while doing retinoscopy.

When a plane mirror is moved upwards the immediate source of light moves downwards while the opposite is true in the case of a concave mirror (Figs. 12.4 and 12.5).

In Fig. 12.4, AB is the plane mirror and O is the object in front of it. The image of O is formed at I. When AB is moved upwards it assumes the position A'B' and image of O is now formed at I', i.e., the image moves downwards as the mirror is moved upwards. The image I' has thus moved in a direction opposite to the movement of the direction of the plane mirror.

In Fig. 12.5, AB is a concave mirror and O is the object in front of it. The image of O is formed at I. Now the mirror is moved upwards so that it assumes the position A'B'. It would be seen in this diagram that the image of O which was at I moves to I', i.e., the image moves upwards as the mirror is moved upwards. The image I' in case of

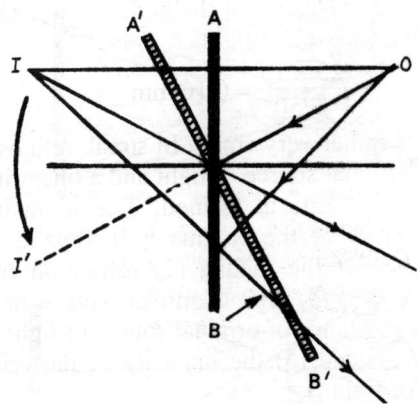

**Fig. 12.4.** Movement of immediate source of light with the movement of plane mirror (opposite direction).

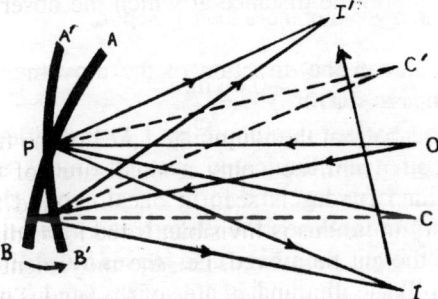

**Fig. 12.5.** Movement of immediate source of light with the movement of concave mirror (same direction).

concave mirror has thus moved in the same direction as the movement of the direction of concave mirror.

The image formed by mirrors acts as the immediate source of light.

When the immediate source of light is moved downwards the illuminated spot on fundus moves upwards (Fig. 12.6). The image of a is formed at a′ on the fundus. When a moves to a position b its image moves upwards to the position b′. This

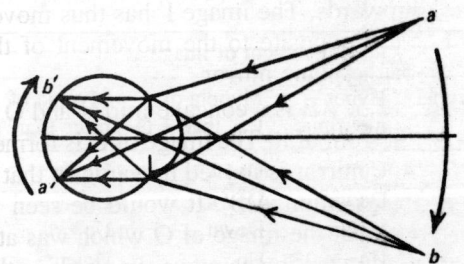

**Fig. 12.6.** Movement of illuminated spot on fundus with the movement of immediate source of light.

movement of illuminated spot of the fundus is opposite to the direction of movement of concave mirror and in the direction of the movement of plane mirror.

In emmetropia the reflected rays from the illuminated spot on the fundus, after refraction by the patient's eye, emerge parallel to each other and meet the observer's eye as such. The observer projects the image in space behind the patient's eye in the direction of the emergent rays (Fig. 12.8). The image of a′ is projected along Na′ to a″ and the image of b′ is projected along Nb′ to b″. Thus when a moves to b (upwards), a″ moves to b″ (also upwards), i.e., in the direction of movement of the plane mirror and opposite to the direction of movement of the concave mirror.

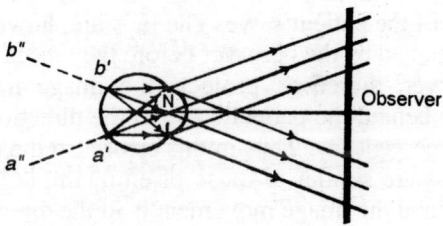

**Fig. 12.7.** Movement of image of illuminated spot of fundus in hypermetropia.

In hypermetropia, the reflected rays from the illuminated spot on the fundus after refraction by the patient's eye emerge divergent to each other and are intercepted by the observer's eye. As in emmetropia the observer projects the image in the space behind the patient's eye in the direction of emergent rays (Fig. 12.7). The image of a′ is projected along Na′ to a″ and the image of b′ is

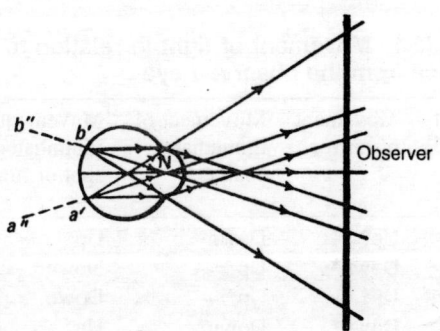

**Fig. 12.8.** Movement of image of illuminated spot of fundus in emmetropia.

projected along Nb′ to b″. Thus when a′ moves to b′ (upwards) a″ moves to b″ (also upwards), i.e., in the same direction. This movement is in the direction of movement of the plane mirror and opposite to the direction of the concave mirror.

In myopia of more than 1 D, the image is formed between the patient and the observer. The movement of the image is in a direction opposite to the movement of the plane mirror and in the same direction as the movement of the concave mirror. However, if the image is not formed between the patient and the observer the conditions simulate those of emmetropia and hypermetropia.

In myopia of less than 1 D when the observer is sitting at a distance of one metre, the reflected rays from the illuminated spot on the fundus, after refraction by the patient's eye, emerge convergent to each other and would meet at a‴b‴ in front of the patient's eye. The rays are, however, intercepted by the observer before they meet. The observer, therefore, projects the image in the space behind the patient's eye in the direction of the emergent ray. Thus in this error also the conditions are similar to those of emmetropia (Fig. 12.9) and the image movement is in the direction of movement of the plane mirror and opposite to that of the concave mirror.

In myopia of more than 1 D, the reflected rays from the illuminated spot on the fundus, after refraction by the patient's eye, emerge convergent to each other and form an image between the observer and the observed eye. The real image is seen by the observer (Fig. 12.10). The image of a′ is formed at a″ and that of b′ is formed at b″. Thus when a′ moves to b′, i.e., upwards, a″ moves to b″, i.e., downwards. The movement is in an opposite direction to the movement of the plane

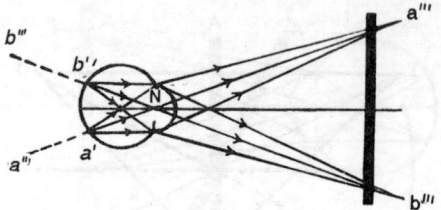

**Fig. 12.9.** Movement of image of illuminated spot of fundus in myopia of less than 1 dioptre

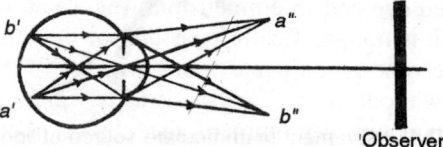

**Fig. 12.10.** Movement of image of illuminated spot of fundus in myopia of more than 1 dioptre.

mirror and in the direction of the movement of the concave mirror.

If the patient is myopic by 1 D the reflected rays from the illuminated spot of fundus after refraction converge and form a real image at the pupillary area. When the illuminated spot on the fundus moves, the image also moves but still fills the pupillary area and is not appreciated by the observer (Fig. 12.11). This is considered as a neutral point. The findings are summarised in Table 12.1.

The neutral point is the point at which the reflected rays from the illuminated spot on the fundus after refraction by the observed eye fill the pupillary plane of the observer's eye. At this stage the observer's eye and the observed eye are conjugate foci.

In case of hypermetropia the punctum remotum is a hypothetical point behind the ob-

**Table 12.1. Movement of light in relation to movement of mirrors if the observer sits at one metre distance from the observed eye**

| Type of mirror | Movement of mirror | Movement of immediate source | Movement of illuminated spot of fundus | Movement of image | | | |
|---|---|---|---|---|---|---|---|
| | | | | Emmetropia | Hyper-metropia | Myopia of less than 1 D | Myopia of more than 1 D |
| Plane | Up* | Down | Up* | Up* | Up* | Up* | Down |
| | Down* | Up | Down* | Down* | Down* | Down* | Up |
| Concave | Up* | Up* | Down | Down | Down | Down | Up* |
| | Down* | Down* | Up | Up | Up | Up | Down* |

* indicates movement with movement of mirror.

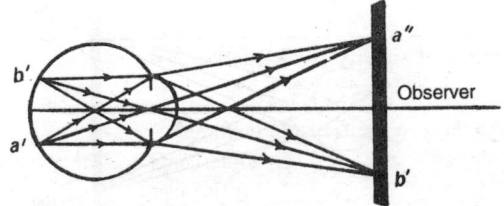

**Fig. 12.11.** Movement of image of illuminated spot of fundus in myopia of 1 dioptre.

served eye and in emmetropia it is at infinity so that it is not practically possible for the observer to become a conjugate focus with the observed eye without the artificial aids as he cannot sit at the punctum remotum of the observed eye. In myopia the punctum remotum of the observed eye is situated in front of the eye so that theoretically the observer can alter his distance in a way that the punctum remotum of the observed eye coincides with the observer. By measuring this distance the state of refractive error of the eye can be estimated, i.e., $100/PR = D$ where $PR$ is the distance of punctum remotum and $D$ the strength of the concave lens required to make the eye emmetropic. This method, however, will be time-consuming and cumbersome.

The other method of estimation can be that the observer sits at a fixed distance from the patient and by placing suitable lenses in front of the observed eye the punctum remotum is made to coincide with the observer. Suitable mathematical calculation can then give the true refractive error. But for the accuracy of this measure the lens should be at the anterior focal point of the observed eye which is rather difficult. One metre is usually chosen as the distance from which the examination is carried out. It is arbitrarily chosen as the mathematical calculations become easier.

$$D_1 + (-1\ D) = d$$

where $D_1$ is the lens which brings the punctum remotum to one metre and $d$ is the refractive error of the observed eye.

If the distance chosen is 66 cm or 2/3 of a metre the formula for calculation will be

$$D_1 + (-1.5\ D) = d$$

Theoretically, the farther away the surgeon is, the more accurate are the results obtained but in practice it is offset with the difficulty in clearly discerning the movements in the pupillary area and changing the lens in the trial frame. The most important observation that has to be made is the point of reversal, i.e., the point at which the punctum remotum of the observed eye corresponds with the nodal point of the observer's eye.

Plane mirror or a concave mirror of more than 1.5 metre focal length is the mirror of choice as with this the illumination of the fundus is adequate and not too brilliant. Concave mirror of more than 1.5 metre focal length for all practical purposes acts as a plane mirror.

### Static retinoscopy

The patient's accommodation for retinoscopy should be either slight or it must be completely relaxed by a cycloplegic. In children under eight years mydriasis and cycloplegia should be achieved by atropine ointment ½ to 1% three times a day for three days. In children between 8 and 14 years or in persons in whom the cycloplegia is not attained by homatropine, atropine 1% drops should be used to produce cycloplegia. In patients between 16 and 45 years 1-2% homatropine eyedrops are sufficient. Both atropine 1% drops and homatropine 2% drops produce a cycloplegia within an hour if instilled every 10 minutes. In patients over 45 years of age the accommodation is usually negligible and no cycloplegia may be necessary. If cycloplegia is desired care should be taken regarding the rise of intraocular tension. Mydriasis and cycloplegia in such persons should be under the supervision of a competent person. In repeat refractions cycloplegia may not be required and mydriasis with epinephrine 5 to 10% drops may be sufficient. Newer cycloplegics which have a quick and short action like cyclopentolate and tropicamide are now available and are quite frequently used.

Short summary of the mydriatics and/or cycloplegics used are given in Table 12.2.

A trial frame (Fig. 12.12) is employed for putting the lens in front of the eye to be refracted. The qualities of a trial frame should be as follows :

- Light.
- Easily adjustable.
- Both the horizontal and vertical adjust-

**Table 12.2. Mydriatics and/or cycloplegics in refraction**

| Drug | Onset of maximum cycloplegia | Duration of activity | Remarks |
|------|------------------------------|----------------------|---------|
| 1. Atropine sulphate | 6-24 hours | 10-15 days | In children |
| 2. Homatropine hydrobromide | 1 hour | 1-2 days | In adolescents |
| 3. Cyclopentolate hydrochloride | 10-45 minutes | 12-24 hours | For office use |
| 4. Tropicamide | 20-30 minutes | 4-10 hours | For office use (effects similar to cyclopentolate) |

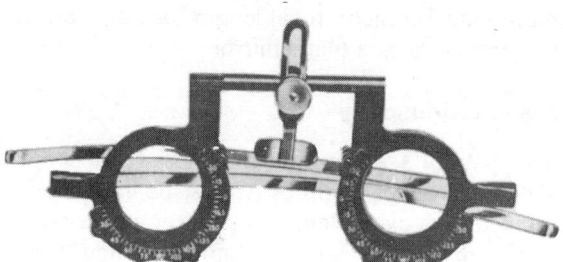

**Fig. 12.12.** Trial frame.

ments should be possible for each eye separately.

- The dial indicating the axes should be truly positioned as otherwise it will introduce errors in prescription of axes.
- The frame should be capable of carrying at least three lenses—a sphere, a cylinder and a Maddox rod or prism.
- The compartment of the cylinder should be such that the lenses are very near each other and also as near the eye as possible as otherwise the principles of homocentric system (Gauss' theorem) are likely to be disturbed.
- The frame should be capable of being tilted to adjust for near vision.

The trial case (Fig. 12.13) is a tray of lenses and accessories used in determining the refractive error of an eye. These lenses are individually marked in the strengths of dioptric power of each lens as well as in the direction of axis of the cylindrical lenses. The trial case consists of the following :

1. A pair of plus spheres ranging from +0.12 to +20.00 dioptres.
2. A pair of minus spheres ranging from –0.12 to –20.00 dioptres.
3. A pair of plus cylinders ranging from +0.12 to +8.00 dioptres.

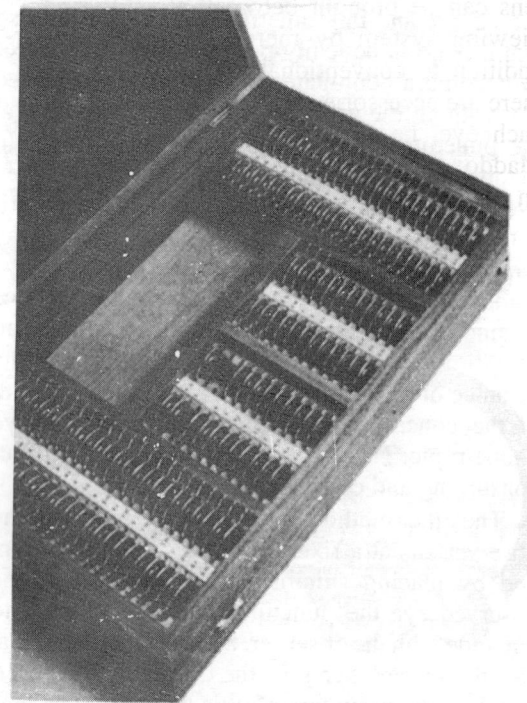

**Fig. 12.13.** Trial case containing the necessary lenses, prisms.

4. A pair of minus cylinders ranging from –0.12 to –8.00 dioptres.
5. Prisms.

The spheres are say 0.12-0.25 and thereafter in 1/4th of a dioptre to 4, ½ dioptres to 6 and then every one dioptre to 8 dioptres in cylindricals and 20 dioptres in spheres; prisms should be up to 10 Δ and some additional ones 15 Δ and 20 Δ.

The accessories such as plano lenses, opaque discs, pinhole and stenopaic discs, Maddox rods, red and green glasses and so on.

For the sake of lightness and thickness the lenses should be of small aperture (down to 15 mm diameter) and have ease of manipulations.

Spheres have a handle and cylinders are without them. Plus and minus lenses have differently coloured rims. The accessories are in a white rim. Refractor or phoropter can be used in place of trial case.

### Refractor or phoropter (Fig. 12.14)

The refractor consists of the entire trial set of lenses mounted on a circular wheel so that each lens can be brought before the aperture of the viewing system by merely turning a dial. In addition to conventional spheres and cylinders there are accessories that may be brought before each eye, i.e., a polarizing lens, a pinhole, a Maddox rod, a working lens for retinoscopy and an occluder.

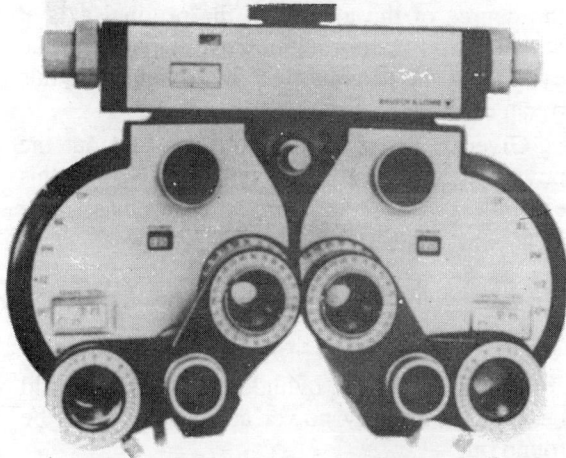

Fig. 12.14. Refractor or phoropter.

A trial frame is adjusted and trial case is within reach. The observer sits at a convenient distance and looks through the aperture of the retinoscope preferably Priestley-Smith type (Fig. 12.15). The light is so adjusted that the face of the patient is in darkness. The patient is asked to look into the eye of the observer and pupillary glow is seen. The mirror is now moved slightly and the movement of the shadow is observed. Suitable lenses are placed in the trial frame till the parallax of the shadow is eliminated. The movement of the shadow gives an indication of the axis in which the error exists. The error is first estimated in the primary axis and then in axis at right angles to it. In simple myopia, emmetropia and hypermetropia the dioptric strength of the

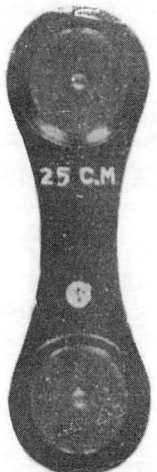

Fig. 12.15. Priestly-Smith retinoscope.

neutralising lens is the same in both the axes (Fig. 12.16).

In astigmatism the dioptric strength varies in the two meridia under scrutiny (Fig. 12.17).

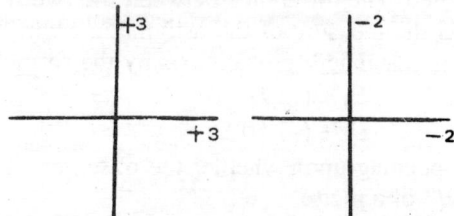

Fig. 12.16. Spherical error in retinoscopy.

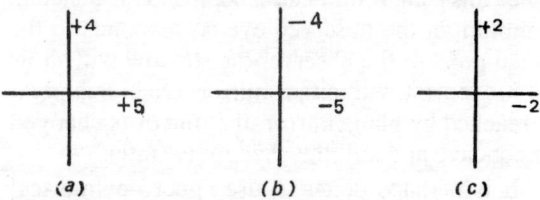

Fig. 12.17. Cylindrical error in retinoscopy. **A** Hypermetropia; **B** Myopia; **C** Mixed.

For the estimation of astigmatism streak retinoscopy gives better results than simple retinoscopy. The optics of streak retinoscope is the same as that of luminous retinoscope (Fig. 12.2) already described except that instead of a circular beam a linear beam is reflected from the retinoscope and this beam can be rotated through 180°. The streak retinoscope of Purvis (Fig. 12.18)

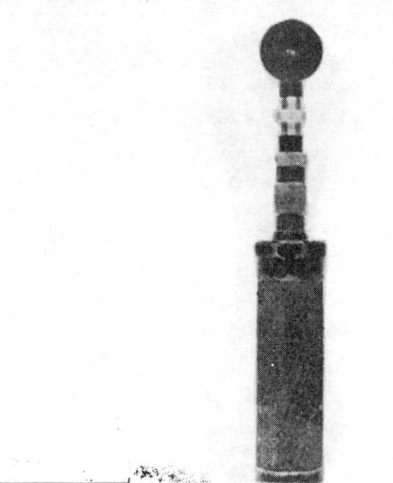

**Fig. 12.18.** Purvis streak retinoscope.

reflects a linear streak of light into the observed eye and the direction of the streak can be easily altered. The streak is rotated into the principal astigmatic meridian and the error is estimated. It is then turned through 90° and the error is again estimated. The difference between the two readings is the measure of the astigmatic error. The error is calculated for each axis by the formula :

$$D_1 + (-1\ D) = d$$
or $$D_1 + (-1.50\ D) = d$$

Depending upon whether the observer sits at 1 or 2/3 of a metre.

The retinoscopic point of reversal obtained by a plane mirror is checked by a concave mirror. Since this point is the neutral point and the punctum remotum of the observed eye corresponds to the nodal point of the observer the shadow will show no movement with either mirror. Once this point is reached by plane mirror, the mirror is changed to concave and still the shadow is static.

It is perhaps better to use sphero-cylindrical combinations in retinoscopy.

One meridian can be corrected with spherical lenses and then the second axis is corrected with addition of cylindrical lenses.

This is easily verifiable and the axis can also be better appreciated.

## Retinoscopy by cylinders

The originator of the concept is Jackson and in his own words : "The shadow test with cylindri-cal lenses is not a thing apart from skiascopy in general, but rather the culmination and full development of skiascopy."

To understand this procedure fully, a few general statements though may not be mathematically accurate but serve as excellent practical principles, are :

1. A cylinder of a known denomination at a known axis has the full denominational value at right angles to the axis and its power varies in other axes. The power of a cylinder in any given meridian can be found out (roughly speaking) by the formula :

$$P_1 = \frac{d \times P}{90}$$

where $P_1$ is the power in the required axis; $d$ is the degree of the axis from the original axis at which the power is sought; $P$ is the power of the cylinder at the original axis. Let us illustrate this by an example.

Given 3 D cyl. at axis 60°, to find out the power of cylinder at an axis of 105°. Now in this example,

$$d = 105 - 60 = 45$$
$$P = 3\ D$$

Hence, $$P_1 = \frac{45 \times 3}{90} = 1.5\ D$$

The power of the cylinder at this axis would be 1.5 D. Similarly power at other axes can be found out.

2. When two cylinders of the same denomination and same strength cross at right angles to each other they form a sphere of the same denomination, e.g., a cylinder of +3 D crosses another cylinder of +3 D at right angles, the resultant power is a spherical lens of +3 D; or +3 D cyl. axis 90° + 3 D cyl. axis 180° = 3 D sphere.

3. When two cylinders are in apposition with each other at the same axis, the resultant is the algebraical summation of the strength of the two cylinders, e.g., +2 D cyl. 90° + –3 D cyl. 90° = –1 D cyl. 90°.

4. When two cylinders of the same sign but of different strength cross each other at right angles the resultant is a sphere and a cylinder. The strength of the sphere is the same as that of the weaker cylinder and the strength of the cylinder

is the difference in the strength of the two with the same axis as that of the stronger cylinder, e.g., +3 D cyl. axis 90° + 2 D cyl. axis 180° = 2 D sphere + 1 D cyl. axis 90°.

5. When two cylinders of the same denomination cross each other obliquely the resultant is a sphero-cylinder and the axis of the cylinder of the resultant combination lies somewhere between the axes of the component cylinders. If the component cylinders are of the same strength the axis of the resultant cylinder is midway between the axes of the component cylinders, e.g., a cylinder +2 D at 90° crosses a cylinder +2 D at 60° then new cylinder will bear an axis of 75°.

6. When two cylinders of opposite denominations cross obliquely, the resultant is a mixed cylinder. The axis of the cylindric component depends on whether the mixed cylinder is given a negative or a positive sign. If a negative sign is given the axis is outside negative component of the cylinder; or outside the axis of the positive component if the cylinder is given a positive sign.

7. If two cylinders of the same sign but of different strength cross each other obliquely then the resultant axis is in proportion of their dioptric strength, e.g., if +4 D cyl. axis 90° crosses a +1 D cyl. axis 40° then the angular deviation between the two is 50°. The new cylinder will have

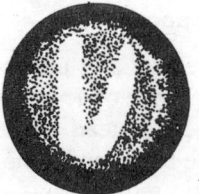

**Fig. 12.19.** Scissors shadows.

an axis in proportion of 4 to 1, i.e., it will cross at 10° from the axis of +4 cylinder or at 80°.

In practical retinoscopy the refraction is determined by the usual methods of retinoscopy. The spherical correction remains in the trial frame and the astigmatism is corrected by a cylinder. If the correcting cylinder is +2 D cyl. at 90° the refractive error of the eye, therefore, in essence is 2 D cyl. axis 90°. Now if we place our lenses of +2 D cyl. at 130° axis it will lead to a combination of lenses of +2 D cyl. axis 90° and a +2 D cyl. axis 130° which can be resolved to an axis of 115°. So that two bands of shadows will move at 15° to either side of the lens and the movement will be with the movement of the mirror. The lens is now slowly moved till these bands disappear which gives an accurate axis. Reflexes produced by streak retinoscopy are illustrated in Figs. 12.19 and 12.20.

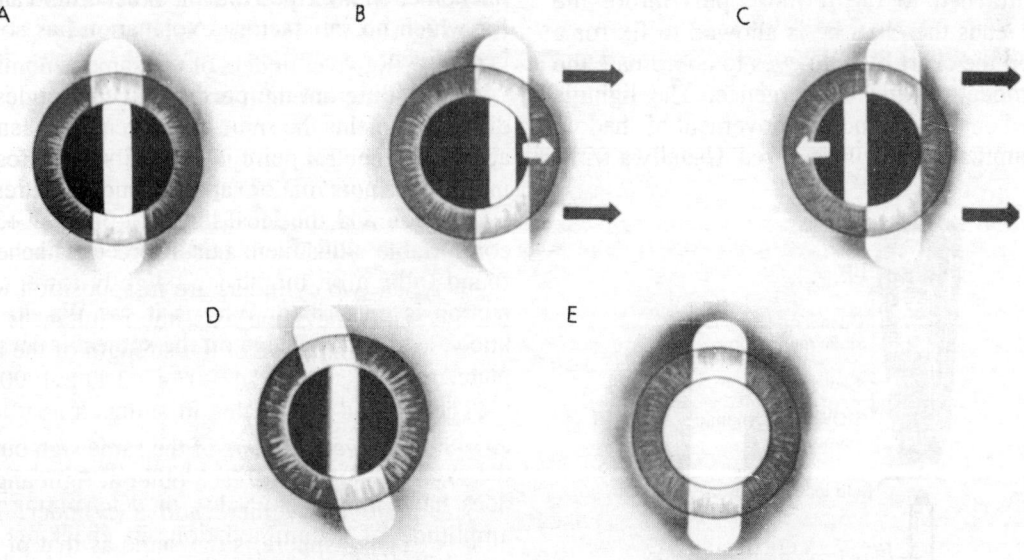

**Fig. 12.20.** Reflexes produced by the streak retinoscope.

### Dynamic retinoscopy

The method is essentially utilised for the determination of amplitude of accommodation. In this method, the eyes, instead of being relaxed as much as possible being under the effect of cycloplegic as in static retinoscopy, are fully accommodating and the refractive error is estimated with the eye accommodating and converging. This examination assists us in measuring the following :

1. The refractive error in a state of accommodation and convergence.
2. The differences in accommodation of the two eyes.
3. The assessment of the near point as well as the degree of negative accommodation.

The technique is rather difficult and requires both practice and experience.

### *Method*

A self-luminous dynamic retinoscope is used (Fig. 12.21). To this retinoscope a fixation chart is attached below the level of the beam of light. A static retinoscopy has been previously carried out and the correction thus obtained has already been placed in the trial frame. To find the negative accommodation, usually a distance of 2/3 of a metre is chosen. The patient is asked to read the chart attached to the retinoscope. Before the patient reads the chart he is allowed to fix for a while on the chart by both eyes to coordinate the accommodation and convergence. The light is reflected on the eye and the movement of shadow in the pupillary plane is observed. Usually a with-

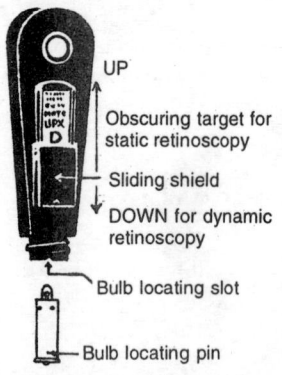

**Fig. 12.21.** Dynamic retinoscope.

UP

Obscuring target for static retinoscopy

Sliding shield

DOWN for dynamic retinoscopy

Bulb locating slot

Bulb locating pin

movement is seen. If an against-movement is noticed, the static retinoscopy is inaccurate and should be re-done. To neutralize the with-movement convex lenses are added till there is no movement of the shadow. Theoretically this point of reversal of dynamic retinoscopy represents the anterior conjugate focus for the accommodating eye. The reduction for the fixing distance gives the static error of refraction but practically it is not so because eyes with sufficient power of accommodation for the purpose will accept additional convex lenses without any alteration in the convergence or, in other words, when this neutral point is obtained (low neutral point), and convex lenses are added binocularly the accommodation gradually relaxes and a wide neutral zone is traversed until the shadow is reversed (high neutral point). This is possible due to negative relative accommodation. The difference between the high neutral point and the low neutral point represents this negative accommodation, i.e., it is the amount of accommodation which can be relaxed while the convergence remains unaltered.

In many instances, at the so-called neutral point, instead of obtaining a neutral shadow with-movement is obtained. A neutral reflex is obtained if the patient either accommodates for an object slightly in front of the mirror or if extra convex lenses are placed in the trial frame. The phenomenon is termed the lag of accommodation for which no satisfactory explanation has so far been given.

For finding out the presbyopic correction the distance remains the same. The strength of lenses at the high neutral point is generally supposed to indicate the point of convergence accommodation association and the lenses should bring about a comfortable adjustment but in practice they are found to be a bit too strong, slightly lower correction is prescribed. Why is it so? We do not know, as the knowledge on the subject is incomplete.

The method is of value in as much as it lays an objective basis for the optical correction when the eye is focused for near vision. The technique does have immediate value in determining the amplitude of accommodation, in checking the possibility of anisometropia for near and in noting the existence of astigmatism at the near point which varies from that found in the static retinoscopy. The method is, however, rarely used.

The near point of the eye and the total amplitude of accommodation can also be measured by this method. This is the distance at which, despite the strongest efforts of accommodation, the shadow is reversed. In this, static correction is before the eye and the patient is asked to fix at a near object 2 and 3 inches away. The target is fixed and the observer starts dynamic retinoscopy at about 15 inches. The movement of the shadow at this distance is against the movement of the mirror. He now gradually moves forward till the movement of the shadow begins to become 'with'. This point is the near point. Suppose it is at 10 cm then the power of accommodation is 10 D. The negative accommodation being known the amplitude can easily be calculated. This method has, however, not found wide acceptance and application in practice.

### Refractometry

Refractometry is used to determine the degree of ametropia with the use of optometers and automated refractors.

Optometers are basically utilising one of the two principles.

In the first, a clear retinal image is formed by an optical system and the degree of adjustment required gives the measure of the ametropia; the clarity of the retinal image is determined by ophthalmoscopic inspection.

In the second, displacement by parallax is the basis of measurement and manoeuvres are made on the instrument so as to superimpose the image to obtain coincidence. Fincham utilised this principle and the same is incorporated in Hartinger's coincidence refractionometer. A refractionometer consists of an illumination system and an observation system. Hartinger's refractionometer (Fig. 12.22) has a single front lens in common between the illumination and the observation system. The system is described as under (Fig. 12.23) :

A filament (X) or bulb is placed at the focus of a light condensing system composed of a combination of lenses (C) which sends parallel rays to meet a reflecting prism P which in turn directs the light to illuminate axially displaceable test

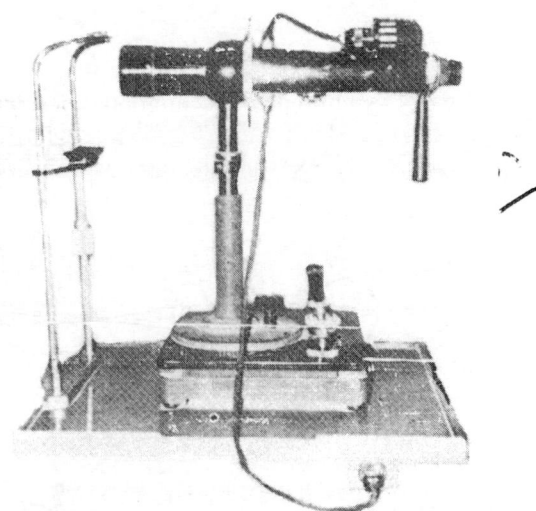

**Fig. 12.22.** Hartinger's coincidence refractionometer.

marks (T). They lie at the focus of an objective ($O_1$). The two images forming bundles of rays from the test marks are refracted in parallel by the objective $O_1$. These rays meet a combination of reflecting prisms or reflecting pentaprisms $P_2$ which form two real images of the test marks in the focal plane of the objective. Each image passes through slit openings in the diaphragm D. The rays through this diaphragm are reflected by the 45° inclined perforated plane mirror (M) and then projected into the patient's pupil by the objective $O_2$ and through the dioptric system of the eye it is projected as a sharply defined image on the retina. The reflected rays from the retina pass back through the objective $O_2$ and through the perforation in the mirror M to reach the objective $O_3$. This concentrates the image at a point S and is observed through the eyepiece E. The perforation in the mirror M lies in the focal plane of the objective $O_3$ so that between it and the eyepiece a telecentric path is produced which causes the emergent rays to maintain the same position relative to the eyepiece when the latter is shifted.

The basic principle of the refractionometer is that the position of the test marks is optically associated with the retina and that the two split images will only coincide with each other when a sharp focus of these is formed on the retina. In emmetropia this normally happens at the setting zero of the instrument. If the target is not in a position which is conjugate to the subject the retinal

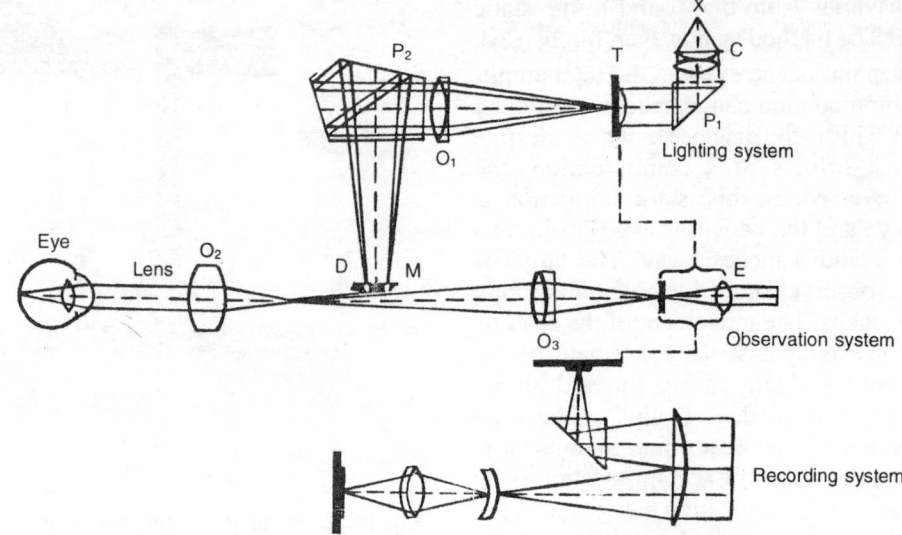

**Fig. 12.23.** Optical principles of coincidence refractionometer.

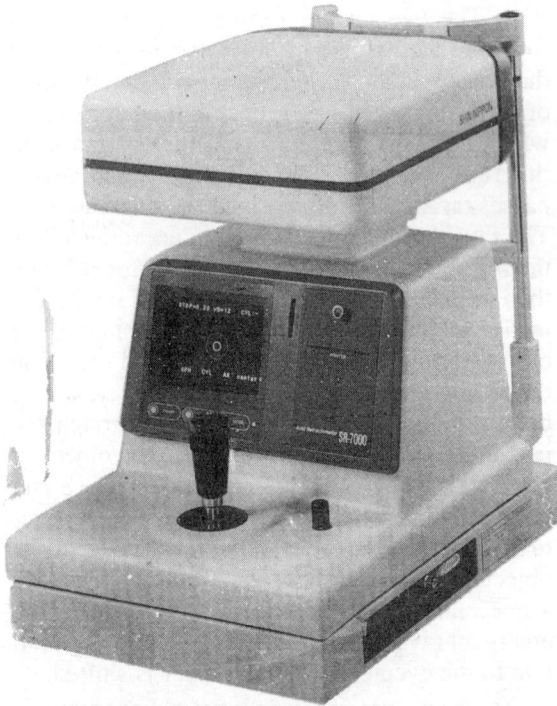

**Fig. 12.24.** Automated refractometer.

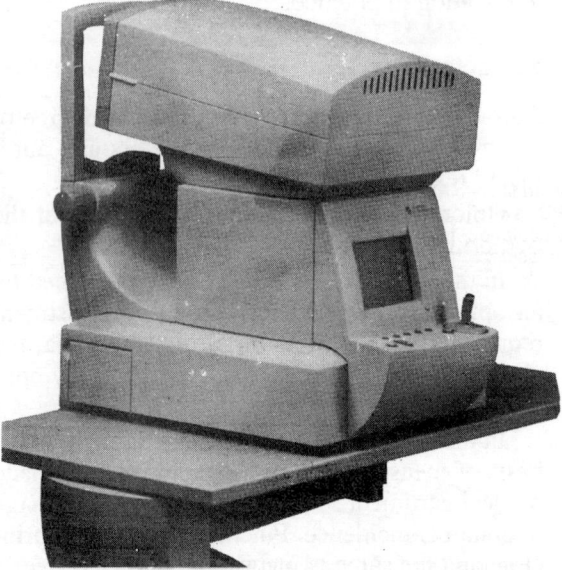

**Fig. 12.25.** Automated refractometer.

so-called tabo-degree scale. The instrument is simple to work with and gives fairly accurate results.

## Automated refractors

Modern automated refractors (Figs. 12.24 to 12.26) give according to some quite accurate readings but in the experience of the author such is not the case. Automated refractor, however, provides enough guidelines for the accurate measurement of ametropia in a patient.

image is displaced from the axis. In ametropia the position of the test mark has to be changed to bring this in sharp focus. This can be mechanically brought about. The movement of the test mark is calibrated on a scale in a way that it gives the dioptric reading which can be read off on the

Bright LED is adopted for a display. When operation is not conducted for five minutes, TV monitor and a display are shut off automatically. Time is indicated on the display.

Measured data can be transferred to the NIDEK Auto optometry system using an IC card. (factory option)

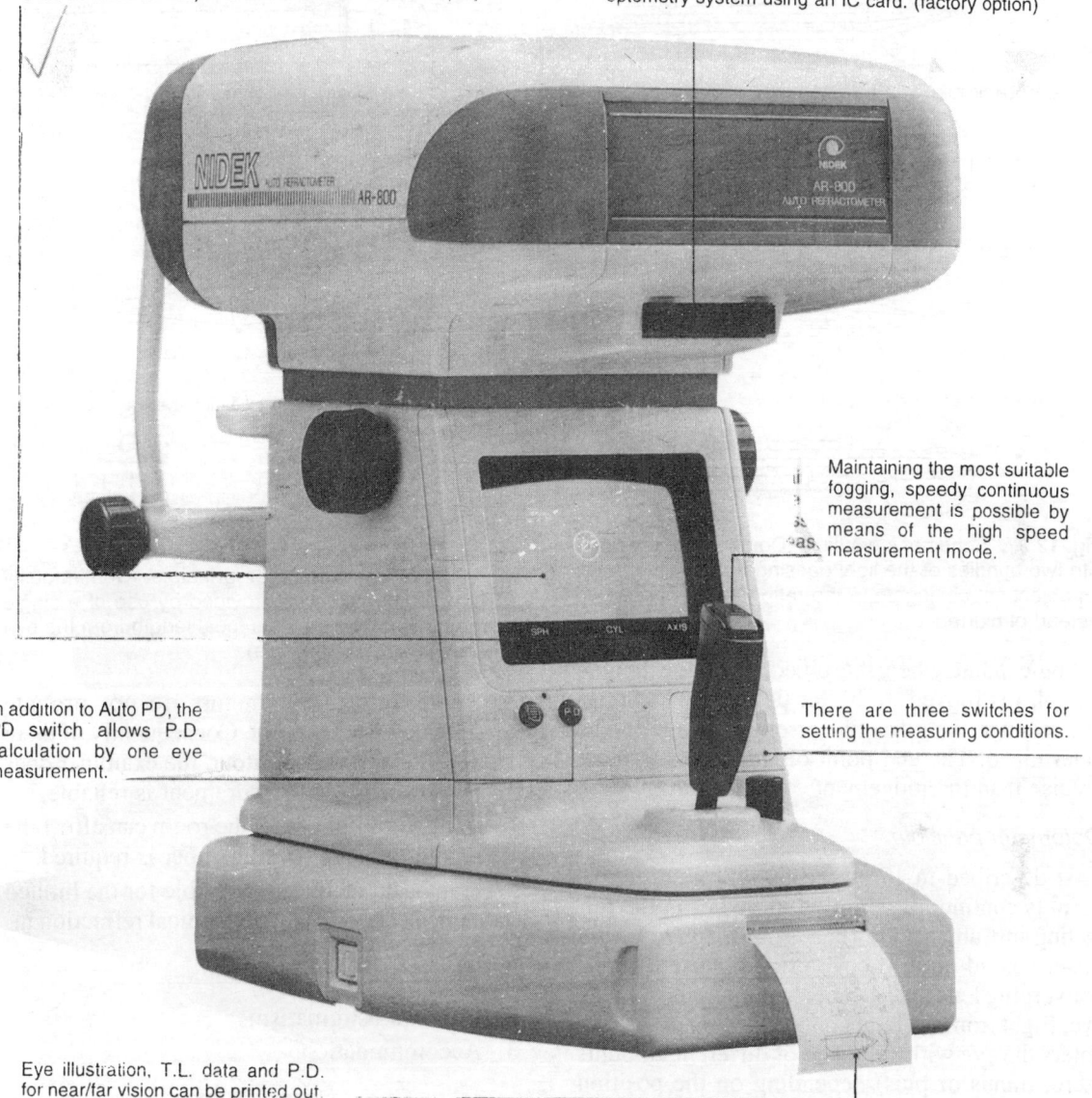

Maintaining the most suitable fogging, speedy continuous measurement is possible by means of the high speed measurement mode.

In addition to Auto PD, the PD switch allows P.D. calculation by one eye measurement.

There are three switches for setting the measuring conditions.

Eye illustration, T.L. data and P.D. for near/far vision can be printed out.

**Fig. 12.26.** Automated refractometer.

Most of the automated refractors utilise infrared light source. The measurement depends on :

1. Scheiner's double pinhole method; or
2. retinoscopic illumination system; or
3. a grating principle.

### Principles

#### Scheiner's principle

In 1619, Scheiner discovered that the point at which an eye is focused could be precisely determined by placing double pinhole apertures before the pupil (Fig. 12.27). The two pinhole apertures limit the rays of light to two small bundles. If the eye is myopic, the ray bundles cross each other before focusing on the retina and two small spots of light are seen. In a hypermetropic eye, however, the ray bundles are interrupted by the retina before they meet and again two small spots of light are seen. The two points of light coalesce to

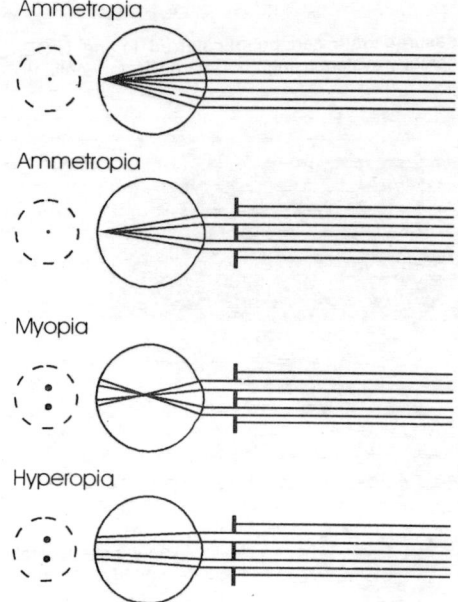

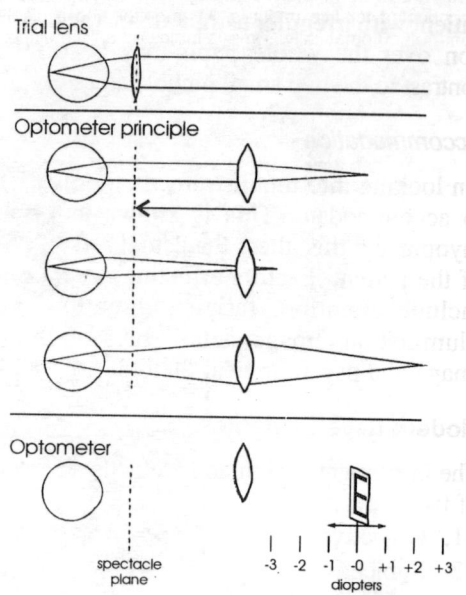

**Fig. 12.27.** Scheiner's principle. Double apertures isolate two bundles of the light passing through the pupil. An object not conjugate to the retina appears doubled instead of blurred.

**Fig. 12.28.** The optometer principle. Continuously variable dioptric power is provided by use of a single converging lens placed at its focal length from the eye (or from the spectacle plane).

a single point when the object (i.e., the double pinhole) is moved to the far point of the eye. In this manner, the refractive error of the eye can be determined. The end point of singleness is more precise than the judgement of least blur.

### Optometer principle

First described in 1759, the optometer principle permits continuous variation of power in the refracting instrumentation (Fig. 12.28). Autorefractometers based on the above principle use a single converging lens placed at its focal length from the eye. Light from the target on the far side of the lens enters the eye with vergence of different amounts (zero, minus or plus) depending on the position of the target. The vergence of the light in the focal plane of the optometer lens is linearly related to the displacement of the target. A scale with equal spacings can thus be made which would show the numbers of dioptres of correction.

### Limitations of autorefractometers

1. The individual patient can accommodate to the instrument.
2. Reflection over the patient's current glasses can occur.

3. Some autorefractometers do not provide vision as an end point. Consequently, if there is an error in the printout, the examiner does not know if the measurement is reliable.
4. Peripheral light from the room can affect the reading; thus a dark chamber is required.

Three basic factors responsible for the limited acceptance of optometers in clinical refraction include :
1. Alignment problem
2. Irregular astigmatism
3. Accommodation

### Alignment problem

As per the requirement of Scheiner's principle, both pinhole apertures must fit within the patient's pupil. If the patient's fixation wanders or he moves his head even slightly, the reading is invalid. Thus, considerable patient cooperation is required.

### Irregular astigmatism

Two small apertures of the eyes' entire optical system are used by the Scheiner's system. In a patient with irregular astigmatism, the best refraction over the whole pupil may be different in contrast to the two small pinhole areas of the pupil.

## Accommodation

On looking into the instrument, the patient tends to accommodate. This is known as instrument myopia and this alters the actual refractive status of the patient. Factors affecting accommodation include attention, fatigue, direction of gaze, illumination, image detail, blur of the retinal image and psychological factors.

## Modern developments

The instrument design and methods are essentially of two types:
  1. Objective
  2. Subjective

### Objective instrument design and methods

The patient's whole pupil is used in this system thus avoiding some of the alignment and partly the irregular astigmatism problems. The operator focuses a single spot of light on the patient's retina and measures the astigmatism by successively focusing the two focal lines. In order to control accommodation, the eye not being refracted is fogged by a trial lens through which the patient fixates at a distant target.

### Automated infrared optometers

The refraction is performed automatically by using infrared light which is invisible to the patient. A visible fixation light is provided in each instrument in order to control the patient's fixation and accommodation.

### Photographic methods

Two photographic methods are available for picture refraction. The advantage of these methods is the very short time required for taking a measurement, i.e., the time required by a single flash exposure.

The method introduced by Howland and Howland uses a special camera lens to photograph the retinoscopic image of a point source of light. The degree of ametropia is estimated by measuring the amount of blur of the photo-graphed image. However, this technique is basically useful in screening and only helps in estimating the gross refraction.

The second method, introduced by Grolman (Fig. 12.29), is more accurate than the first and uses an array of point sources of light spaced at varying dioptric distances from the patient's eye and flashed simultaneously. One end of a separate fibreoptic bundle is conjugate to each point source and receives the image point source as reflected from the patient's fundus. The images received by all fibreoptic bundles are recorded in a common plane on a strip of photographic film. The refractive error is judged by identifying the two sharpest ellipses and their orientation on the film.

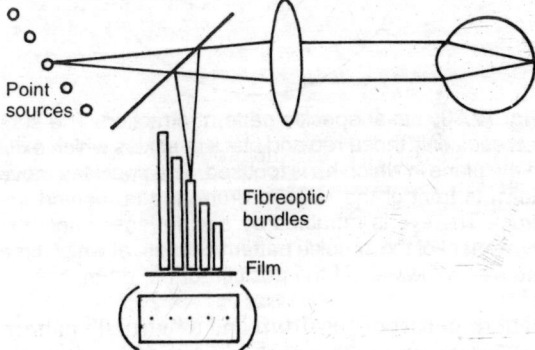

**Fig. 12.29.** Grolman photographic system for objective refraction.

### Electrophysiological methods

This uses the visually evoked response for estimating automated clinical refraction. An advantage of this method is that it tests the entire visual system, from the cornea to the visual cortex. Spherical correction to the nearest 0.25 dioptres is relatively easy to obtain. However, it does not measure the astigmatism very effectively.

### Subjective instrument design and methods

A variety of subjective instrument designs and methods are available and are explained below.

### Laser speckle pattern refraction (Fig. 12.30)

The beam of light from a continuous wave gas laser is diverged with lenses onto the surface of a slowly moving drum. The reflected laser light sets up a random interference pattern, a "real"

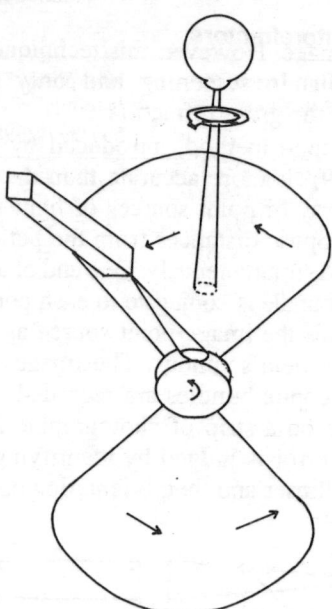

**Fig. 12.30.** Laser speckle pattern refraction. The subject sees only those red and black speckles which exist in the plane in which he is focused. The speckles move down in front of the rotating drum and up behind the drum. The eye is refracted by adding lenses until the movement of the speckle pattern ceases, at which time the eye is focused at the position of the drum.

pattern in part of the drum and a "virtual" pattern behind the drum. The surface of the drum appears to be covered with red and black speckles to the patient. The speckles appear to move in one direction or the other, depending on whether the patient is myopic or hyperopic with respect to the position of the drum. Various meridians may be refracted by introducing lenses before the patient's eye until the movement of the speckle pattern ceases. A given meridian is easily refracted with a precision of ±0.25 D. However, an effective method for locating a cylinder axis has not been devised.

### Meridional refractometry

By measuring the spherical correction for three arbitrary meridians, complete refractive correction can be determined by mathematical calculation.

Meridional refractometry is best suited for objective instruments which can refract multiple meridians either very quickly or simultaneously. A higher accuracy is obtained by refracting four or six arbitrary meridians instead of three. However, sophisticated calculations are required for the four or six meridian approach.

### Computer actuated refraction

A computerised system to perform subjective refraction using conventional refraction optics and conventional refracting techniques is used. The binocular refractor consists of a full range of trial lenses and accessory optical devices for each eye. The spherical and cylinder lenses, cross cylinders, prisms and Maddox rods, filters and pinhole apertures are arranged in four disks within each half of refraction. The disks are driven by stepping motors in response to commands from the computer. A variety of slides for visual acuity and refraction, both for distance and near, are presented using random-access slide projectors. The patient responds with a single push-button box held in the lap as the computer follows a series of flowcharts to arrive at the refractive correction and corrected visual acuity.

### Instruments having continuously variable spherocylindric power

Various cross cylinders in combination with a pair of standard spherical optometers have been used. However, continuous variability of this instrument is not a significant advantage over conventional refractors.

### Comparison of subjective and objective instruments

The comparison of subjective and objective instruments has been summarized in Tables 12.3 and 12.4.

### 1. Infrared vs. visible light

The objective refractors use low levels of invisible infrared light, the advantage being the absence of any visual lines from the measurement procedure which could stimulate accommodation. However, a refractive difference is generally seen between the infrared refraction obtained by the instrument and the visible light refraction that is desired. The refractive difference can be attributed to the chromatic aberration of the eye and the fact that infrared light is reflected not from the photoreceptors but from a different layer of retina. The difference in refraction is substantial, being 0.75 to 1.5 D and has individual variation. The calibration of the instrument for the measurement of the zero error of the objective refractors must be based on empirical data which

**Table 12.3. Comparison of different commercially available autorefractors**

| | Cannon | Nidek | Shin-Nippon (SR 7000) | Humphrey (Models 597/597k/598/599) |
|---|---|---|---|---|
| 1. Vertex distance | 0/12/13.5 mm | 12 mm, 13.75 mm | 0, 12, 13.5, 15, 16.5 (1.5 mm steps) | 0 and 10.5-16.5 mm in 1.5 mm steps |
| 2. Measurable range | | | | |
|   Sphere | −20 to +20 D | −18 to +23 D | −22 to +22 D | +20 D to −17 D |
|   Cylinder | 0 ± 10 D | 0 ± 8 D | 0 ± 10 D | ± 7 D |
|   Axis | 1 to 180° | 0 to 180° | 1 to 180° | 0 to 180° |
|   Pupil distance | Max. 85 mm (increment 1 mm) | Max. 85 mm (increment 1 mm) | 30 to 90 mm | — |
|   Cylinder sign | −, +, +/− | −, +, +/− | −, +, +/− | |
| 3. Steps | | | | |
|   Sphere | 0.12 or 0.25 | 0.25, 0.12, 0.01 D | 0.12 or 0.25 | 0.12, 0.25 D |
|   Cylinder | 0.12 or 0.25 | 0.25, 0.12, 0.01 D | 0.12 or 0.25 | 0.12, 0.25 |
|   Axis | 1° | 1° | 1° | 1° |
| 4. Cylinder sign | −, + or ± | −, + or ± | −, + or ± | −, + or ± |
| 5. Measuring time | — | 0.3 sec. | 0.15 sec. | — |
| 6. Minimum pupil diameter | 2.5 mm | 2.9 mm | 2.9 mm | 2.9 mm |
| 7. Display | 5″ TV monitor | LED digital display | 5″ TV monitor | 5″ CRT |
| 8. Dimensions (in mm) | 300 × 525 × 996 | 260 × 475 × 440 | 310 × 505 × 487 | 457 × 305 × 406 |
| 9. Weight | 19 kg | 18 kg | 20 kg | 22.6 kg |
| 10. IOL implanted eye measurement | Possible | Possible | Possible | — |
| 11. Power saving function | Power for monitor, lamp and motor turns off where operating is interrupted for approx. 5 min. | Present | Works if device is unused for 10 mins. | — |
| 12. Power supply | | | | |
|   Voltage | 110/120 V, 220/240 V, 230 V | 100/120 V, 200-220/230-240 VAC | 100-240 V | — |
|   Frequency | 50/60 Hz | 50/60 Hz | 50/60 Hz | 90-265 VAC |
|   Consumption | 70 VA | 80 VA | 45 VA | — |
| 13. Data output | RS-232C provided; connectable to personal computer plotter, auto-phoropter | RS-232C interface | RS-232C interface video terminal | RS-232C and video |
| 14. Print | Thermal line printer; prints measurement, date, time, serial No., eye diagram | Date, time, patient's number, objective measurement values, far PD, near PD, eye illustrations | Thermal printer (up to 10 measurements of each eye can be recorded and printed out) | — |
| 15. Standard accessories | R-30 main unit, power supply cable, chin rest paper (100), printing paper (2 rolls), dust cover and blower brush | Spare fuses (2), spare printer paper (3), chin rest paper (1), power supply cord (1), dust cover (1) | Schematic eye (1), power cable (1), paper roll (2), spare fuse (2), dust cloth (1), chin rest paper (100), frame for PD measurement (1) | — |

**Table 12.4. Comparison of subjective and objective autorefractors**

|  | Objective | Subjective |
|---|---|---|
| 1. Source of light | Infrared light | Visible light |
| 2. Time required for measurement | 2-5 min. | 5-10 min. |
| 3. Patient cooperation | Less | More |
| 4. Ocular factors |  |  |
| (a) Macular disease with clear media | Better |  |
| (b) Hazy media (equivalent to 6/18) | Comparable | Comparable |
| (c) Hazy media (equivalent to > 6/18) |  | Better |
| Examples | 1. Safir ophthalmetron<br>2. 6600 autorefractor<br>3. Dioptron | 1. Vision analyzer<br>2. SR III subjective refraction system |

correlates the objective findings with the clinical results obtained by the conventional methods.

### 2. Time required for measurement

The actual measurement time required with the objective refractors is within seconds; the greatest portion of time required for refraction is spent in positioning and instructing the patient. It is usually complete in 2 to 5 minutes. The subjective refractors require about 5-10 minutes; nevertheless they provide more information.

### 3. Patient cooperation

Less cooperation is required for measurement of refractive errors by objective refractors as compared to subjective refractors. In objective refraction, the patient stays still and looks straight ahead at a target during the automatic refracting procedure. However, the subjective refractors require the patient to turn the knobs to focus various targets.

### 4. Ocular factors

In the presence of macular disease with clear media, objective refractors give better results. With hazy media, the performance of objective and subjective instruments is comparable up to a media haze equivalent to 6/18 visual acuity. With a greater media haze, the objective instruments usually do not function properly, but only rough estimations can be made even with subjective instruments.

### Accuracy of measurement

The accuracy of automated refractors is related to how closely the instrument measures the true refractive status. Subjective refinement with the Jackson cross cylinder is usually considered to be the most accurate method of refraction. However, many artifacts are present in the cross cylinder technique. Distorting effects of cross cylinder are present with letter charts, such that the patients tend to prefer taller rather than flatter letters, thereby causing erroneous testing. These artifacts with letter charts not only produce power errors but also axis errors. Visual acuity is also not a true measure of refractive status, as several different refractive corrections give equal visual acuity but different levels of ocular discomfort. Thus, no reliable standard for measure of true refractive correction exists. Certain amount of variability is therefore expected when comparing the results of automated refractors with those of conventional clinical techniques of refraction.

Several clinical trials have been reported for objective refractors, whereas the subjective refractors have not been properly evaluated. Objective refraction produces refractions which are equivalent to those from good retinoscopies, i.e., retinoscopies with cooperative patients having adequate pupils and clear media. When compared with subjective refractions, one can expect an agreement of ±0.25 D sphere, ±0.25 D cylinder and ±5° axis (for cylinder powers > 0.50 D) in approximately 2/3rd of the eyes.

# CHAPTER 13

# Subjective Examination

In subjective examination the refractive status of the eye is determined by obtaining response from patient to a change in the power of lenses. This method of examination determines the combination of lenses which appears to give the patient maximum visual acuity. In this method the correct estimation of astigmatism is actually very difficult. Even the precise determination of sphere is, more often than not, troublesome. The accommodative effort which cannot be relaxed may not only give an erroneous impression about the spherical correction but also astigmatism may also be concealed. It may be worth mentioning that many refractionists still are under the impression that asthenopia in many refractive errors is due to an excessive use of accommodation particularly so in hypermetropia. This concept is not entirely true. Accommodation effort may produce asthenopia but it is neither necessary, nor desirable nor even always possible to totally relax accommodation. Generally speaking, the basic guiding principle should be to prescribe the strongest plus lens or the weakest minus lens which the patient accepts to achieve maximum possible acuity of vision. The tendency to load the patient with plus lenses may in itself introduce new sources of asthenopia not previously implicated. Similarly, loading patients with minus lenses may precipitate asthenopia due to accommodation which the patient was not experiencing before the use of these glasses. Generally speaking, the smaller the circle of least confusion, the sharper the visual acuity.

The greatest problem in subjective assessment of refractive errors is the indeterminate factor of accommodation.

Several methods are used but they are usually not reliable. They are :

## 1. Under cycloplegia

The method offers no advantage over the method of retinoscopy and acceptance under cycloplegia and post-mydriatic test. As in the objective method this subjective technique is employed to inactivate accommodation which is the biggest hurdle in the precise measurement of both the spherical and astigmatic correction. The disadvantage of more than one visit is not eliminated. The method, at best, can be described as a trial and error method because unlike in retinoscopy the examiner has no starting point for the focus of the retina may be at infinity (emmetropia), in front of the retina (myopia) or behind the retina (hypermetropia). Similarly in an astigmatic eye both the foci may be in front or both behind or one in front and the other behind the retina.

## 2. Fogging technique

It is most perfect non-cycloplegic control of accommodation. The method makes an attempt to induce relaxation of accommodation by artificially producing myopia or leaving residual myopia and blurring the distant vision with a high convex lens. As in true myopia accommodative effort cannot correct myopia, the same is relaxed. This technique is constant for assessing acceptance under cycloplegia, post-mydriatic prescription or for non-cycloplegic routine. In this method a plus lens stronger than the maximum correction of either meridian in hypermetropia or minus lens weaker than the minimum correction in myopia is put in the frame in front of the eye to be examined. Gradually minus lenses are added till the vision becomes distinct thus revealing the correct number. In this method a minus cylinder is always employed which is arrived at by the interpretation of astigmatic charts (vide infra). It has the advantage of proceeding in an orderly fashion from one step to the next despite the nature of the refractive error. Though this method is not accurate yet it is a good procedure for determining the refractive error under reasonable and habitual physiological circumstances. It does give a correction within tolerable limits of wearability and of correcting all but the most resistant accommodation effort. The method is recommended for acceptance under cycloplegia, post-mydriatic test and where objective assessment by retinoscopy under cycloplegia is not possible due to circumstances beyond one's control.

### 3. Astigmatic fan

Amongst the various charts available for the subjective determination of astigmatic error astigmatic fan is perhaps the most useful (Fig. 13.1). Similar devices used in the literature are fixed clock or sunburst dials, movable or rotating dials.

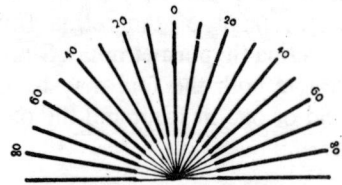

**Fig. 13.1.** Astigmatic fan.

On looking at an astigmatic fan if the vertical lines are clear the diffusion ellipses on the retina are vertical indicating that the horizontal meridian is emmetropic. This will mean that the subjective testing should be performed with the cylinder in horizontal axis, the axis in which the cylinder should be placed one after another till the lines are equally distinct. Similar effects can be seen by rotating the stenopaic disc with a slit in front of the eye.

### 4. Technique of binocular fogging with the use of astigmatic fan

The technique is conducted in stages, one monocular and one binocular and in each eye the cylindrical power and axis is determined first and then the spherical power. The binocular test consists in finding out a balanced prescription for achieving the best visual acuity.

The proper amount of fog is determined by placing a lens before the eye so that both principal meridians become myopic, the vision will become blurred and the power of accommodation will be relaxed. As the power of the lens is reduced, the meridian closest to the retina will begin to approximate the retina, and some lines on the astigmatic fan will become visible and successively more dominant. At a certain point these lines will focus on the retina and the other will focus in front of it by the interval of Sturm and will provide the point of greater contrast. By placing further lenses the focus of this meridian is disturbed and subsequently when the other meridian is fully in focus after covering the interval of Sturm, the previous meridian will be focused behind the retina, and once again a contrast will be obtained. In this situation there is always a possibility of the accommodation becoming active and producing inaccurate results. The optimum position for measuring the astigmatism would be at the first point of greater contrast. Some observers, however, feel that the proper step at which fogging procedure should be stopped is at a point short of exercising the accommodation, yet close enough to the visibility of the clear lines, to provide critical contrast.

The next step is to determine the axis of the cylinder. The patient is asked to point out the blackest or a group of blackest lines. The blackest line or the centre of the group of blackest lines represents the axis of the plus cylinder or the axis of minus cylinder which lies 90° from the meridian of this line. On this meridian, the movable V of the fan is shifted and the patient is asked to state if the two limbs of the V are equally black. If it is so the determined axis is correct.

Once the principal meridians have been determined and the axis of the correcting cylinder preferably minus cylinders is located, the correction consists simply of increasing the cylinder until the contrasted lines become equally black. In this as in the correction of sphere the weakest minus cylinder making the contrasting black lines appear equally black should be chosen. Another important method of determining the end point is to ask the patient whether all the lines of the astigmatic fan are equally black. If the lines of the principal meridians are blacker than the lines of meridians in between, it gives an information that the astigmatism is irregular.

Once the astigmatism has been adequately corrected by the minus cylinder, further testing should be done on Snellen's letter chart. Plus lenses are placed in front of the eye till the vision is less than 6/18. The fog is slowly reduced till 6/18 line is clearly read. The power of the lens achieving this is noted. Further reduction in power of lens improves the acuity till the best possible line can be read with the maximum plus lens or weakest minus lens. A reduction in power of lens in fogging method means an increase in the dioptric power of minus lenses or a decrease in the dioptric power of plus lenses.

### Duochrome test

The test is based on the principles of chromatic aberration. It is usually seen that the patient chooses yellow as the criterion for normal vision and that variations in refraction should be judged from the standpoint of the relative focus of colours other than yellow; the blue being myopic and the red end hypermetropic.

The test (Fig. 13.2) consists of opaque letters graded from Snellen's 18 to 5 which are placed before each of the box one half of which is covered by red and the other half by green. In emmetropia the two appear equally clear or equally blurred. When a hypermetrope sees the chart the green letters are more distinct than the red while to a myopic the red letters are more distinct than the green.

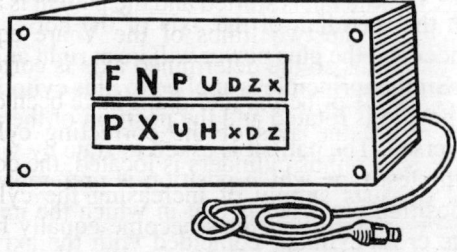

**Fig. 13.2.** Duochrome test.

In the fogging method the patient is requested to compare the two charts to determine whether the letters are clearer in one or the other colour. With the maximum fog the red colours seem

better. The plus power is consequently reduced until the two charts appear equal or makes the green chart just better. With further reduction of the power the green becomes brighter and brighter.

This method was originally devised to check the spherical refraction but it has a much wider application now and it is being employed in conjunction with the usual routines of refraction as a check upon the subjective response. The results should be, however, cautiously interpreted and the test carefully performed to ensure that accommodation does not lead to transference of the focus for the green to the red and vice versa.

### Cross cylinder of Jackson (Fig. 13.3)

The cross cylinder is essentially a mixed cylinder in which the spheric component is one half of the power of the cylinder component with axes at right angles. With its use the cylindrical correction can be altered at the same time as the spherical correction is proportionately changed in the opposite sense. It is carried on a handle set at an angle of 45° from the axes of the cylinders so that when it is held before the combination in the trial frame and rapidly rotated around the axis of the handle the cylinder is changed from one direction to the other at right angles.

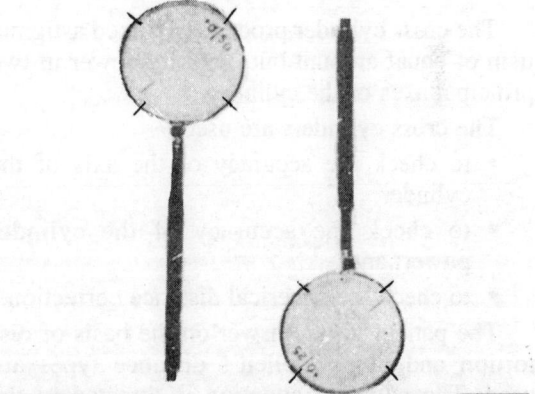

**Fig. 13.3.** Jackson's cross cylinder.

Suppose in the trial frame we have +1 D sph. with +1.25 D cyl. axis 120° and by subjective test it is discovered that the vision can be improved with putting a –0.50 D cyl. at an axis of 30°. This means that we are actually correcting the vision with +0.50 D sph. with +1.75 D cyl. at an axis of 120°

Now take another situation where the vision improves by adding +0.50 D cyl. at an axis of 30°. This means that we are actually correcting the vision with +1.50 D sph. with +0.75 D cyl. at an axis of 120°.

A combination of –0.25 D sphere with +0.50 D cyl. actually means that the cross cylinder has the following dioptric strengths. –0.50 D cyl. in one axis and +0.25 D cyl. in another axis at right angles to the first axis. Similarly a combination of –0.50 D cyl. in one axis and +0.50 D cyl. in an axis at right angles to the first axis.

Let us mathematically depict this.

$$\frac{-0.25 \text{ D sph.}}{+0.50 \text{ D cyl.} \rightarrow 180°}$$

$$= \frac{-0.25 \text{ D cyl. axis } 180° \quad -0.25 \text{ D cyl. axis } 90°}{+0.50 \text{ D cyl. axis } 180°}$$

$$= \frac{-0.25 \text{ D cyl. axis } 90°}{+0.25 \text{ D cyl. axis } 180°}$$

A combination of –0.25 D sph. with +0.50 D cyl. is commonly used. Another combination in common use is –0.50 D sph. with +1.00 D cyl. The axis of the plus power is indicated by white dots or white lines and the minus power by red dots or red lines.

The cross cylinder produces a mixed astigmatism of equal amount but opposite power in two principal axes of the cylinder.

The cross cylinders are used
- to check the accuracy of the axis of the cylinder;
- to check the accuracy of the cylinder power; and
- to check the spherical distance correction.

The patient gives answer on the basis of distortion and blur. Snellen's distance types are used. The patient's attention is directed to the letters on two lines above the line of best visual acuity with corrections.

### Checking the accuracy of the axis

The principle of oblique cylinders is usefully employed to check the axis by the crossed cylinders. Usually a combination of +0.50 and –1.00 is used.

The proposed cylinder is placed in the trial frame in front of the eye to be tested at an axis which the examiner feels is the correct axis. The above combination of the cross cylinder is held before the trial frame alternatively so that each axis lies at 45° to the major and minor cylindrical axis. The cross cylinder is, therefore, held in front of the trial frame with its handle in the axis of the cylinder in the trial frame, testing first with one face and then twirling it through 180° to evaluate the second position. Visual improvement is then noted in one or the other axis, the correcting cylinder is turned slightly in the direction of the cylinder of the same sign (+ or –) in the cross cylinder. The process is repeated till the position of the trial cylinder is such that in either position of the cross cylinder there is no alteration in distinctness. It is always better to focus the attention of the patient to a letter on the Snellen's chart at two lines above the lines which he reads distinctly with the correcting lens in the trial frame.

### Checking the accuracy of the cylindrical power

The power of the lens can be checked quite easily provided the axis has been located correctly. The handle of the cross cylinder is shifted 45° from the located axis so that the cross cylinder now lies in a manner that one axis is in the axis of the cylinder in the frame and the other axis is perpendicular to the axis of the cylinder. In case of minus cylinder, minus of the cross cylinder will be in the meridian of the axis of the correcting cylinder and the plus power will lie at right angles to it. Similar principle is applied to plus cylinders. The handle is rotated and the position of the axis is reversed. The patient is asked to state by viewing the test type which position is preferable. If the position preferred is that in which the minus of the cross cylinder coincided with the axis of the minus cylinder or the plus of the cross cylinder coincided with the axis of the plus cylinder the power of the cylinder is increased and the test repeated. If the preferable position is the opposite, then the power is reduced. If none of the positions is preferable, i.e., are equally good, or are equally bad, the power of the correcting cylinder is accurate

### Checking the accuracy of the distance spherical correction

The patient is seated before the astigmatic fan and wears on the trial frame the final prescription. Now the cross cylinder is placed with the axis of the plus cylinder at 90° if the correction is plus sphere but if the correction is minus sphere the minus of the cross cylinder is placed at 90°. The patient is fogged, the plus sphere is reduced and the patient is asked at each step as to which lines on the fan appear clearer than other. If the vertical lines appear darker before the horizontal the plus power is reduced until the lines appear equally bright. If the horizontal lines appear darker, additional plus power is required. In this technique an assumption has been made that the astigmatism has been completely and properly corrected.

## MALINGERING

It attempts to mislead wilfully with regard to the existence or the seriousness or the origin of a disease or disability in order to gain desired end. There are several types of malingering :

- *Simulation* which is the feigning of a non-existent disease or disability.
- *Exaggeration or aggravation* which is the pretence that a condition is worse than it is.
- *False attribution* which is the assignment to a disease or injury due to a cause which is not real.
- *Dissimulation* which is a pretence that

though it actually is present, a disease or injury does not exist.

### Tests for malingering

A large number of tests are employed for the detection of malingering.

### *Tests for functional and simulated defects*

*These tests are to assess*

- *Pupillary reflexes :* Presence of both direct and consensual light reflex.
- *Menace reflex :* When an object is suddenly approximated and not gradually, there is a reflex closure of lids.
- *Attitude of patient :* He avoids all obstacles while approaching the observer.
- *Objective fixation test :* By covering one eye and allowing the patient to fix with the other. In this a 6 Δ prism is suddenly inserted and the patient on uncovering the covered eye fixes to avoid diplopia even momentarily.
- *Opticokinetic nystagmus.*

### *Tests for simulation of binocular blindness*

- *Diplopia test :* The tests aim at producing diplopia by prisms. The suspected eye is covered and diplopia elicited in the good eye by bisecting the pupil with the base or preferably the edge of a strong prism. The suspected eye is then quickly uncovered and simultaneously the prism slipped over the whole pupil of the other. If diplopia still exists it is a case of malingering.

There are so many other tests for malingering.

# SECTION IV

# Errors of Refraction

# CHAPTER 14

# Errors of Refraction

## General consideration

In normal individuals, parallel rays meeting the eye are focused on the retina to form a circle of least diffusion. Such a state of refraction is termed as emmetropia. The far point is at infinity. If in a state of rest of the eye the parallel rays are not focused on the retina and do not form a circle of least diffusion, the eye is said to be in an ametropic state. The normal refractive power of an emmetropic eye is about +60 D.

If the rays are brought to a focus behind the retina the error is hypermetropic due to lesser refractive power of the eye and if the rays are focused in front of the retina the error is myopic due to more refractive power of the eye. When the rays of light from more than one meridian are brought to a focus at different points, i.e., the refractive system is not concentric and no single focus is formed, the eye is in a state of refraction which is termed astigmatism.

At birth the child is hypermetropic and it is only with gradual growth that the child becomes emmetropic. An emmetropic condition of the eye, though ideal, is hard to attain and is rather rare in the strictest sense. Some degree of astigmatism is not uncommonly seen. The attainment of emmetropic state is dependent upon the exactitude of the length of the eyeball, the curvature of the refracting surfaces, the relative positions of the refracting media, the refractive indices of the media and the position of percipient elements. One or the other or all of them may be altered leading to ametropia. The focus of rays from infinity in different refractive states is shown in Fig. 14.1. Etiology of ametropia may be considered as under. The far point in these refractive errors is shown in Fig. 14.2.

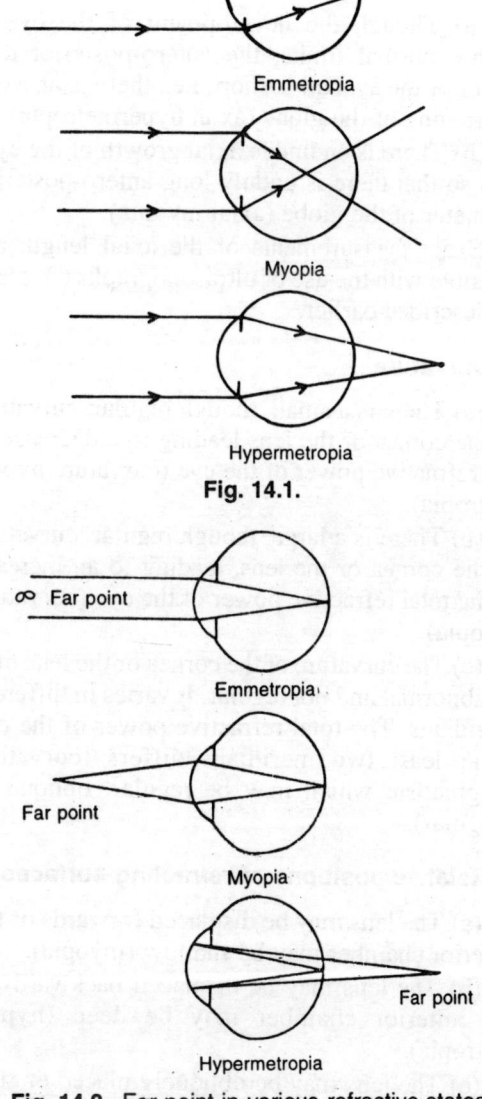

Fig. 14.1.

**Fig. 14.2.** Far point in various refractive states.

### 1. Axial (Fig. 14.3)

In this system the percipient elements are either situated behind or in front of the focus of rays The total refractive power of the eye remains unaltered.

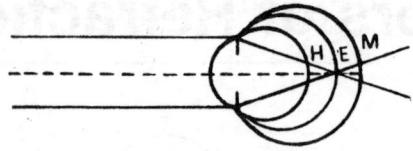

**Fig. 14.3.** Axial length in refractive error.

(a) Though the development of the eye is within normal limits, the antero-posterior diameter of the eyeball is short, i.e., there is an axial shortening of the globe (axial hypermetropia).

(b) There is an undue axial growth of the eyeball so that there is unduly long antero-posterior diameter of the globe (axial myopia).

Exact measurements of the axial length are possible with the use of ultrasonographs (A-scan) as described earlier.

### 2. Curvature

(a) There is a small, though regular, curvature of the cornea or the lens leading to a decrease in the refractive power of the eye (curvature hypermetropia).

(b) There is a large, though regular, curvature of the cornea or the lens, leading to an increase in the total refractive power of the eye (curvature myopia).

(c) The curvature of the cornea or the lens may be abnormal and not regular. It varies in different meridians. The total refractive power of the eye in at least two meridians differs (curvature astigmatism which may be regular, oblique or irregular).

### 3. Relative positions of refracting surfaces

(a) The lens may be displaced forwards or the anterior chamber may be shallow (myopia).

(b) The lens may be displaced backwards or the anterior chamber may be deep (hypermetropia).

(c) The lens may be obliquely placed or subluxated (astigmatism).

(d) The retinal elements may be obliquely placed (astigmatism).

### 4. Index

It is due to anomalies of refractive index of one or more media.

(a) *Aqueous humour :* If the refractive index is too low, hypermetropia results; if the refractive index is too high, myopia results.

(b) *Vitreous :* If refractive index of the vitreous is too high it causes myopia and if it is too low it causes hypermetropia.

(c) *Lens :* If the refractive index of the lens is too low hypermetropia results, if it is too high myopia results. In cortical sclerosis the refractive index of the cortex approximates that of nucleus while in nuclear sclerosis the difference between the two is accentuated so in the former hypermetropia results while in the latter myopia occurs.

### 5. Absence of elements

If the lens is absent (aphakia) there is high hypermetropia.

### Distribution of refractive errors

In a survey done by the National Society for Prevention of Blindness, India, in primary school children, higher secondary students, college students, industrial workers and in urban and rural population it has been found that the prevalence of refractive errors is 22.35%. The distribution of refractive errors is given in Table 14.1.

### Distribution in various ages

At birth the child is hypermetropic up to by +2.0 to +5.0 D. Hypermetropia usually decreases with age though in very small percentage of cases it may show an increase. In about 90% of the cases the refraction ranges between +0.25 and +5.0 dioptres. In about 40% of hypermetropic newborns and 25% of the myopic newborns there is astigmatism.

In pre-school children the hypermetropia present at birth starts to decline till at two to five years of age it is reduced to about +2.0 dioptres in a large majority.

In school children the hypermetropia decrea-

**Table 14.1. Distribution of refractive errors (in percentage) in various groups of population**

|  | Males | Females | Total |
|---|---|---|---|
| Primary school children (5-12 years) | 14.9 | 18.12 | 17.33 |
| Higher secondary school children (13-18 years) | 23.45 | 27.32 | 25.12 |
| University students (19-25 years) | 26.19 | 30.14 | 28.36 |
| Adult population |  |  |  |
| Rural | 16.1 | 18.99 | 17.01 |
| Urban | 23.53 | 28.22 | 25.77 |
| Industrial |  |  | 19.77 |
| Bus drivers |  |  | 25.00 |
| Total | 21.19 | 24.55 | 22.35 |

ses and is about +1.0 D less than that present at birth.

If myopia was present at birth it usually increases with increasing age in school children. Even if the child was hypermetropic at entry to the school he may gradually develop myopia. When compared to the white population where myopia ranges from 25-60% at the age of 21, the percentage of myopia in India seems to be less (27%). When seen over a period of time in this country myopia seems to be showing an increasing trend. There is also a difference in myopia between school-age individuals who are in the rural and urban population and those going to school and not going to school. There is more myopia in girls than in boys which is a trend similar to one seen in other countries. If myopia is associated with increasing demands of near work this is a paradox as the percentage of girls attending school in this country is much lower than that of the boys. If the degree of hypermetropia is between +1.0 D and +1.5 D at school-going age it is likely that the child will become emmetropic. If the child has hypermetropia of less than one dioptre or myopia he is likely to become myopic. If the hypermetropia is more than +1.5 D he is likely to remain hypermetropic.

**Heredity and refractive errors**

Refractive errors are frequently inherited but the exact mechanism of this inheritance is ill-understood. What laws of inheritance the transmission of refractive error obeys need to be elucidated. Due to the multiplicity and variability of factors responsible for producing ametropia, it is not possible to apply simple numerical laws of heredity to refractive errors. As a general rule several principles are clear, i.e.,

1. The refractive states are frequently hereditarily transmitted not only within a family but also in races.

2. That the mode of transmission of lower errors is different from the mode of transmission of higher errors.

3. That along with the higher errors some other ocular pathology like night blindness, nystagmus, microphthalmos, vitreous degeneration, retinal detachment etc. may also be inherited. It is difficult to say that they are through a single gene or different genes. It is also stated that in myopia the inheritance factors are multiple and not always consistent.

4. Environmental factors may modify the genetic influence. The refractive properties of the eye may be considered to be determined more by genetic than by environmental factors and that the refractive state and its components generally follow a pattern set up by a number of genes with additive effects. Since myopia and myopic degeneration is on the increase in India, the possibility of mutation of genes due to environmental factors cannot be ruled out.

**Clinical symptoms**

The most important symptoms of refractive errors are asthenopia and/or diminution of visual acuity.

Asthenopia is defined as uncomfortable, painful and irritable vision. These symptoms include headaches, fatigue, eye strain, photophobia and irritation of eye.

Asthenopia in refractive states is due to their being uncorrected leading to formation of indistinct images, difficult to interpret as in astigmatism and myopia. Sometimes it may be the result of accommodative strain due to an effort to correct the refractive state as in hypermetropia. Eye strain is more common in smaller errors of refraction than in higher errors

In high errors of refraction the most prominent symptom is a failure of vision.

When a refractive error is small the patient is able to rectify it to a greater or lesser extent by muscular effort and this a patient continually does to the best of his ability. The constant strain thus unconsciously imposed upon him brings in muscular and nervous fatigue with its attendant train of reflex symptoms. Most of the time the visual acuity recorded is normal and when the patient is asked to get his refractive state checked or prescribed glasses after a full check up he resents it and usually does not accept it but if he can be persuaded to wear the correction it will frequently bring an equally unexpected and dramatic relief.

Asthenopia, as described earlier, is a symptom complex visual and ocular and under which referred and functional symptoms are complained of.

## Visual symptoms

Visual acuity is not a true guide to the assessment of asthenopia. As already stated above, asthenopia is mainly caused by muscular effort which is able to compensate for the diminution in visual acuity. Asthenopia is essentially due to the effort to compensate for optical and muscular imperfections. The visual symptoms get marked in times of temporary deterioration of general health when a sense of confusion and blurring of vision results.

## Ocular symptoms

These are due to the increased muscular work which the defect invokes and discomfort of the resultant muscular fatigue which may lead to a permanent vascular congestion.

The eyes feel tired and uncomfortable. There is hyperaemia of the conjunctiva. There is mild, dull aching pain but sometimes it may be severe and acute. There may be vague but generalised headache. There is lacrimation. Rubbing of the eyes gives temporary relief. This may lead to congestion and low grade of conjunctivitis. It may also result in repeated styes or chalazia. Chronic irritation may also lead to blepharitis.

On the whole the eyes may characteristically look watery, suffused and bleary.

## Referred symptoms

Mostly refractive errors lead to headaches and vertigo. Headache occurs in almost every possible variety and may be referred to any part in the distribution of the ophthalmic division of the V cranial nerve (trigeminal). It may sometimes have a migrainous characteristic. Usually it is localised around the regions of the eye.

Refractive errors are not usually associated with vertigo or giddiness but sometimes correction of oblique astigmatism may produce vertigo probably due to the difficulty in adjustment to new visual values as a result of this correction.

## Functional symptoms

The optical anomaly may lead to psycho-pathological states, particularly in women. The patients depict abnormal sensitivity to light and they prefer to go about in dark glasses. The patient may become neurotic and treatment of visual conditions may not offer relief. On the contrary treatment of psychological state may result in visual relief as well. In such cases visual relief should always follow and not precede psychological treatment.

# CHAPTER 15

# Hypermetropia

Hypermetropia or hyperopia is the refractive condition of the eye wherein either the total refractive power of the eye or the length of the eyeball is diminished and the rays of light are not focused on the retina but behind it until and unless extra accommodative effort is made. The posterior principal focus of the refractive system of the eye is located posterior to the retinal plane. It may be stated that in hypermetropia the retina is situated in front of the posterior principal focus of the dioptric system of the eye. By the voluntary effort of an individual it is possible to increase the refractive power of the eye and focus the rays on the retina. This voluntary effort of accommodation puts considerable strain on the ciliary muscles of the eye leading to ocular symptoms indicating the presence of this refractive state.

In recent years axial alteration as a cause of refractive errors in a significant number of cases is being doubted. This is particularly so in the case of hypermetropia. Hypermetropia is by far the commonest refractive error.

## Classification

The types of hypermetropia can be classified as follows :

1. *Simple :* It is produced by normal biological variations, i.e., axial and refractive.

2. *Pathological :* It is caused by congenital and acquired elements that are outside the normal variations, i.e., deformational, curvature, index, absence of lens as in aphakia, and displacement of lens, and other elements.

3. *Functional :* It is due to paralysis of accommodation.

In hypermetropia the rays of light are focused on to a point behind the retina (Fig. 15.1) and this can be corrected, if small, by voluntary accommodative effort (Fig. 15.2). Even in high errors some of the refractive error can be corrected in this way but in view of its not being able to relieve the symptoms of failure of vision it is seldom exercised.

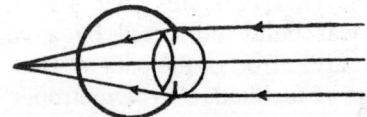

**Fig. 15.1.** Focus of parallel rays in hypermetropia.

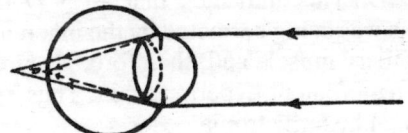

**Fig. 15.2.** Correction of hypermetropia by voluntary effort of accommodation.

The degree of hypermetropia corrected by the patient's accommodative effort is *facultative hypermetropia*. The remaining uncorrected hypermetropia is termed *absolute hypermetropia*. If the voluntary accommodative effort of the patient is abolished, the total degree of hypermetropia after abolition of accommodation is termed *manifest hypermetropia*. As age advances and accommodative effort cannot be sustained hypermetropia becomes absolute till the effort of accommodation fails to correct any hypermetropia or the facultative hypermetropia is abolished and becomes absolute hypermetropia and no difference remains between the absolute and manifest hypermetropia. This means that all manifest hypermetropia becomes absolute hypermetropia with the abolition of the facultative hypermetropia due to gradually weakening and later total failure of the accommodative effort to correct any hypermetropia.

Besides the above some of the hypermetropia is corrected by the inherent tone of the ciliary muscle, which is called *latent hypermetropia*. The degree of latent hypermetropia is high in young individuals but it becomes gradually less in older persons. The latent hypermetropia can be abolished by producing complete cycloplegia. The hypermetropic error estimated under complete cycloplegia is *total hypermetropia*.

Let us illustrate this by an example. If the patient subjectively shows that he has +3 D hypermetropia, it is the value of absolute hypermetropia. The patient continues to see 6/5 up to +5 D hypermetropia by relaxing his accommodative effort. This indicates that +2 D hypermetropia was being corrected by a voluntary accommodative effort of the patient. Hence +2 D is the value of facultative hypermetropia and +5 D represents manifest hypermetropia. Now under full cycloplegia the hypermetropic error detected is +6.5 D. This indicates that +1.5 D hypermetropia was being corrected by the inherent tone of the ciliary muscle and, therefore, it represents the degree of latent hypermetropia. Thus +6.5 D is the total hypermetropia.

(a) Absolute hypermetropia    +3 D

(b) Facultative hypermetropia    +2 D (i.e., corrected by voluntary effort of accommodation)

(c) Manifest hypermetropia    +5 D (a + b)

(d) Latent hypermetropia    +1.5 D (i.e., corrected by the tone of ciliary muscle)

(e) Total hypermetropia    +6.5 D (c + d)

The accommodative effort can be measured by the fogging method or dynamic retinoscopy. It is unusual to find a hypermetropic who does not show an increase in ciliary tone over the normal ciliary tone.

In simple hypermetropia as stated above :

- The globe may be shortened to the extent that it is too short for the rays to be focused onto the retina in spite of the fact that the total refractive power of the eye is the same

as of normal eye. The axial hypermetropia may be considered to be an error of under-development of the eye.

- The refractive simple hypermetropia is defined as the condition in which the refractive system of the eye is too weak for the anterior-posterior length of the eye. This may be due to changes in the

  - Refractive indices wherein the refractive index of lens cortex or vitreous is too high or that of aqueous, lens nucleus or cornea is too low.

  - Changes in curvature of cornea or lens is unduly low due to flattening of surfaces.

  - Decrease is depth of anterior chamber also leads to hypermetropia.

The pathological hypermetropia may be due to :

- deformational changes in the globe (microphthalmos, retinal oedema, tumours, etc.); or

- changes in curvature as in cornea plana; or

- changes in the refractive index of various media because of metabolic changes; or

- absence of lens as in aphakia; or

- anterior displacement of lens.

As is the case with other refractive errors, a dominant inheritance is the cause of simple hypermetropic errors. The dominance may be irregular.

Hypermetropia is physiological in very young children and shows variations with age. At birth the child has +2 D to +5 D hypermetropia which diminishes as the age progresses until after puberty the refraction becomes normal and remains stationary. In old age a further tendency to hypermetropia is evident. At this stage the hypermetropia is mainly of index type and some of it is also due to curvature changes in lenticular fibres. As the lens grows with age newer and newer fibres laid down at this stage are less curved.

In old age, in hypermetropes more and more hypermetropia becomes absolute. Both facultative and latent hypermetropia become less and less. The diminution in facultative hypermetropia is due to inability to sustain a voluntary effort of accommodation and the diminution in latent

**PLATE I**

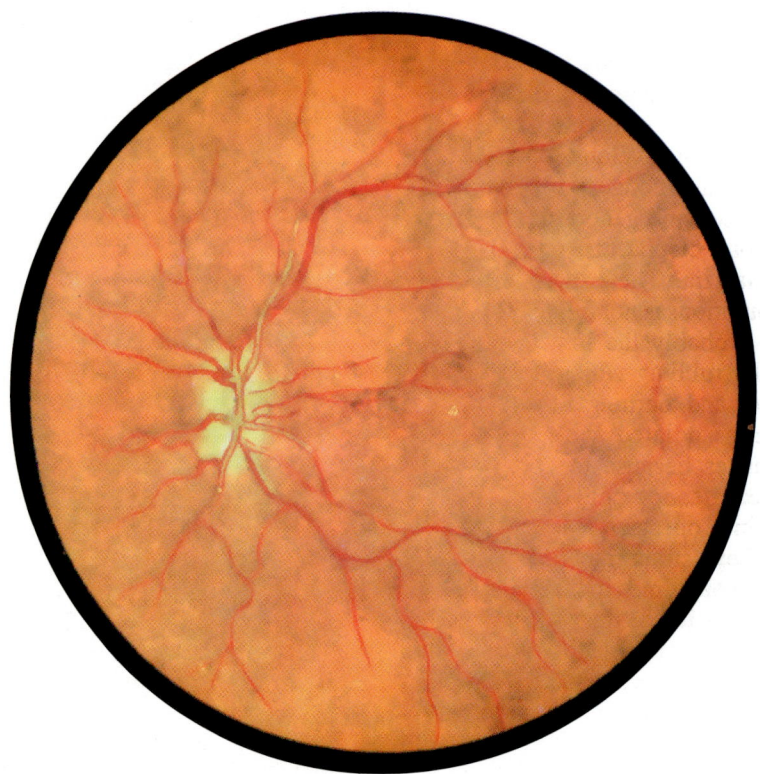

**Fig. 15.3.** Pseudoneuritis in hypermetropia.

hypermetropia is due to a decrease in the inherent tone of ciliary muscle. A point may be reached when all hypermetropia becomes absolute.

**Clinical considerations :** The symptoms vary over a wide range. The patient can correct, in young age, a low and moderate hypermetropic error by sustained effort of accommodation and symptoms of visual failure may be totally absent except when this effort breaks down as in bad general health or periods of general stress, visual acuity falls and patient complains of dim vision. Due to sustained accommodative effort asthenopia occurs. There is a state of ocular stress leading to vague headaches especially frontal or frontotemporal in location. Sometimes the headache may be occipital. It may sometimes show migrainous tendencies or even develop cephalgia. There is tearing, smarting and congestion. There is also photophobia, nausea and general fatigue. It may lead to squamous blepharitis, recurrent styes and recurrent chalazia. The exact causal relationship of these conditions is not fully known and is ill-understood. Probably the infection is introduced in the eye by rubbing which is often done to relieve itching and burning sensation. Most complaints are associated with visual demands at near distances because the accommodation must compensate not only for focal demands of near point, but also for hypermetropia. Symptoms of eye strain may be absent if near work is avoided. Sometimes in these cases the visual acuity is better without than with correcting glasses as the patient is unable to relax the accommodative effort he has so got used to. It is not uncommon to find some young children with low hypermetropia presenting themselves as a case of myopia. In these cases the compensating accommodative effort overshoots the mark. The child then holds objects nearer than usual.

The symptoms increase towards the evening. The patient after some continuous work likes to close his eyes for a few minutes and palm them before starting again.

Usually a hypermetrope can make himself comfortable for near vision by holding the object as far away as possible. When the degree of error is very high the object may be held by the patient quite near the eyes and this may give a deceptive idea of myopia. He keeps the objects near so that the image formed on the retina is large and he is able to see the objects.

Hypermetropia, especially in children, may be associated with convergent strabismus which may be due to an alteration in AC/A ratio (accommodation convergence/accommodation ratio).

In high hypermetropia the eye is small, the chamber is shallow, the angle of the anterior chamber is narrow and the cornea is small. Due to a regular increase in the size of lens, with age, these eyes become prone to an attack of angle closure glaucoma. This point should be borne in mind while instilling mydriatics.

The fundus may be normal or may show a peculiar sheen causing a reflex effect called shot silk appearance. It may show a characteristic appearance which may resemble optic neuritis or papilloedema (Fig. 15.3) which bears no relationship to the degree of hypermetropia. The margins are indistinct and irregular. The disc assumes a dark greyish red colour and there may be grey radial striations emanating from it. There may be greyish areola around it, accentuating the irregularity of disc margin. The reflexes on the vessels may be accentuated which in some cases may even be misinterpreted as arterio-sclerotic changes. The vessels may not uncommonly show

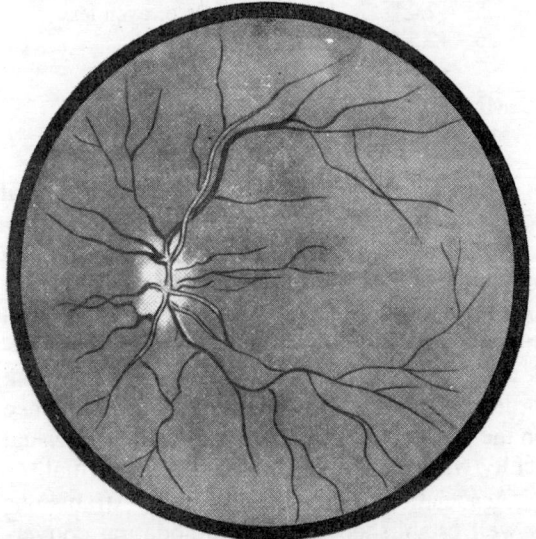

**Fig. 15.3.** Pseudoneuritis in hypermetropia. (*See also* Plate 1)

undue tortuosity or abnormal branchings. The macula is usually situated at an abnormally greater distance from the eye and the cornea is decentred so that the visual axis cuts the cornea considerably to the inside of the optic axis making a large positive angle alpha, i.e., the angle at which the visual axis joins the optic axis is greater than normal. A large angle alpha gives a false impression of divergent strabismus. True divergent squint in relation to hypermetropia is very rare indeed.

**Visual acuity :** In low degree of hypermetropia the visual acuity recorded may indeed be normal. The uncorrected visual acuity, however, varies with the degree of the refractive error and how far the accommodative effort is active. The relationship can thus be expressed in terms of absolute hypermetropia and not the true refractive state. The visual acuity attained in the presence of absolute hypermetropia has been worked out as under :

**Table 15.1.**

| Dioptric error of absolute hypermetropia | Visual acuity |
| --- | --- |
| 1.  +0.5 D | 6/9 |
| 2.  +0.75 D | 6/12 |
| 3.  +1.0 D | 6/12-6/18 |
| 4.  +1.5 D | 6/24 |
| 5.  +2.0 D | 6/24 or even less |
| 6.  +2.5 D | 6/60 |
| 7.  +3.5 D | 4/60 |
| 8.  +4.5 D | 3/60 |

There is proportional diminution of visual acuity as the error in terms of absolute hypermetropia increases. The corrected visual acuity may not reach to normal, particularly so in higher errors of refraction, due probably to perceptual factors but sometimes may be due to underdevelopment of the retina. It has been seen that judicious prescription of glasses and persistence on the part of the wearer leads to increased visual acuity which may eventually become normal.

Association of hypermetropia with strabismus is well established and accommodation convergent squint with consequent unilateral amblyopia is not unknown. The condition should be diagnosed and treated early. To improve occlusion of the normal eye may have to be resorted to. Sometimes, even in the absence of squint occlusion gives good results if there is partial amblyopia.

**Treatment**

The treatment consists in prescribing convex lenses so that the rays are brought to a focus on the retina (Fig. 15.4). In Fig. 15.4, it would be seen that in uncorrected hypermetropia the parallel rays are brought to a focus at a, i.e., behind

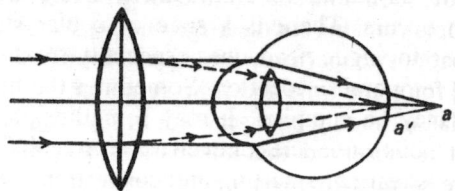

**Fig. 15.4.** Correction of hypermetropia by convex lens.

the retina. When a convex lens of appropriate power is inserted in the pathway of light, it can be brought to a focus at a′, a point near the retina. In general, the principle of correction of hypermetropia should be inhibition of any ciliary muscle contraction for distance except that resulting from inherent tone of the ciliary muscle. The second guiding principle is comfort to the patient. If patient is complaining of no symptoms of accommodative asthenopia, has normal visual acuity and shows no significant muscular imbalance no treatment is necessary. Ocular asthenopia is due to compensatory efforts of the accommodation mechanism. Due to a sustained and prolonged tonus of ciliary muscles it is difficult to relax it all at once. The aim, therefore, should to be correct all astigmatism and a part of hypermetropic error. The glasses prescribed are such as can be worn with comfort in the first instance. Gradually increase the correction at adequately placed intervals (3 to 6 months) till the patient accepts full manifest hypermetropic correction. The final aim remains to be to prescribe the maximum of convex lenses required for the full correction. The procedure is both laborious and time-consuming besides exercising the patience of the refractionist and the patient. Some persons do advise full hypermetropic correction in the first sitting but this is usually inadvisable as the glasses are seldom tolerated, particularly so if in the post-mydriatic test the patient is not comfortable with them. They are seldom worn. It is important to remember that in children hypermetropia diminishes with the growth of the child. Children who have been prescribed hypermetropic glasses should be examined once a year and if necessary the correction should be weakened. It will be seen that in not a small number of cases there does not remain any necessity of such glasses. If the degree of hypermetropia remains small, a trial should be given to the patient to perform his visual functions unaided for some time and if no symptoms develop the glasses should be discarded. In several instances it is observed that the patient initially has severe symptoms even when the refractive error is small but after an initial use of glasses the symptoms disappear and do not reappear even when visual functions are performed unaided.

In practice, however, each individual should be dealt with on its own merits. It would be advisable to determine the manifest hypermetropia and order lenses on this basis. The aim should be to correct the patient as near to his manifest hypermetropia as possible. Of course, due regard should be given so that the patient remains within the limits consistent with comfort and good vision. Correcting hypermetropia is a tricky problem and all different factors like age, state of accommodation, muscle balance and general physical and nervous states as well as vocation should be fully kept in view. The author prefers to perform retinoscopy in all hypermetropes under cycloplegia even if it is a repeat refraction cautiously keeping in view the possibility of glaucoma.

When a person does not accept the full correction for his hypermetropic correction a few ophthalmologists favour prescribing bifocals even in young individuals with a view to relax accommodation when working for near and reduce asthenopic symptoms. The experience shows that such bifocal prescriptions more often than not add to the complexities of the symptoms and seldom, if ever, give relief. Such a step is neither advisable nor helpful. A full correction of hypermetropia in the presence of discomfort with wearing correction is advisable only in two situations.

1. In the presence of accommodational spasm to rest the ciliary muscle.
2. In the presence of latent or intermittent convergent strabismus to relieve convergence indirectly, by relieving accommodation.

### Pathological hypermetropia

This is a rare condition and is almost always due to deformation of the globe. The inheritance is usually recessive. It may be axial or curvature in type. It is only in flattening of the cornea that help can be rendered by prescribing contact lenses or resorting to refractive surgery or excimer or holmium laser therapy.

### Aphakia

Aphakia means the absence of lens from the eye but from the optical point of view it may be considered to be a condition or conditions in which the lens is absent from the pupillary area. In most of the cases it is due to operative removal of the crystalline lens. In some of the cases lens may dislocate in the vitreous chamber. Rare causes are absorption, traumatic extrusion, and congenital absence of lens.

### Optics of aphakia

Aphakia is an extreme form of hypermetropia. After removal of the lens the total refractive power of the eye is reduced to 43.05 D. There being only one main refracting element, i.e., the cornea, this is more near to the concept of Donders' reduced eye. The two principal points are almost at the anterior surface of the cornea. The nodal points are very near each other and about 7.754 mm from the anterior surface of the cornea which shows that both the principal points have shifted forwards in the uncorrected eye. The nodal points also shift. In the uncorrected eye they shift backwards. In the corrected eye, however, they shift forwards. The parallel rays of light are brought to a focus about 31 mm behind the cornea while the eye is 23-24 mm long. In aphakia the anterior focal point is at 23.22 mm (normal is 17.05 mm). The dioptric system of the eye must, therefore, be supplemented by a strong converging lens. If the eye was emmetropic before the development of the cataract the correction required is about 10 dioptres. The relationship of aphakic refraction to preoperative ametropia is not straightforward. If ametropia is of index type, e.g., myopia in nuclear cataract, the post-operative refractive error would be identical with an operated emmetropic eye. Axial ametropia, however, makes a difference. The power of lenses required after operation can, roughly, be calculated by the formula +10 D sph. + ½ the dioptric power of the pre-existing glasses. For example, for myopia of –10 D the new number required would be +10 D + (½ of –10 D, i.e., –5 D) or +10 D – 5 D = +5 D and for –20 myopia it would be +10 – 10 D = 0.00 D. For hypermetropia of +5 D it would be +10 D + (½ of +5 D or +2.50 D) or +10 D + 2.50 D sph. = +12.50 D. This is only a guideline and may not eventually be true because of varying factors in the aetiology of the error.

However in some clinics these days axial length of the eyeball is determined by using ultrasonic methods employing computerized determination.

Corneal astigmatism is always present and is attributed to the operative scar. It is against the rule and is +8 to +10 dioptres about a week post-operatively and is gradually reduced to about +2 D in six weeks time. The downward trend may continue for as long as 3 months or so. If there be a pre-existing error of astigmatism it gets added algebraically. Since the ultimate astigmatism due to operative scar is unpredictable, it is not possible to mathematically calculate the astigmatic error. In view of this it is not advisable to prescribe glasses earlier.

If glasses are insisted upon they should only be temporary and preferably only spherical. Temporary correction has the advantage that the patient can somewhat adapt himself to the new vision. For distance the average correction is +10.00 D sph. (sometimes +11.00 D sph.). Correction is also needed for reading distance which varies from +3.00 to +4.00 dioptres depending upon individual needs of the patient.

Spectacle frames should be well fitting, otherwise the weight of thick convex lenses would sag them down thus changing the effective power of the lens. The precise distance between the cornea and the back of the trial tens should be supplied to the optician. The weight of the glass can be reduced if hardened plastic lenses are used. The plastic lenses have a disadvantage of being scratchable.

The aphakic eye has several handicaps as a visual apparatus.

1. **Size of the image :** The image size increases by about 30%. It has been stated earlier that if the correcting lenses are worn at the anterior principal point the size of the retinal image is uninfluenced by a correcting lens. This statement does not hold good for aphakics. The size of the image varies in comparison with that of an emmetropic eye by an amount depending on the difference between their anterior focal distance. On calculation the ratio works out to be 1.36 to 1, i.e., the image in the aphakic eye will be about 1/3 larger than in an emmetropic eye even when in each case the lens is worn at the anterior focal distance. This will be true for all cases where the anterior focal distance will get varied. The increase in the size of the image is larger if the eye was previously myopic and there is lesser increase in the size if the eye was hypermetropic pre-operatively.

2. **Vision in aphakia :** A large image falsifies the visual acuity recorded on the Snellen's chart. The vision recorded is theoretically better than the actual visual acuity in terms of visual angles. A vision of 6/9 in a corrected aphakic eye should be regarded as equivalent to 6/12 in an emmetropic eye or in an eye whose optical system is unaltered.

3. **Accommodation :** Due to absence of lens it is totally abolished. It is impossible to prescribe lenses which could permit a visual range from infinity to near point. In practice one prescribes

1. a pair of glasses for distant vision and another pair for near vision, or
2. some persons prefer to prescribe one for distance and the other pair for bifocal for near and intermediate distance.

The author prefers to follow the first alternative. The patient learns to achieve some elasticity by increasing or decreasing the distance at which the lens is worn by shifting the spectacle frame.

4. **Aberration :** There is a spherical aberration. The phenomenon is termed as pin-cushion

distortion. In this the straight lines become curves and the linear world becomes one consisting of parabolas which continually change their shapes when the patient moves the eyes. When the objects are viewed through the periphery, they look enlarged, nearer and elongated in radial direction. When the objects are moving they appear to be moving faster.

On lateral movement there is a prismatic effect, and more than 2 to 3 prism dioptre effect is rarely tolerated.

When the objects or lights are viewed from the periphery of the lens there is also a chromatic aberration.

Aspherical lenses though mitigate these effects yet seldom are the answer to these problems. Conoid cataract lenses, which have an ellipsoid of revolution as the front surface and optically correct the aberration inherent in spherical lenses, can be employed. In these lenses the power gradually reduces from the centre to the edge.

### Field of vision

The useful monocular and binocular field of vision is limited and is about 50° all round. The patient is, however, more concerned about a roving ring scotoma usually described as the jack-in-the-box phenomenon (Fig. 15.5).

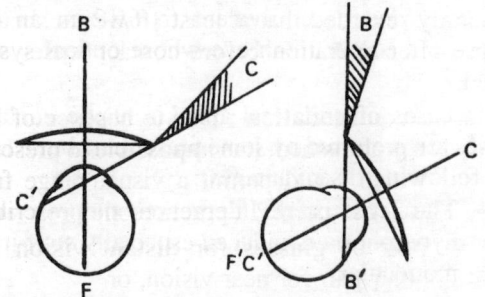

**Fig. 15.5.** Roving ring scotoma in aphakia (jack-in-the-box phenomenon).

In Fig. 15.5, when the eye is in primary position (Fig. 15.5A) there is a ring scotoma (C) of approximately 15°. When the eye moves to the side, the scotoma moves in the opposite direction (Fig. 15.5B), it takes up the position B (that is towards the fixation point). It follows that if while the eye is in primary position (Fig. 15.5A), an object in the region attracts attention and the eye is moved to fixate it, it thereupon disappears (Fig. 15.5B). In Fig. 15.5A, B is visible and C is not visible (scotoma); as the eye fixes the object at C, B becomes invisible (shifting of scotoma). Depending upon the position, objects in this position, therefore, appear and disappear in the most disconcerting way.

A ring scotoma of 15° is caused by the prismatic effect at the periphery of the correcting lens when it is placed a short distance in front of the eye and the eye is in the primary position. The scotoma tends to move with an against motion to the motion of the eye. As the eye moves to the peripheral lens position, the scotoma moves to a more central one opposite to the direction of the movement of the eye. In this way when the patient sees an object, and turns his eye towards it, the scotoma may move a sufficient distance inwards to occlude it. Upon shifting his eye from it, the scotoma again shifts and the object becomes visible again as to pop in and out of view.

From the above it is evident that an aphakic patient has to face with a very peculiar type of vision. He should be forewarned. With patience and perseverance he must try to adapt himself to these new environments. In course of a few weeks or months the patient comes to know that he has not to move his eye in relation to spectacles, but to move the head as a whole; he becomes aware of the apparent slant of an even floor, and can climb up and down the staircase, which was a great problem in the beginning. His higher centres get adjusted to a new judgement, and movements of overshooting or undershooting gradually become finer and finer.

It is not difficult to determine the refractive error in aphakia. Keratometric readings are valuable because astigmatism is entirely corneal. The pupil can be dilated by phenylephrine and cycloplegic is not required. In retinoscopy the shadow is faint and it moves with the movement of the mirror. With bigger colobomas confusion may be produced by peripheral shadows. To obviate it either concentrate on neutralization in central zone, or use a pupillary disc in the trial frame.

## Binocular vision and aphakia

To attain binocularity in unilateral aphakia is a problem. Even in binocular aphakia binocularity is not always present. Worth's four-dot test many a time reveals suppression or diplopia in such cases. If binocularity has existed before in life it can be restored. It is unwise to fix the operation of the second eye, in bilateral cataracts, after a long time, i.e., the inter-operation interval should not be long. In this interval as the eyes are dissociated, convergence becomes poorer and exophoria or even exotropia may result. In such cases orthoptic exercises, relieving prisms and even muscle surgery may be needed.

In monocular aphakia with an emmetropic other eye, which has active accommodation, i.e., young patients with aphakia after traumatic or congenital cataract, the major hindrance to binocularity is aniseikonia of 30% due to aniso-metropia. It ordinarily prevents fusion though in rare instances fusion in the central field has been found to be present and is possible. The problem is not only due to magnification but also to the varying prismatic effect, while seeing through different parts of the periphery of lenses. Other hindrances are a tendency to suppression and muscular imbalances. A neglected patient of this type develops deviation of the operated eye and the only use of such an eye is a wider field of vision. Both prism prescription and/or muscle surgery are often unsuccessful. There are differing views with regard to the advisability of operating on such eyes. Some people believe that the effect of leaving cataracts unoperated is prolonged occlusion which leads to further weakening of existing fusion and that post-operatively sufficient fusion for good usage does occur if the cataracts are removed early. The author and many others believe that the extraction of an opaque lens from an eye, when its fellow retains good vision, is inadvisable. It should only be undertaken if there is absolute necessity for a full field of vision or if the cataract is becoming hypermature or if an intraocular lens implant is planned.

Recent trends in optics of aphakia are mainly channelized to eliminate or considerably diminish aniseikonia and to attain binocularity. In spite of all recent advances the goal seems to be still distant. Aniseikonia with spectacle glasses placed 15 mm in front of the cornea is about 30%, with contact lenses 10-13%, with Strampelli's anterior chamber implants 5% and with Ridley's type posterior chamber implants it is 0.2%. Aniseikonia up to 6% is commonly tolerated but higher limits can be reached by selective suppression of dissimilar peripheral parts of the two images. It also depends upon the visual acuity and the extent of confused peripheral vision with which the patient feels satisfied.

Contact lenses are better tolerated in monocular aphakia and have following advantages over spectacles :

- Less aniseikonia, hence more chances of binocularity.
- Elimination of various aberrations and prismatic effect of spectacle glasses.
- Bigger and better field of vision.
- Eyes can move more freely as the relative position of the contact lens remains constant.
- Cosmetically better.

Two types of contact lenses are used :

1. Haptic or
2. Corneal.

As with spectacle lenses, enough time must elapse for the cornea to have taken on a fixed curve before contact lenses are prescribed. It is generally regarded that at least 10 weeks should elapse after operation before contact lenses are fitted.

In cases of unilateral aphakia haptic contact lenses are preferred by some prescribers but it has the following disadvantages :

- The lens usually depresses the eye and hyperphoria is induced especially so if it is monocular.
- The lens may rotate due to its weight being mostly in temporal part.
- The lens rides slightly outwards and may induce exophoria and excyclophoria.
- In monocular fittings they provide a poorer cosmetic appearance and a lighter retinal image size.

The corneal contact lenses have been found to be better tolerated by our patients and are usually prescribed by the author. They also have the following disadvantages :

The lens usually rides low and introduces prismatic effect with base down leading to hyperphoria in varying degrees. Even the contact lens wearer will require spectacles for many occasions which are not served by contact lenses. We do not prefer bifocals hence additional specs are required for reading purposes.

Corneal type of contact lenses are the most effective visual aid in monocular young aphakics where 10 L implant is not contemplated.

In my practice I have found that some contact lenses are quite effective and tolerated well. However, if a patient finds the wearing and taking out of these lenses too cumbersome, trial can be given to extended wear lenses.

## Intraocular implants or pseudophakos

Aphakic glasses present problems as described above. Use of contact lenses reduces these problems but add some of their own like taking them out daily and keeping them sterile to prevent the deterioration of ocular hygiene. The difference in the size of image still remains to the level of 10-13% between the normal eye and the aphakic eye wearing contact lenses. With intraocular lenses particularly the post-chamber implant, the lens being almost near the normal position, the magnification defects are reduced (0.2%). In all three states, however, the absence of accommodation persists. It has become almost a routine procedure.

Intraocular lens implantation is another step forward to achieve binocularity and do away with glasses.

Ridley's posterior chamber implant was an innovation in which the artificial visual device was put in a natural position of the lens.

It is, therefore, pertinent to describe the ophthalmic optics of aphakia in terms of pseudophakia, i.e., with intraocular lens implantation (IOL). With intraocular lenses the problems of retinal image are almost, if not, totally eliminated and the question of peripheral distortion of images does not arise. Phenomena like jack-in-the-box are totally eliminated. The quality of vision has thus changed to approximate near normal except the accommodation.

The size of image in the normal eye and the aphakic eye are shown in Figs. 15.6 and 15.7.

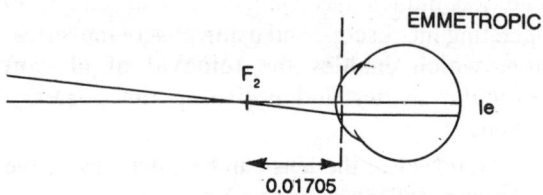

**Fig. 15.6.** Size of image in normal eye.

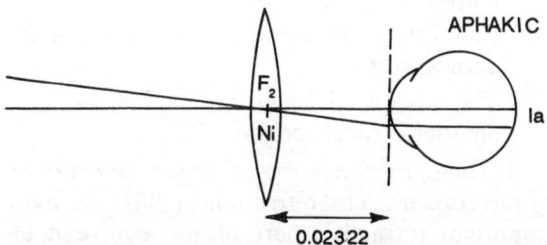

**Fig. 15.7.** Size of image in aphakic eye.

In Fig. 15.6, $I_e$ is the size of retinal image in emmetropic eye and in Fig. 15.7 the size of the retinal image is $I_a$ and they are related as their respective focal distances, i.e., 0.02322 is to 0.01705, or 1.36 : 1.

There are two places where IOLs are inserted, anterior chamber and posterior chamber (Figs. 15.8 and 15.9).

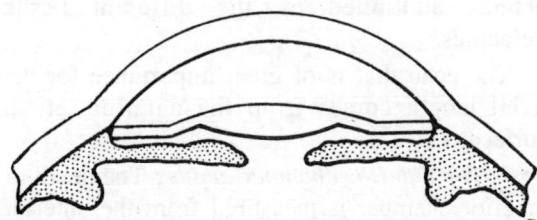

**Fig. 15.8.** Anterior chamber angle fixated intraocular lens.

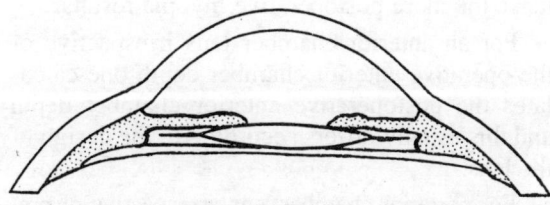

**Fig. 15.9.** Posterior chamber intraocular lens.

For a proper choice of intraocular lens, the determination of the power of the lens is required. The techniques have been refined under an operating microscope and using phacoemulsification, which enables the removal of all soft lenticular matter and polishing the posterior capsule.

The power of the lens can be calculated if the following values are known :

1. The refraction of the anterior surface of the cornea.
2. The distance of the retina from the anterior corneal surface.
3. The anticipated distance of the IOL from the anterior corneal surface.

1. *The refraction power of the anterior surface of the cornea :* The refraction of this, the most important refractive part of the eye, can be obtained by measuring the radius of curvature of the anterior surface of the cornea (K). The commercially available ophthalmometers show not only the radius of the anterior surface of the cornea but also the refractive power of the cornea.

2. *Measuring the axial length of the eye :* As described earlier the axial length of the eye, from the apex of the cornea to the macula, is measured by an A-scan ultrasonographic apparatus. The results are depicted in Fig. 15.10. What we measure actually is the time interval between echoes multiplied by the different tissue velocities.

The echo that is of great importance for the axial length comes from the anterior retinal surface.

3. *The anterior chamber depth :* The depth of anterior chamber is measured from the anterior surface of the cornea to the anterior surface of the lens (or IOL). This distance greatly influences the refractive power of the eye. The lesser the distance the more postoperative myopia results.

For an anterior chamber lens irrespective of the operative anterior chamber depth one calculates the postoperative anterior chamber depth and this usually differs according to the design of the lens.

For posterior chamber lens, irrespective of pre-

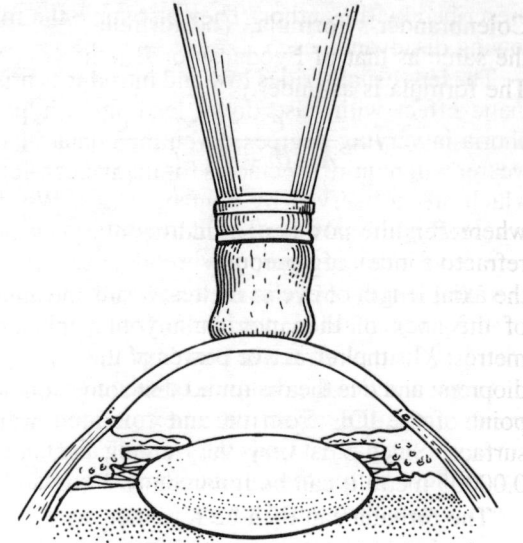

**Fig. 15.10A.** Compu-Scan transducer.

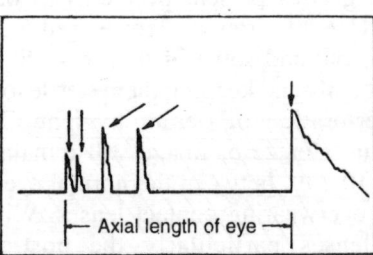

— Axial length of eye —

**Fig. 15.10B.** Axial length of eye with ultrasonograph.

operative measurement, a postoperative anterior chamber depth of 4 mm is employed for calculation.

**Calculation formulae**

The variables used are :

1. Refractive power of the cornea based on K.
2. Axial length of the eyeball as measured by A-scan.
3. Assumed values of the anterior chamber depth.

This information is fed into a variety of formulae. These formulae are grouped into two.

**Theoretical formulae**

These are based on assumptions of the anterior chamber depth. These are essentially included in

Colenbrander's formula. The formula is almost the same as that of Fyodarov or Binkhorst et al. The formula is as under :

$$P = \frac{C}{A-(b+d)} - \frac{C}{\dfrac{C}{K}-(b+d)}$$

where $P$ is the power of IOL required; $C$ is the refractive index of aqueous/vitreous = 1.336; $A$ is the axial length of eye in metres; $b$ is the distance of the apex of the anterior surface of IOL in metres; $K$ is the refractive power of the cornea in dioptres; and $d$ is the distance of second principal point of the IOL from the apex of its anterior surface. Since $d$ is very very small, i.e., about 0.00005 metre it can be ignored.

The formula can then be rewritten as

$$P = \frac{1.336}{A-b} - \frac{C}{\dfrac{C}{K}-b}$$

### SRK-I formula

The most widely used formula is the SRK-I (Sanders, Retzlaff and Kraff) formula which is based on the bulk experience of surgeons looking retrospectively. It takes into account the axial length and keratometric readings except individual specifics IOLs. The formula is based on empirical values. It has only questionable advantage over the theoretical formula given above.

It can be expressed as

$$P = A - 2.5\,L - 0.9\,K$$

where $P$ is the implant power to produce emmetropia; $L$ is the axial length of the eye; $K$ is the average keratometer reading; and $A$ is the specific constant for each lens type/or manufacturer.

There are many modifications and variations of these formulae.

It seems the determination of the power of IOL is much easier if, instead of calculations, we read the power from a nomogram (Fig. 15.11).

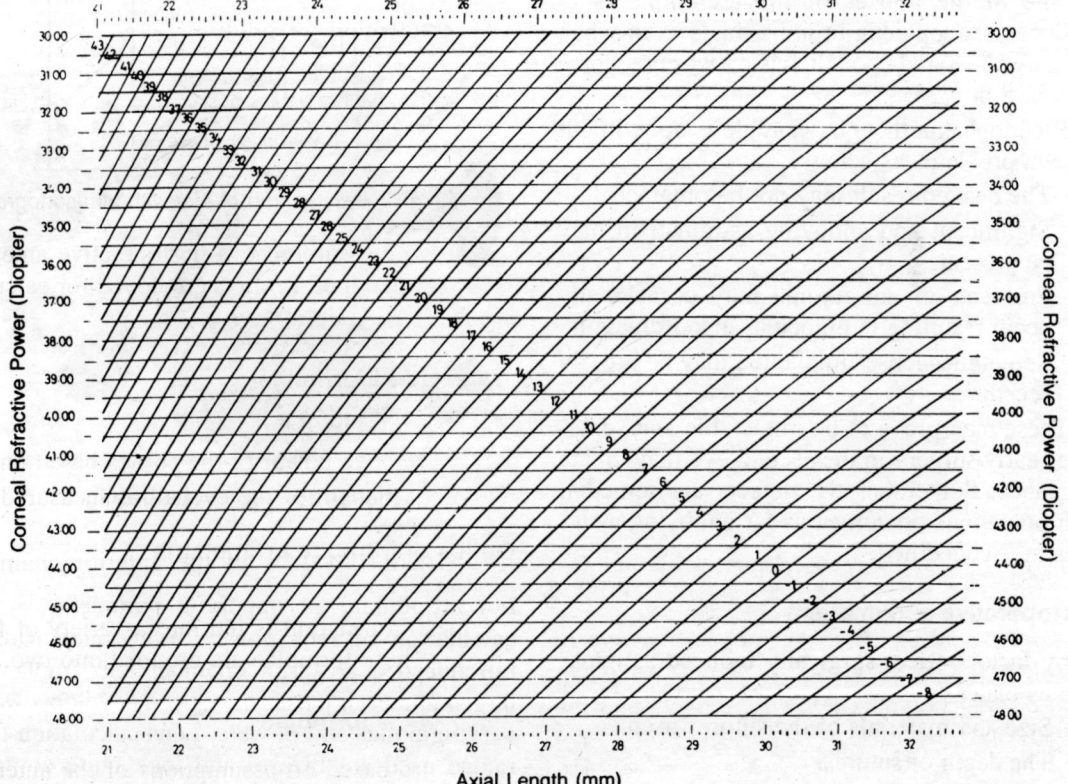

**Fig. 15.11.** Nomogram for the determination of the emmetropia lens calculated from the axial length, the refractive power of the cornea, and the assumed distance of the IOL from the corneal surface of 3.5 mm oblique curves. Pseudophakos (dioptre).

Nowadays computerised instruments are available which are programmed to give a much more accurate reading than the nomograms. Many ultrasound apparatuses are also available which are compatible with programmed computers.

Digital ocular computer can be coupled with ultrasonic measuring tools. In them $K$ readings can be fed and it will automatically give the IOL power.

We can calculate power of IOL which can produce post-operative emmetropia or variations of desired hypermetropia or myopia.

### Aims of lens implantation

The basic aim of pseudophakia is to produce emmetropia as far as possible, remove the drawbacks of aphakia correction and allow maintenance of binocular function even in monocular aphakics especially in young adolescents and adults. Use of both eyes for near vision is also the aim.

One of the abuses of the technique is to produce pseudophakia in individuals even when in the eye operated upon the vision was not worse than 6/18 or 6/24.

Pseudophakia though desirable is not without its own problems as below :

1. The desired result may not be obtained.
2. Significant and annoying astigmatism may be present.
3. Problems of aniseikonia may occasionally occur resulting in binocular incoordination.
4. Sometimes lenses implanted may be grossly eccentric.

These may prove to be intractable and sometimes early surgery in the second eye may create a balance. Sometimes the defects are remedial with operations on cornea as far annoying astigmatism is concerned.

### Postoperative astigmatism

Many factors effect surgically induced astigmatism as under :

1. Size and materials of the sutures used.
2. The depth of sutures.
3. The size of bites.
4. Tightness of sutures.

5. Size of the wound and nearness to the cornea the larger the incision, the more the chances.

The astigmatism caused by sutures is fortunately corrected rapidly with the judicious removal of sutures. One should, however, be careful not to remove the sutures too early as it would cause gaping of the wound resulting in astigmatism itself or compounding the already existing postoperative astigmatism. In suture created astigmatism it is not possible to correct it without removing the sutures which should be done 8 to 12 weeks or more after surgery.

It is better to prevent astigmatism by

- regulating suturing through intraoperative keratometry (Zeiss keratometer) (Fig. 15.12);
- resorting to small incision surgery with foldable lenses with or without sutures (proper bevelled incisions are required);
- preliminary suturing with 8-0 sutures through 12 o'clock methylene blue track followed by 10-0 nylon sutures and removal of 8-0 sutures.

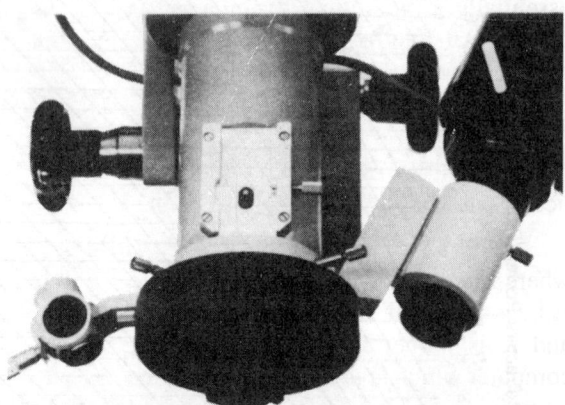

**Fig. 15.12.** Zeiss keratometer.

### Optics of intraocular implants

For artiphakia, an important parameter is the calculation of lens power. Ever since Ridley introduced a posterior chamber lens implant a large number of lenses have been developed with varying optics and powers. Lens calculation formulae used are bizarre and look quite complicated. Mostly they are dependent upon the axial length, the corneal power and the position of intraocular lens. Fritz (1981) analysed these formulae and came to the conclusion that most of them can be resolved into a common equation as under :

$$P = \frac{N}{A - D - g\,(t)}$$
$$= \frac{N}{\dfrac{N}{K} - D - g\,(t)}$$

where $N$ = index of refraction of the cornea;

$A$ = axial length;

$D$ = position of the intraocular lens;

$K$ = corneal power;

$P$ = the power of the intraocular lens (IOL); and

$g\,(t)$ = function of IOL thickness and vertex.

For purposes of calculation of the power of IOL the axial length is measured by immersion ultrasonographic method. Most satisfactory results are obtained if different parameters are fed and computer is programmed to calculate from emmetropic to any ametropic IOL power. This is essentially a theoretical formula but is found to be quite satisfactory for practical purposes and is commended by Langston (1982).

While several enthusiasts have evolved different regression formulae for calculating the power of intraocular lenses to be given to a particular case but now all seem to converge to :

$$P = A - 2.5\,(A.L.) - 0.9\,(K)$$

where $P$ is the power of the lens to be implanted; A.L. is the axial length; $A$ is the corneal power; and $K$ is numerical constant generated by the computer which is in the neighbourhood of 115.6.

These regression formulae are based on measurement of axial length by applanation methods. If similar techniques are used these regressions can be usefully employed. The experience of a fair number of IOL implant experts, however, does not find greater accuracy in regression formula than in theoretical formula.

## When to expect stable visual result

Whatever the mode of surgery for removal of cataract, vision takes time to settle. The larger the size of the incision the longer it takes to settle. It is for this reason that small incision non-suture surgery with or without phacoemulsification is resorted to. The result also depends upon the method of suturing, the tightness of sutures and the materials used. The details of these are beyond the scope of this book but have briefly been mentioned above.

In cases where implants are not given it takes about six weeks to 3 months for the vision to settle down. In the interim period a temporary lens in a round frame, power differing from +9.0 D sph. to +12.0 D sph. adopting a cafeteria approach can be given. Some surgeons prefer to use temporary bifocals with addition of +3.5 D sph. to the distant correction picked up by the patient. Bifocals should not be routinely prescribed but should only fulfil the felt need, if there be any.

Unfortunately this settlement of vision depends upon competent surgery. Inadvertent and incompetent surgery like ragged wound, inadequate wound closure, inclusion of vitreous strands or capsular remnants in the wound lips, leaving behind of large amount of soft lenticular matter all contribute to delay or permanent visual defects particularly astigmatism.

In pseudophakia also the vision takes time to settle and changes go on taking place because of

- movement of intraocular lens due to shrinkage of capsular bag;
- posterior capsular thickening;
- finer adjustments at the wound level.

These are, however, not very consequential.

In cases where cutting of sutures does not produce the desired results corneal surgery of some type may be needed (refractive surgery).

# CHAPTER 16

# Myopia

Myopia is the refractive state of the eye in which with normal tonic accommodation, the parallel rays of light are brought to a focus on a point in front of the retinal plane (Fig. 16.1) when the eye is at rest.

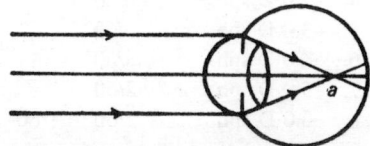

**Fig. 16.1.** Focus of rays from infinity in myopia.

In myopia the eyeball is usually deformed; the deformation occurs at the posterior part of the globe only (Fig. 16.2), the anterior part is normal. The eyeball is usually large and looks prominent. When adducted the equator can be seen.

Myopia may be classified into simple or pathological.

## Simple myopia

It is usually not progressive but sometimes the error may show a mild increase during the years of growth.

1. **Axial :** It may be axial, in which the eye is relatively too long for its refractive status. In this the total refractive power of the eye may be the same as in any normal eye but due to increased length of the eyeball the parallel rays are brought to a focus in front of the sentient layers of the retina.

2. **Refractive** in which the dioptric power of the eye is too strong for the axial length; in this case the axial length may be the same as in any normal eye.

The refractive myopia may be further considered as :

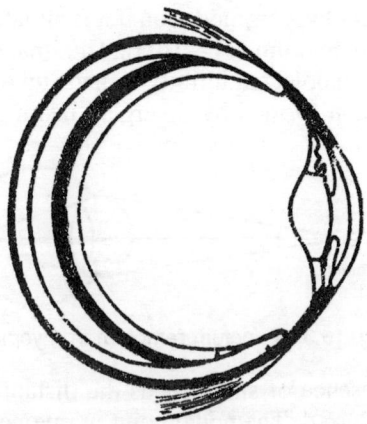

**Fig. 16.2.** Enlargement of globe at posterior pole.

(a) **Curvature** in which the cornea is more curved than the normal as in megalocornea or buphthalmos or there may be an increase in the curvature of lens.

(b) **Index :** This may be due to change in index of refraction of the lens (diabetes and cataract). It may be high refractive index of aqueous, lens nucleus and cornea or low refractive index of lens cortex or vitreous.

3. **Functional** where there is an excessive use of accommodation.

In terms of axial myopia the eye should be considered as an overdeveloped eye in which the processes of growth have exceeded the normal limit. According to Sorsby 35% of myopes remain stationary and 15% show only slight progress. Even in those cases where there is progress of myopia the eye remains healthy and the visual acuity can be corrected to normal with appropriate lenses. The border line between the simple and degenerative types is ill-defined. Simple myopia like simple hypermetropia is autosomally dominant but there are a number of reports which claim that recessive mode of inheritance is the commonest form of inheritance. The type of occupation also has some influence in causation of myopia and lends support to the concept that environmental factors are important in the aetiology of myopia.

## Optics of myopia

In myopes a near object may be focused without any effort of accommodation if it is situated at the punctum remotum (Fig. 16.3). The image on the retina of an object at infinity is made up of circles of diffusion formed by divergent beam. In view

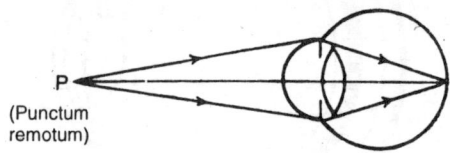

P
(Punctum remotum)

**Fig. 16.3.** Punctum remotum in myopia.

of the absence of sharp focus the distant objects appear blurred. The nodal point in myopes is farther away from the retina and the image formed is larger in size which partly compensates for the blur due to absence of sharp focus. Accommodation is of little value to myopes, as any exercise of accommodation would only accentuate his visual problem. It would neither increase his vision nor reduce his myopia. In higher errors of refraction the amplitude of accommodation is small. The patient has no incentive to improve it and convergence does not get an accommodative influence. All these factors result in fatigue of accommodation and eye strain. Due to dissociation of convergence and accommodation exophoria commonly occurs and this may ultimately break into exotropia.

The eye of simple myopia is large and prominent. The chamber is deeper than normal and the pupil reacts sluggishly to light. The macula is slightly nearer to the disc than in a normal eye. The visual axis gets so altered that in some cases the angle alpha becomes slightly negative which gives an impression of a convergent squint (apparent convergent squint). In myopia more commonly one sees a divergent strabismus.

## Clinical picture

In myopes the main symptom is inadequacy of visual performance. The visual acuity beyond the far point is severely affected. In view of various adaptations by the patient it is difficult to accurately guess the unaided visual acuity but the visual acuity and the degree of error are usually correlated as seen in Table 16.1.

**Table 16.1.**

| Degree of myopia | Visual acuity |
|---|---|
| 1. −0.5 D sph. | 6/9 to 6/12 |
| 2. −1.0 D sph. | 6/18 |
| 3. −1.5 D sph. | 6/24 to 6/36 |
| 4. −2.0 D sph. | 6/36 |
| 5. −3.0 D sph. | 6/60 |
| 6. −4.0 D sph. | 3/60 |
| 7. −5.0 D sph. | 2/60 |
| 8. −6.0 D sph. | 2/60 to 1/60 |

Some of the patients improve their naked eye vision by screwing their eye or making the interpalpebral aperture into a stenopaic slit. In such cases the visual acuity may fail to show any correlation with the refractive error.

There are usually no symptoms of eye strain except in small errors. Occasionally patients complain of photophobia which is not infrequently associated with dilated pupil. Due to this dilatation of pupil an excessive quantity of light, to which the retina is not adapted, gains access and produces glare. The dilatation of pupil is itself due to a lack of pupillary tonus because of inadequacy of accommodation. All myopic patients can reduce the annoying photophobia and can also improve the visual acuity by screwing the eye thus taking advantage of the phenomenon of stenopaic slit. The screwing of lids may sometimes lead to headache. In smaller degrees of error symptoms of eye strain may occur. The myopic patient usually takes the blurring of vision for granted, concentrates his energy into indoor activities and develops little, if any, interest in outdoor work. He becomes introvert and self-centred. He is usually intelligent and has always proved himself to be a bright student. He is a front-bencher until he reaches a higher class where there is no allocation of seats. He then finds that he cannot see the black board clearly if he sits on a seat in one of the back rows, thus becoming conscious of his defect. He usually seeks optical aid at this time. In middle age when accommodation starts weakening he has the advantage of not requiring glasses for near work. In this country there are proud men who narrate stories of how their elders never needed glasses. The fact is that they never needed the acuity of vision in young age and always were unaware of their limitations and in middle and later stages their failing accommodation did not pose a problem as the eye was always adapted for near work.

There is ocular asthenopia due to dissociation between convergence and accommodation. The punctum remotum of a myopic eye is located at a distance which corresponds in metres to the reciprocal of the dioptric value of its refractive error. The patient converges for a point for which he may not have to accommodate. For all points of near work the patient has to converge as any emmetrope but does not have to make commensurate efforts of accommodation. This adjustment is usually fatiguing and annoying particularly if quick changes in working distances are constantly required. This leads to a dissociation between convergence and accommodation. Sometimes to keep pace with the convergence an over-accommodation results which may ultimately lead to spasm of accommodation which in turn artificially increases myopia and establishes a vicious circle. More frequently there is an attempt at convergence which gives rise to muscular imbalance. Fusion becomes weak and binocularity is affected. The patient starts suppressing one eye and relying on the other. The suppressed eye deviates usually outwards. If this occurs in young age sometimes the eye may deviate inwards.

## Pathological myopia

It is variously termed as degenerative, progressive, malignant and pathological. Pathological myopia is accompanied by degenerative changes in the posterior pole of the eyeball. It is an aberration in the axial growth of the eyeball though not always so. Agarwal and Khosla have shown that degenerative changes and growth are independent of each other but may be closely related.

They have advanced the theory of multiple gene defect inheritance as the cause of variable picture in progressive myopia. Degenerative myopia is the most important of refractive errors which caused much visual disability and may ultimately lead to blindness. In western countries it is one of the commonest causes of economic blindness.

Pathological myopia may be associated with congenital anomalies like colobomas, staphylomas, choroidal degeneration, optic and choroidal atrophy. Or, it may be disease acquired development as in goitres, tuberculosis, measles and other debilitating diseases. Or, it may also be seen in developmental degenerative changes with loss of vision due to rapid axial growth and persistent progression of myopia after puberty.

To explain this axial growth several theories have been advanced from time to time. These theories are :

1. Based on mechanical concepts in which it is believed that there is mechanical stretching of the posterior part of globe owing to weakness of the sclera and that external and internal environments as determined by the habit and health of the individual influence the growth of the eyeball; or

2. Biological concept of differential growth which is probably genetically determined. Now it is generally believed that biological rather than mechanical factors are more important and that the environment plays a part of insignificant importance.

## Mechanical concepts

Since myopia commences at the school going age when a child is put to close work and progresses throughout the years of school life, near work and reading were considered to be the primary causal factors, but now generally this is not accepted as a possible cause. This as a cause remains statistically unauthenticated.

## Anatomical factors

It is believed by some that the depth of the orbit has a determining influence on the axial growth of the eyeball. Some statistics are available in the literature which seem to support this contention but on closer analysis no significant relationship can be unequivocally determined.

The distension of sclera may be due to abnormal accommodation. The pull of intra- or extraocular muscles leads to congestion and softening of the sclera but such an association is not very common. The treatment of progressive cases by bifocal glasses has been produced as an evidence in favour of accommodation as a causative factor. These authors think that in at least some of them accommodation influences the progress for when accommodative activity is relieved by a suitable lens the progress of myopia is arrested. These authors further contend that correction with bifocals leads to considerable diminution in the rate of the progress of the disease. These arguments stand fully refuted. It has also been argued that abnormal accommodation should produce changes in the anterior segment of the eyeball but most of the changes seen in myopia are limited to the posterior pole. The experimental data available negates the hypothesis. Accommodation, on the balance of evidence available, does not seem to play a major role in the production or progression of myopia.

The distension of sclera may be due to a pull at the posterior pole by a short optic nerve. The shortness of the nerve may be absolute or relative. Such a view is not unequivocal. Shortness of optic nerve has not been reliably demonstrated or found to be associated with progressive myopia.

The softening of the sclera may be due to the congestion of eyeball produced by excessive convergence, gravity, manual labour and eye strain but none of them seems to offer any satisfactory explanation. There is increasing belief that we are paying a penalty of civilization but such an assumption is hypothetical and lacks statistical proof, unless mutation of genes is considered as a possibility.

The stretching of sclera may be due to weakness caused by autolysis of the local tissues. Whether such an autolysis takes place is rather doubtful.

There is frequent association of myopia with glaucoma but the configuration of buphthalmic eye is totally different from that of a myopic globe. It is extremely doubtful if intraocular tension or insidious chronic simple glaucoma has

any role in the causation or progression of myopia.

The extraocular muscles are said to exert pressure on the globe particularly the medial recti in convergence or the pressure by intraocular muscles as in excessive accommodation have been blamed from time to time but they have hardly anything to commend.

However, Hardia believes that the sclera cannot even withstand normal intraocular pressure in cases of progressive myopia. He, therefore, performs a drainage operation to stem the progress of myopia before doing radial keratotomy on such patients (children of growing age).

Nutritional deficiencies like those of calcium and vitamins are sometimes believed to be responsible for scleral weakness but biochemical and clinical data have failed to substantiate such an assumption.

There are some who believe that aberrations of growth in endocrinal system, particularly in the parathyroids, may be responsible for the weakness of the sclera. The detailed studies negate this hypothesis.

An intrinsic weakness of the sclera (scleromalacia) has been postulated by some but whether such a condition exists is doubtful.

From a large number of inexplicable and often contradictory theories, two important factors emerge—excessive close work and general debility. Both of these are doubtful causes of progressive myopia but at best these can be considered to be contributing factors.

**Biological concepts**

As most growth processes myopia seems to be hereditarily determined. Each coat of the eye, i.e., the retina, choroid and the sclera, has its own growth potential. Retina is determinant in developing myopia. The overgrowth of retina produces incongruity. The sclera due to its distensibility follows the retinal growth but the choroid becomes susceptible to degenerative changes due to this stretching. The choroid undergoes degeneration. The outer retinal layers are dependent for their nutrition on choriocapillaris. A degeneration of choroid results in degeneration of retina.

It has been suggested that the retinal pigmentary epithelium may be of paramount importance. The suggestion has been made on the basis of early oculographic changes in high myopia. Such a deduction is not without its pitfalls.

So far no satisfactory hypothesis has emerged to explain the aetiology of myopia. It is, however, unexceptionably linked to heredity and the processes of growth. Agarwal and Khosla suggested that the heredity is multiple gene defect; axial length, degenerative changes, vitreous changes and pathological complications are determined by different genetic influences. Each factor is carried by a different gene. That there is a related genetic influence of one factor on the other cannot be denied.

That progressive myopia is inextricably linked with the processes of growth cannot be denied. The lengthening of the posterior segment of the globe commences and ends only with the beginning and termination of period of growth.

Myopia is, therefore, predominantly due to genetic factors which influence the processes of growth. Nutritional deficiencies, debilitating diseases, indifferent general health and endocrinal aberrations may be contributing factors but certainly not the determining ones. The linking up of close work with the aetiology of the disease is uncalled for. It is incidental and has no aetiological relationship.

### Clinical features, pathology and complications

1. There is considerable failure in visual functions. In pathological myopia the error is usually high and the vision is usually not correctable to normal. When the error is corrected the objects look smaller in size, they are well defined and look brighter than normal which is annoying and fatiguing.

2. There are multitude of muscae volitantes and floating opacities which are attributed to liquefied vitreous. These cause anxiety to the patients so much so that they may develop an obsession about the impending and imagined dangers.

There is contraction of visual fields for white and colours and in some ring scotomas may be seen. These visual inadequacies are related to choroidal atrophy. These should not be confused with glaucomatous field changes.

The light sense is subnormal and sometimes in very high myopes there is night blindness. The electro-retinogram and electro-oculogram are also subnormal and on the basis of these it has been suggested that these changes are related to chorio-retinal and pigment epithelium degenerative changes.

The eye usually looks large in size and is prominent. When adducted, the equatorial part may be seen in the palpebral aperture.

The cornea is flatter than normal and the anterior chamber is deep. The pupil is somewhat dilated and reacts sluggishly to light.

The changes in the optic disc are seen as an obliquity of its entry. Myopic crescent (Fig. 16.4) usually appears at puberty and in the early stages it is seen as a white sharply defined area on the

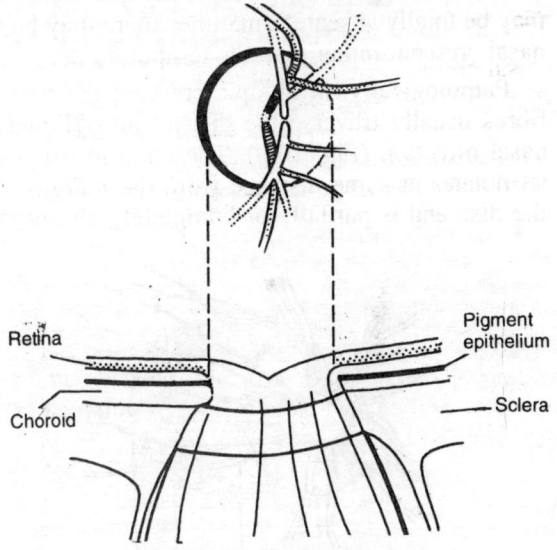

Retina

Choroid

Pigment epithelium

Sclera

**Fig. 16.4.** Myopic crescent.

temporal side of the disc. The crescent may be present superiorly or inferiorly; sometimes it may be annular (Fig. 16.5). In some cases the scleral canal is directly seen and the optic nerve shows an oblique entrance. The sharp edge is sometimes pigmented. The presence of a crescent does not necessarily mean that the patient is myopic. Though there is generally a close relationship

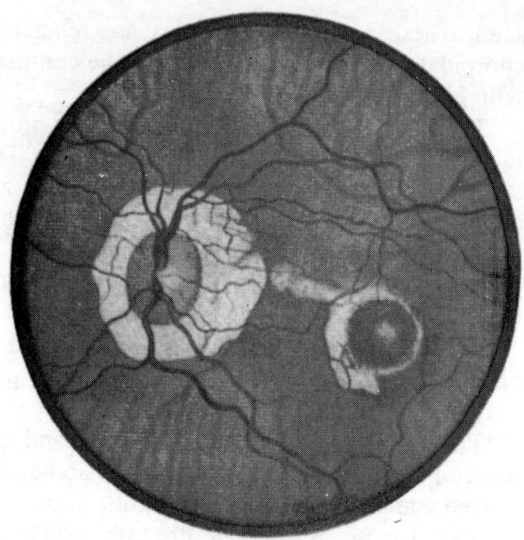

**Fig. 16.5.** Annular crescent. (*See also* Plate 2)

between the form, frequency and extent of crescent with the degree of myopia yet it is not invariably so and in many high degrees of myopia crescent may be totally absent. Sometimes there may be a nasal crescent rather than the temporal one.

Pathologically, in myopic crescent the nerve fibres usually traverse the disc in an obliquely nasal direction (Fig. 16.6). The choroid usually terminates at some distance from the margin of the disc and is partially or completely absent in

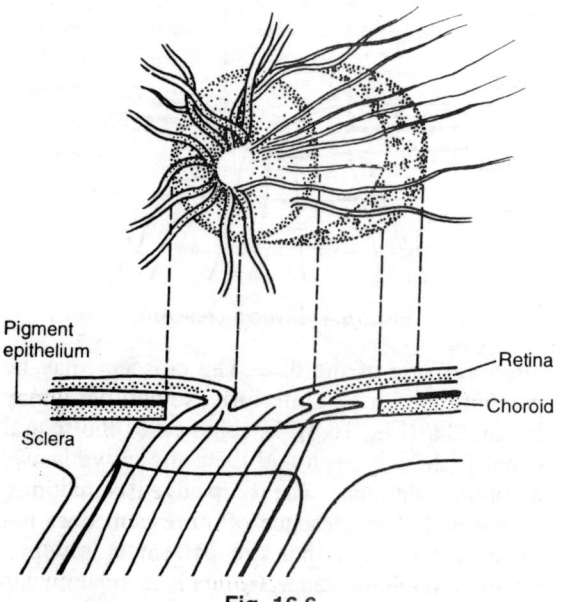

Pigment epithelium

Retina

Choroid

Sclera

**Fig. 16.6.**

the area of the crescent. Bruch's membrane may also terminate at the same point as other layers of choroid. The outer retinal layers and the pigment epithelium are usually absent at the crescent area though the inner layers of the retina continue.

Supertraction of the retina occurs over the nasal side of disc and encroaches over the disc causing a blurring of the nasal margin. The retinal vessels emerge about halfway across the papilla bending over the curved edge of the covering retina.

Pathologically, in supertraction, the choroid stops at the edge of the disc and the retina overlaps it. Sometimes the choroid also overlaps the disc but always to a lesser extent than the retina.

Atrophy of choroid is almost always present. The choroid at the posterior pole gets atrophic especially in higher grades of myopia. The changes are essentially degenerative and not inflammatory in nature. The larger vessels become visible and the smaller meshwork disappears. There is attenuation of retina and the pigment epithelium. There is loss of pigment from the pigment epithelium which makes the choroidal vessels prominent and gives a tigroid appearance to the fundus. In later stages there is even total disappearance of choroidal tissue so that circumscribed white area of sclera becomes visible ophthalmoscopically. The patches later become pigmented at their borders due to proliferation of choroidal pigment. The area gives an appearance of a patch of chorio-retinitis (Fig. 16.7) and is hardly distinguishable from the end result of an inflammatory condition in spite of its being essentially degenerative in nature. These changes tend to occur most frequently in the centre and at the periphery.

The changes are most marked in the neighbourhood of the macula. There is chorioretinal atrophy, disturbance of pigment and alterations in vessels which aggregate into tufts. These appear as small red spots which are erroneously regarded as thrombotic or haemorrhagic spots. Later actual and local extensive haemorrhage may occur. Due to haemorrhages in the macular area there is gross diminution of vision which incapacitates the patient. A central circular dark spot (Förster-Fuchs's spot—Fig. 16.8) forms an occasional characteristic feature at the macula which is due to proliferation of pigment epithelium and is possibly associated with choroidal haemorrhage.

# PLATE II

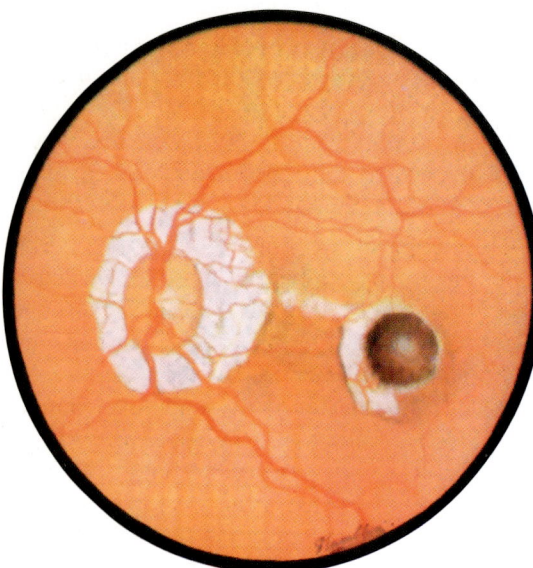

**Fig. 16.5.** Annular crescent

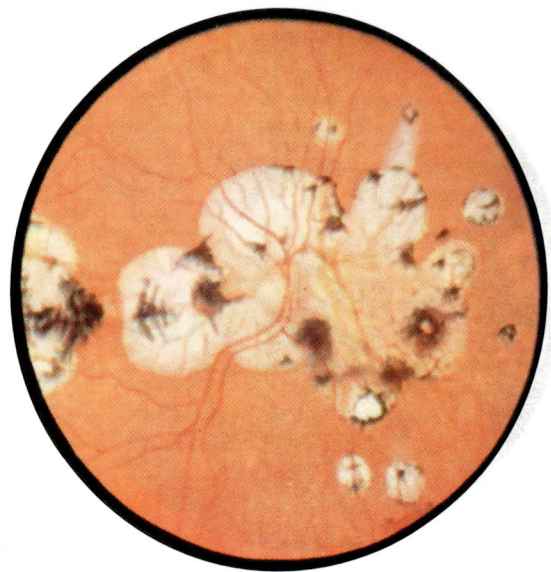

**Fig. 16.7.** Advanced degenerative changes.

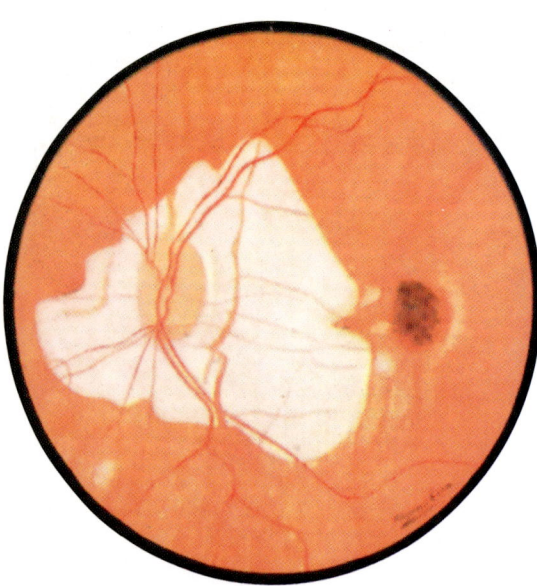

**Fig. 16.8.** Spread of degeneration around the disc towards the macular area at which there is a Förster-Fuchs's pigmented spot.

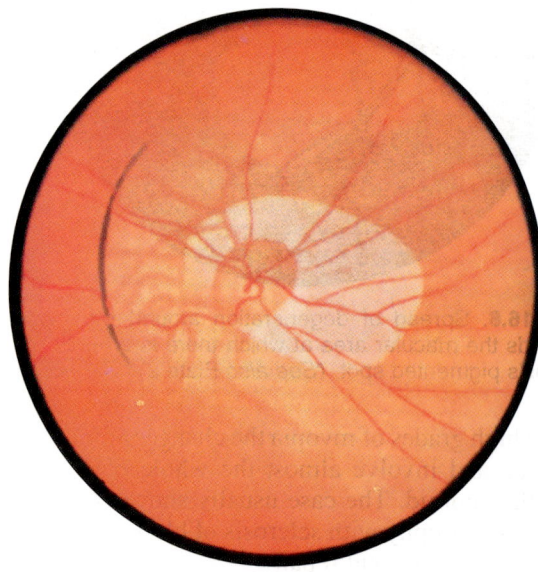

**Fig. 16.9.** Posterior staphyloma with a sharp ridge on the nasal side.

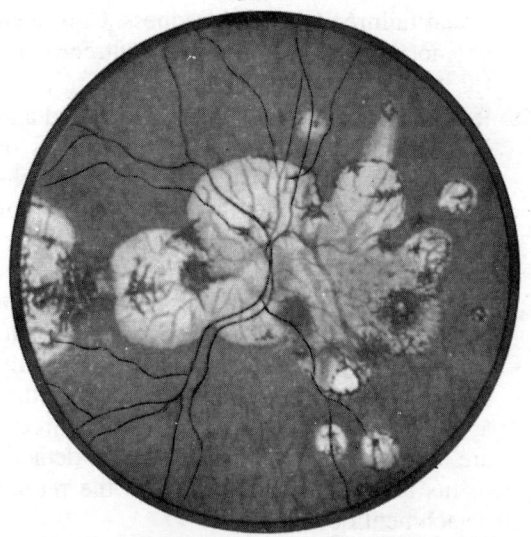

**Fig. 16.7.** Advanced degenerative changes. (*See als*
Plate 2)

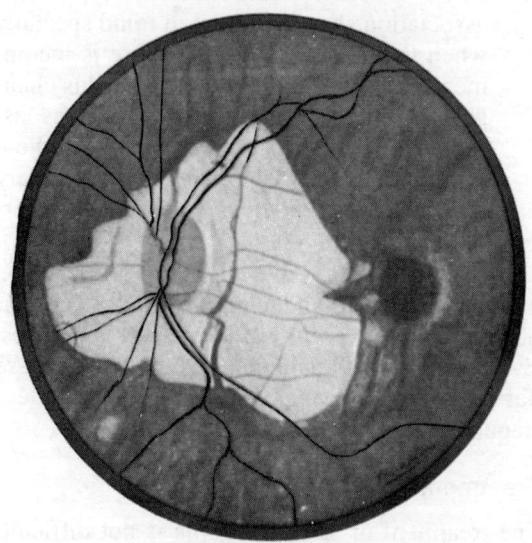

**Fig. 16.8.** Spread of degeneration around the disc
towards the macular area at which there is a Förster-
Fuchs's pigmented spot. (*See also* Plate 2)

In high grades of myopia the changes are more
marked and involve almost the whole of retina
and the choroid. The case usually shows diffuse
choroidal atrophy with sclerosis of blood vessels.
The lesion is beyond repair.

Similar changes appear at the periphery of
retina and are characterised by small patches of
atrophy and pigmentary proliferation anterior to
the equator. The retina may become adherent to
the vitreous by fibrous bands, traction by which
may result in a retinal hole, or, as is more
common there occurs a cystoid degeneration of
the retina which may give way leading to the
formation of a retinal hole.

The myopic changes take the form of tears and
haemorrhages in the retina and its extensive detachment. This may occur spontaneously and is usually
associated with lattice type of degeneration, snail
track lesions which are pulled off by the detached
vitreous which also shows degenerative changes.

The sclera shows ectasias and difference in
refraction at various parts of the fundus. In many
cases there is a localized ectasia near the disc and is
termed posterior staphyloma (Fig. 16.9). There is
an abrupt edge. It is ophthalmoscopically recognised as a dark line over which the retinal vessels
show a sudden kinking as they dip over its edges
and sometimes disappear from view as at the edge
of a glaucomatous cup. Sometimes ectasia extends
to the nasal side and presents as a sharp crescentic
linear shadow on the nasal side of the disc.

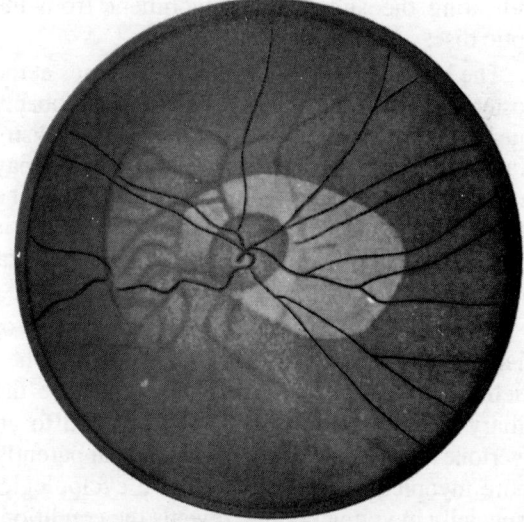

**Fig. 16.9.** Posterior staphyloma with a sharp ridge on
the nasal side. (*See also* Plate 2)

Vitreous degeneration commonly and almost
constantly appears in myopia. The vitreous shows
microfibrillar degeneration (Fig. 16.10) leading
to liquefaction and formation of micellar and

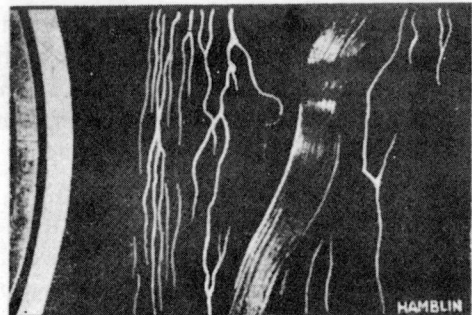

**Fig. 16.10.** Microfibrillar degeneration of vitreous.

bizarre shaped floating opacities. These give rise to disturbing entoptic phenomenon. The vitreous may show hyaloid holes and posterior detachment which can be detected ophthalmoscopically and more easily with biomicroscopic techniques. The detachment presents as reflex streak of Weiss which is a brilliant, crescentic, finely striated line on the nasal side of the disc but many a time can be demonstrated on the temporal side or even as a circular streak surrounding the posterior pole. In the posterior pole the vitreous face may show a condensation forming a grey membranous opacity frequently taking the form of a ring indicating the site of its detachment from the optic disc.

The lens may sometimes show opacities at the posterior pole. The lenticular changes are probably due to an aberration of lenticular metabolism. Nuclear changes are also not uncommon and may lead to aggravation of the myopic refraction. The lens may sometimes be tremulous which is probably due to overstretching of the zonular fibres.

As stated earlier myopes show a blurring of distance vision and comfort in near work. When such a patient is corrected for this distance the ciliary muscle is exercised and may lead to an overtone which makes an individual apparently more myopic. A correction under a cycloplegic, especially in young people, reveals the condition. In many previously uncorrected cases there is a lack of tone of ciliary muscles which pathologically presents as an atrophic change.

The complications of myopia are :

1. Choroidal thrombosis and haemorrhages, which are not uncommon, lead to gross visual failure and even blindness. Choroidal haemorrhage may leak into the vitreous and fill it with blood.

2. Retinal detachment is the most dreaded and one of the most common complications of myopia. The complication of retinal detachment like other factors and changes of myopia may be of genetic origin and independent of myopia itself. The exact mechanism of retinal detachment in myopia is ill-understood. It is in no way related to the degree of myopic change. It is essentially related to degenerative changes in the retina and the vitreous. The features of detachment are similar to other degenerative detachments as in senility. In myopes the retinal detachment occurs earlier.

3. Myopia is also associated with chronic simple glaucoma in some cases. The glaucoma is slow, insidious and of chronic type. This association should be kept in mind specially when the degree of visual failure is incommensurate with the degree and fundus changes of myopia. They are conditions associated with each other probably without any causal relationship. Both are hereditary and are independently genetically determined.

Myopia seems to have inhibitory influence on hypertensive and diabetic retinopathies. Vascular obstructions also occur less frequently in myopes. Even papilloedema is much less marked in these persons and angle closure glaucoma is less frequent.

**Treatment**

The treatment of simple myopia is not difficult. All it requires is a proper retinoscopy and correction of error by suitable glasses so that the rays which were convergent and focused in front of the retina are brought to a focus on the retina, i.e., from a to a' (Fig. 16.11).

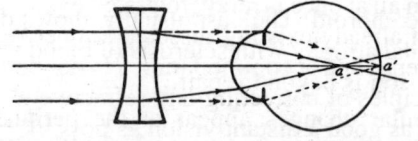

**Fig. 16.11.** Correction of myopia by concave lens.

An attempt should also be made to exclude the possibility of the disease being degenerative, a proposition by no means easy. Both simple and degenerative myopia may be hereditary. Perhaps ultrasonic measurements of the length of the eyeball at frequent intervals may provide the answer. For the time being heredity and rapid progress of the disease are important parameters. Besides these, disproportionate loss of vision, accentuated foveal reflex and disproportionate vitreous degeneration should arouse one's suspicion. A close follow-up of these cases should be done. The error should not be undercorrected. As far as possible, subject to the patient being comfortable, a full correction should be ordered. In the beginning constant wearing of spectacles should be ordered, but if after a lapse of considerable time it is established that it is stationary and simple, constant use of spectacles need not be insisted upon. Even for near work the use of glasses in earlier stages is important. This helps the eyes to perform the functions under normal relationship of convergence and accommodation.

The treatment of progressive myopia is difficult. There is no unanimity on the line of treatment to be adopted. Each prescriber treats the condition according to his own concepts of its etiology. Besides the correction of optical condition, the progress of the disease and its complications have to be considered, and attempts are necessary to prevent them if possible. Since the genesis of the disease is little understood and varied factors like heredity, nutrition, near work, endocrinal aberrations and general debility, singly or in combination, are said to contribute towards the progress of disease, the problem of treatment becomes more difficult. The most important amongst the lines of treatment is the correction of optical error.

### Correction of optical error

Should optical error be corrected in full? All are not agreed on this point. Full optical correction if given all at once is rarely tolerated by myopes due to an already existing dissociation between convergence and accommodation. No doubt the basic principles of correcting any refractive error is to give as good a distant vision as possible with the least degree of accommodative effort. A full cor-

rection of myopia is likely to produce excessive ciliary activity and may indirectly aid in the progress of myopia. Many young myopes are not comfortable for near work with full myopic correction. If the error is under-corrected the patients are left with a degree of myopia which may precipitate visual symptoms and it leaves behind lack of visual clarity. The patients are also not helped in coming out of their introvert personality. Some people are of the view that bifocals can be prescribed for near work. Neither seems to be the correct approach. The full correction of the refractive error should be the aim as it would aid mental and educational development by opening out the world for these young individuals besides giving them a proper orientation of their surroundings. The advocacy does not imply that full correction should be ordered at once but this may be achieved in two or three stages within six months to a year after fully explaining the problem to the patient and his parents. It is, therefore, advisable to begin with undercorrection and gradually build up the prescription to full correction. In the beginning the lenses which give the best vision with greatest comfort should be prescribed. Bifocals are not advocated as the full correction is intended to be prescribed in stages.

In very high myopes, where diminution in size of image and optical aberrations of correcting glasses make it difficult for the full corrections to be prescribed for work, contact lenses should be prescribed. These are more optically efficient. They comparatively increase the size of the image and help to eliminate the distortions and aberrations produced by high concave lenses. These have been found to be more effective in macular degeneration. In high myopes, due to the motivation of the patients, their tolerance is good and they are worn by them with comfort.

In cases which show considerable retinal damage and which show insignificant visual improvement either with conventional correcting spectacles or with contact lenses, it may be advisable to order for low vision aids like telescopic spectacles.

**Heredity :** In view of irrefutable evidence that myopia has a strong genetic bias, the hereditary transference to disease may be avoided by advising against marriage amongst two individuals with progressive myopia and if they marry they should be warned about their children having the possibility of developing progressive myopia. Theoretically it sounds excellent but it is seldom practised and the advice is almost never heeded. Consanguineous marriages should also be avoided in recessive hereditary traits. The children of myopes should be closely supervised and early treatment instituted.

**Nutrition :** Adequate care with regard to the diet of the myopes should be taken. It should be rich in vitamins, proteins, calcium and other minerals. The child should be advised to consume adequate amounts of vitamin D, green vegetables and milk.

**Near work :** Many people believe that near work, which requires both convergence and accommodation, favours the progress of the disease. Their assumption has no authentic proof and in all probability is incorrect. Limitation of near work leads to disruption and retardation in the educational progress of children and seems to be totally unjustified. Myopia schools were in vogue in some countries where an attempt was made to educate children by the cultivation of associated memory and sharpening of senses other than the visual sense. Sending of children to myopia schools creates in them a feeling of inferiority complex from other children going to normal schools, a state not conducive to well-being in the present competitive world. An adequate therapeutic regime would be development of good ocular and general hygienic habits. For near work there should be good and adequate illumination, avoidance of glare, easy and natural posture and clarity of print to avoid ocular fatigue. Children should be allowed to do near work. Adequate care should be taken to avoid stress and excessive near work. Care should be taken that children maintain good general health. Relaxation and open air

exercises are absolutely essential. In the modern world there is tendency to work in artificial light even when abundance of sunlight is available. Myopes should be encouraged to utilize more and more of sunlight for their work. Children's books should not be printed on highly reflecting paper like art paper. Small prints should also be discouraged.

**Endocrinal therapy :** Some people advocate that parathyroid hormone be given as it would help in better absorption and utilization of vitamin D. They feel that it will help in maintaining of calcium and phosphorus metabolism and balance. Placental implants and injections have been used by some workers and they claim good results in stemming the progress of myopia but in the hands of the author they have given disappointing results and they did not appear to stem the progress of the disease. No hormonal therapy is of any use in the treatment of myopia.

### Operative treatment

The two most important operative treatments consist of either removal of lens or the shortening of the eyeball. More recently support of the sclera and flattening of the cornea have been attempted. Details are given in chapter of refractive surgery (Chapter 18).

### Prognosis

If the degree of myopia is limited to not more than –6 D at 21 years of age further advance is unlikely. The prognosis of older cases is dependent upon the degree of degenerative changes.

Myopia stops progressing at the period of cessation of growth. In myopic women, with every pregnancy, myopia may advance further due to disturbed metabolic balance.

# CHAPTER 17

# Astigmatism

Astigmatism is defined as the optical condition of the eye where the power of refraction in two or more meridia differs. The light consequently cannot be brought to a point focus on retina. This is due to the presence of toroidal instead of spherical curvatures of the refracting surfaces of the eye and the change of curvature is gradual from one meridian to another and in uniform increments. Each meridian has a uniform type of curve (regular astigmatism). If, however, the curvature in different meridia is irregular and conforms to no geometrical figure the astigmatism is irregular. Irregular astigmatism may be due to one or more of the several factors.

**Corneal factors :** Keratoconus and old corneal scars due to ulcer or injuries produce irregular astigmatism. It can be easily seen when examined with a Placido's disc.

*Placido's disc :* It is a flat disc on which has been painted alternating black and white concentric rings which encircle a white aperture with a small lens (Fig. 17.1). The patient is placed with a strong light behind one shoulder, the cornea is observed through the central hole in the disc. The lens serves to magnify the image. The reflections of the ring are free of distortions if the cornea is normal curved otherwise there is distortion of rings (Fig. 17.2). For convenience of controlled illumination an electric Placido's disc has been designed. Photographic attachments have also been used to obtain keratographs.

**Optical densities :** Irregularity in optical densities of lens as in incipient cataract and irregularity in vitreous densities as in diabetes mellitus, produce irregular astigmatism.

**Choroidal neoplasms :** These, if situated in the macular area, may cause irregular astigma-

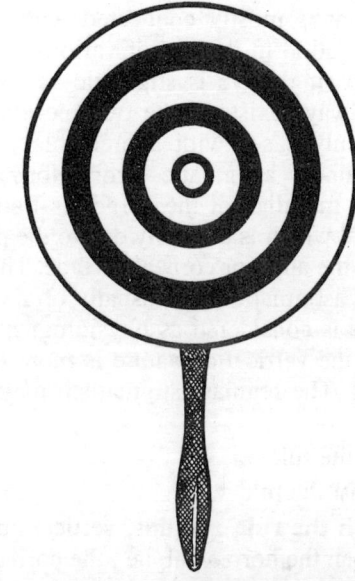

**Fig. 17.1.** Placido's disc.

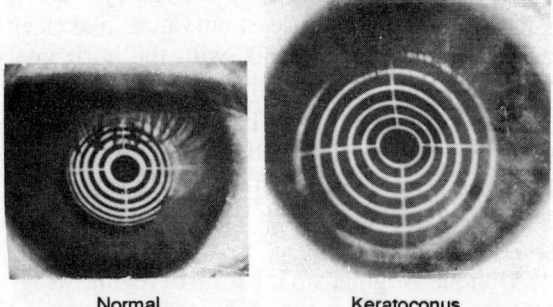

Normal        Keratoconus

**Fig. 17.2.** Pattern on cornea in normal and keratoconus.

tism due to an angular incidence of light rays on the retinal surface.

**Obliquity of retinal elements :** This may lead to an irregular astigmatism as is sometimes seen in posterior staphyloma.

## Regular astigmatism

In regular astigmatism there is a different refraction by the eye in two meridians at right angles to each other. Such a refractive state can be corrected by suitable spectacle lenses.

Regular astigmatism may be curvature or refractive in origin. Alterations in curvature of cornea (mostly the anterior surface), lens and decentring of optical systems of the eye account for a very large percentage of cases. Refractive astigmatism is mostly connected with the lens due to variation in density of various laminated zones. No single eye is stigmatic as some difference always exists in the two meridia but in practice only cases with appreciable error are included under astigmatic error. Normally the horizontal meridian of the cornea is flatter than the vertical which is probably due to the pressure of lids on the anterior corneal surface. This leads to a small astigmatic error, usually of about 0.12 D but this is considered as physiological. It implies that the vertical curvature is more than the horizontal. The regular astigmatism may, therefore, be

1. with the rule, or
2. against the rule.

1. **With the rule :** In this, vertical curvature is more than the horizontal, i.e., the correction of this astigmatism will require the prescription of a concave cylinder at 180° or a convex cylinder at 90°. If the meridian of least curvature makes an angle of not more than 30° with the horizontal plane the astigmatism is still with the rule.

2. **Against the rule :** In this, the horizontal curvature is greater than the vertical curvature, i.e., the correction of astigmatism will require the prescription of a concave cylinder at 90° or a convex cylinder at 180°.

Oblique astigmatism is a form of regular astigmatism where two meridia are not horizontal and vertical though still at right angles to each other. If the axes are not at right angles to each other yet the difference is seen only in two meridia, the error should be termed as bi-oblique.

The optical conditions in astigmatism obey the principles of differential refraction. The images formed in different position of the retina are given in Fig. 17.3. A line appears distinct to an astig-

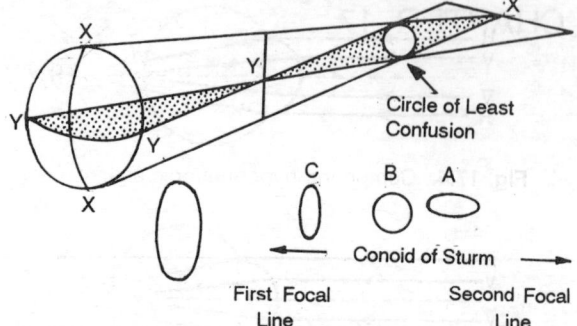

**Fig. 17.3.** Astigmatic interval of a sphero-cylindrical lens.

matic eye when it is parallel to the meridian of the eye which is ametropic to its distance and is indistinct when it has the same direction as the meridian which is emmetropic to its distance. The phenomenon is easy to explain. If either of the principal meridians is emmetropic to its luminous point the latter forms in the retina a line or diffusion image or a focal line which is perpendicular to the emmetropic and parallel to the ametropic meridian. The line is distinct in the ametropic plane because elongated images of diffusion of all points composing the line coincide with the line image itself. On this principle is based the subjective examination of astigmatism though an objective assessment of the refractive state is desirable. Instead of a focal point there are two foci in the form of the lines, i.e., the two focal lines. The interval between the two focal lines represents the focal interval. The focal interval is the degree of measure of astigmatism. Astigmatism is further classified according to the position of retinal percipient elements in relation to these two points. If the retinal percipient elements are situated at a position between the two focal lines, the astigmatism is classified as mixed. Otherwise it is either myopic or hypermetropic. Based on this the regular astigmatism is classified as :

**Hypermetropic :** When the retinal percipient elements are situated in front of the focal lines. If they are in front of both the focal lines the astigmatism is called compound hypermetropic astigmatism (Fig. 17.4). If the retinal percipient elements are situated at one of the focal points and in front of the other focal point, the astigmatism is termed simple hypermetropic astigmatism (Fig. 17.5).

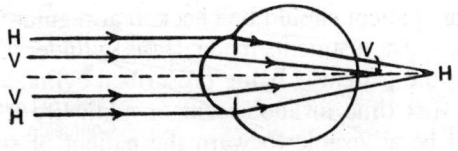

**Fig. 17.4.** Compound hypermetropic astigmatism.

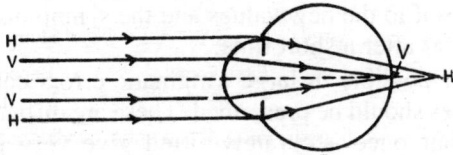

**Fig. 17.5.** Simple hypermetropic astigmatism.

**Myopic :** When the retinal percipient ele-ments are situated behind the focal lines. If the retinal elements are situated on one of the focal lines and the other focal line is in front of these elements the astigmatism is termed simple myopic astigmatism (Fig. 17.6).

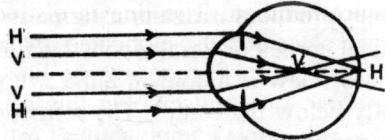

**Fig. 17.6.** Simple myopic astigmatism.

If both the focal lines are in front of the retinal elements, the astigmatism is termed compound myopic astigmatism (Fig. 17.7).

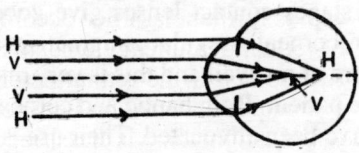

**Fig. 17.7.** Compound myopic astigmatism.

**Mixed :** In mixed astigmatism one of the focal lines is in front of the retina and the other is behind the retina (Fig. 17.8).

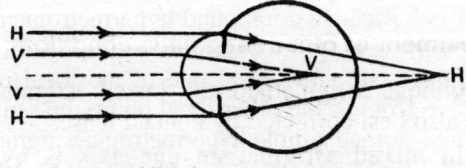

**Fig. 17.8.** Mixed astigmatism.

Regular astigmatism like other refractive errors is inherited but the mode of inheritance is not certain. It is generally believed to be autosomal dominant with incomplete penetrance and variable expressibility.

### Incidence

Astigmatism occurs with equal frequency in both sexes and in about 50% of all cases of refractive errors provided physiological astigmatism is not taken in the computation of these figures. The most common type of astigmatism is compound myopic astigmatism, followed by compound hypermetropic, mixed and simple myopic astig-matism. In most of the cases astigmatism is less than 1.5 D. Higher degree of astigmatism is not more than 20% of all cases of astigmatic errors. In 60% of the cases it is between 1 and 1.5 D.

Frequently a symmetry of astigmatism be-tween the two eyes exists. This relates not only to the degree of the refractive error but also to the axis. Mostly the axes of both eyes are parallel to each other or alternatively the sum of the two axes is 180°. Astigmatism is more frequently with the rule in the younger and against the rule in the elder population.

Accommodation may alter the nature of the image appreciably by varying the position of focal lines. An increase occurs in amount of astig-matism and a change in axis on accommodation. The increase in degree of astigmatism is about 10%. The exact mechanism by which this takes place is by no means unequivocally established.

### Clinical picture

The chief complaints of astigmatism are visual disability and severe eye strain with varying degrees of headache which is due to constant effort to see clearly. In low grade of astigmatism the visual disability is minimal but in higher grades there is dimness of vision, blurring and even distortion of objects leading to considerable visual disability. The patient makes an attempt to focus one meridian clearly and the meridian nearest to emmetropia is chosen. More often than not patient exhibits a preference for the vertical meridian. To obtain distinct vision in low grades of astigmatism efforts of accommodation put a considerable strain in the eyeball, and lead to symptoms of asthenopia. There is drowsiness, headache, dull pain in and around the eyeball, dizziness, nervousness and sometimes nausea. In a few cases even convulsions may appear. In higher errors of astigmatism since efforts of the patient are not likely to ameliorate the visual disability, no such attempts are made, the patient suffers only from visual disability and there is complete absence of asthenopic symptoms. In low errors besides the symptoms already described, there may be burning and itching sensation in the eye. The patient may constantly rub the eye which may result in the falling of the lashes, hyperaemia of the lids and squamous blepharitis. The constant rubbing may introduce infection leading to occurrence of recurrent chalazia and styes. An occasional head tilt may be seen in the direction of the axis of the cylinder to reduce distortion of objects caused by the obliquity of the axis. This habit may result in permanent torticollis. In all the cases there is a tendency to close the lids partly to produce a stenopaic slit to improve the visual performance. Patients wearing corrections have a tendency to wear the lenses inclined to the plane of the eye at some odd angle.

## Treatment

The basic principles of correction of refractive errors like myopia and hypermetropia are equally applicable to the correction of astigmatic errors. Small errors produce symptoms. Meticulous subjective and objective testing should be done and a full correction ordered. In larger astigmatic errors there are considerable difficulties in effecting corrections. Asymmetric corrections between the two eyes leads to an artificial heterophoria when looking through lenses in any position except through the centre of the lens. In cylindrical errors there is a change in the size of image depending upon whether it is a plus lens (magnified) or a minus lens (diminished). There is also a distortion of image in the meridian of greater power besides their rotatory displacements. The difficulties are accentuated if the axes are oblique which may lead to distressing feelings. In order to diminish these the patient resorts to cyclotorsions, aniseikonic compensations in fusion and psychological indifference. In high astigmatic

errors patient should be checked at regular intervals and adjustments made. If the cylinder is high or if the patient is being prescribed cylinders for the first time in adolescent or adult life it may well be advisable to warn the patient of spatial distortions like ups and downs in the floor, and tilting of horizontal surfaces. The patient adjusts himself to the new values and the symptoms disappear after a short time.

If possible in large astigmatic errors contact lenses should be prescribed. These are difficult to fit but once accurately fitted give very good results provided the astigmatism is corneal in origin.

## Irregular astigmatism

This is usually seen in pathological conditions of the cornea and in curvature type of astigmatism. Index type of irregular astigmatism is due to lenticular changes especially during the process of maturation of cataract. Tilting of lens also sometimes produces irregular astigmatism.

Conical cornea or keratoconus from the optical point of view is a conical bulge whose apex is slightly below the centre. The refraction is irregular and usually a high degree of irregular myopic astigmatism is present. The condition is usually progressive and presents difficulties in optical correction.

## Treatment of keratoconus

In early stages contact lenses give good optical results in corneal irregular astigmatism but later on they are of no avail and this is very disappointing to the patient. Both haptic and corneal contact lenses have been advocated. Their use is credited with arresting the progress of keratoconus but this seems unlikely. In case contact lenses fail to provide relief and corneal opacities prevent optical correction keratoplasty is the only treatment in spite of indifferent results in some cases. Excimer laser therapy is useful.

## Treatment of other astigmatic conditions

Bi-oblique astigmatism and mixed astigmatism are also best corrected by contact lenses.

In mixed astigmatism one axis is hypermetropic and the other is myopic. It does present certain difficulties in prescribing glasses. Two sets can possibly be prescribed. Either the myopic or the hypermetropic axis is first corrected by a suitable spherical lens. Other axis is then corrected by an appropriate cylindrical lens.

Let us illustrate this by an example.

Horizontal axis +3 D and vertical axis –2 D.

Now if we correct the horizontal axis first by a +3 D spherical lens we make the vertical axis more myopic by an identical strength over and above its original error, i.e., the vertical axis now becomes –5 D which can be corrected by placing a concave cylinder of 5 D with its axis in the horizontal direction. The prescription will read as :

$$\frac{+3 \text{ D sph.}}{-5 \text{ D cyl.} \rightarrow 180°} \qquad ...(\text{i})$$

In the other set of glasses if we correct the vertical axis by a suitable sphere of –2 D this will result in an increase in hypermetropia in the horizontal axis by the like strength. This can be corrected suitably by a convex cylinder placed in the vertical direction. The prescription will read as :

$$\frac{-2 \text{ D sph.}}{+5 \text{ D cyl.} \downarrow 90°} \qquad ...(\text{ii})$$

Looking at (i) and (ii) one can realise that given the one the other can be easily worked out. This change from one to the other is termed transposition of the lenses. This can be achieved by the following formula.

"The power of new sphere is the algebraical summation of the power of the old sphere and the old cylinder (i.e., a sum of +3 D and –5 D = –2 D) and the new cylinder has the same power as the old cylinder but has the opposite sign (i.e., –5 D cyl. becomes +5 D cyl.) and is placed at right angles to the axis of the old cylinder (i.e., instead of at 180° the new cylinder is placed at 90°).

Surgery for astigmatism is being attempted and gaining some popularity (see Chapter 18).

# Refractive Surgery

Attempts have been made to correct the refractive state of the eye by resorting to either surgical or laser therapy. Hypermetropia, myopia and astigmatism all have been subjected to these interventions. Only short references are given and the reader is referred to refractive surgery books for greater details.

## SURGERY FOR MYOPIA

The surgical interventions for myopia are basically divided into two groups :

### Operations on the cornea

#### Keratomileusis

The aim of the operation is to carve out on the exposed substantia propria of the cornea a frozen parallel placed lamellar corneal disc removed from the patient's ametropic eye a tissue lens of the exact value and opposite to the ametropia and its interlamellar replacement are fashioned and implanted. As a hundredth of a millimetre is the unit of tolerance, it is evident that this operation requires great care and mathematical precision. It is claimed that it can correct 15 to 20 dioptres of myopia.

The disc removed is immersed in a special solution for 3 minutes with its epithelial side in contact with a lathe base to which it is firmly fixed and hardened by freezing. The disc is then carved out by lathe cutting and it is thawed by gentle irrigation with isotonic physiological solution at room temperature and is then reattached.

It is a difficult operation and requires very expensive instrumentation and great skill. It has almost been abandoned. Even where these cryolathe machines were purchased they are stacked in ophthalmic museums.

#### Keratophakia

The second operation on the cornea is keratophakia. The purpose of this operation is to carve, by the same technique as keratomileusis, a corneal tissue lens which may be either concave or convex, from the centre of donor's cornea. Epithelium and Bowman's membrane are removed. Sections of 7.5 mm and 0.25 mm in thickness are preferred for correction of myopia.

The cornea is incised, and with a circular corneal knife an intralamellar space is cleaved of sufficient diameter to accommodate the corneal tissue lens. After insertion of this the corneal incision is closed by 10/0 sutures.

This operation can also be done for hypermetropia where a graft of 8.0 mm diameter and thickness of 0.38 to 0.45 mm is utilised.

#### Epikeratophakia

The operation is similar to keratophakia except that instead of an intralamellar pocket, a pocket is fashioned under the edge of the epithelium where the cryolathed donor homograft is inserted.

In the market pre-shaped lenticules are available.

#### Keratectomy and homoplastic surgery

In this operation a partial keratectomy is followed by replacement of corneal lenticule of appropriate dioptric power, from where epithelium has been removed, is prepared by the surgeon as for keratomileusis. Pre-shaped corneal lenticules are also available.

It is claimed that this can correct up to 25 D myopia. The results are, however, not as satisfactory as with autografts.

## Corneal inlays

Intracorneal acrylic implants into the stroma have been used for the purpose. They are specifically shaped implants. These inlays can also be made of polysulphones or hydrogels.

## Radial keratotomy

Radial keratotomy is becoming more popular as an operation for correcting myopia. It aims at flattening the anterior corneal surface for the purpose of decreasing myopia and astigmatism.

For the operation to succeed the cuts should be as deep as possible yet macro-perforations should be avoided. In best hands micro-perforations do occur which prove to be of little consequence. The incisions must be at least to 2/3 depth of cornea.

With refinement of pachometers and their computerization the corneal depth measurements have become more precise. These measurements help the surgeon to go to the desired depth. Similarly with the use of sharp calibrated diamond knives clean cut incisions can be made. The calibration of these knives is so designed that once adjusted it will not go beyond the desired depth.

The surgery is performed under topical anaesthesia with a wire lid speculum in place. The corneal diameter is measured. The visual axis is located and the optical zone of the cornea marked (Fig. 18.1). The corneal thickness is measured by an ultrasonic pachometer in four positions on the

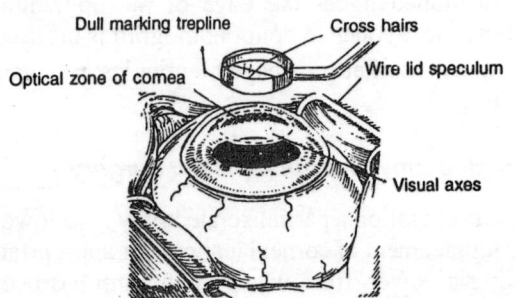

**Fig. 18.1.** Marking of optical zone (Stage 1 of radial keratotomy).

circular mark around the clear zone. The knife is set at the thinnest of these paracentral readings (Figs. 18.2, 18.3 and 18.4). The surgeon fixes the globe with a double-pronged forceps and marks

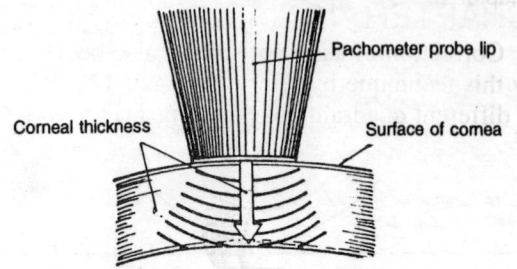

**Fig. 18.2.** Pachometry (Stage 2 of radial keratotomy).

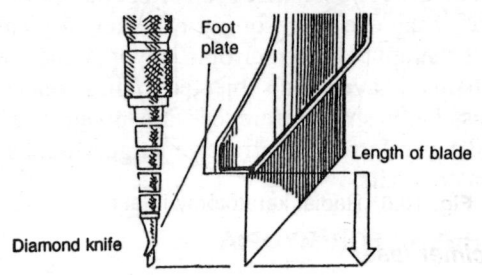

**Fig. 18.3.** Setting of diamond knife at thinnest zone of cornea (Stage 3 of radial keratotomy).

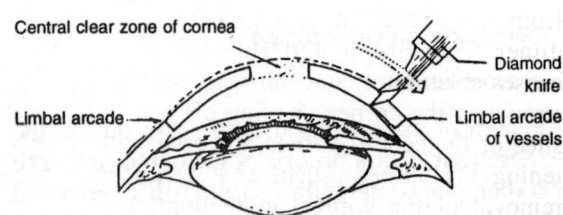

**Fig. 18.4.** Cutting of the deepest part of cornea without perforating it (Stage 4 of radial keratotomy).

4 to 16 radial cuts as desired (Fig. 18.5). These cuts extend from central clear zone to the limbal vascular arcade.

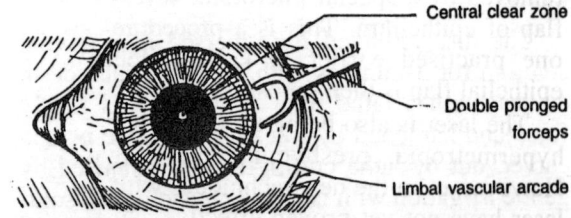

**Fig. 18.5.** Making 4 to 16 radial cuts in cornea (Stage 5 of radial keratotomy).

Earlier 16 or more cuts were made but several surgeons now make only 4 cuts. There is, however, no limit to the number of cuts and it is left to the judgement of the operating surgeon.

Correction of astigmatism has also been done by this technique by altering the number of cuts in different quadrants of the cornea (Fig. 18.6).

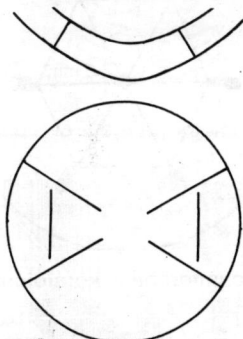

**Fig. 18.6.** Radial keratotomy in astigmatism.

### Excimer laser

It is a surface-ablating and tissue-disruptive laser.

This laser operates at 193 nm ultraviolet light from the excitation of argon-fluoride (excited dimer from argon and fluorine gases). This causes ablation of concentric areas of superficial stroma of the cornea shaving off a microscopic slice of the central cornea and reshaping it flattening the corneal surface. It is applied after removal of the corneal epithelium. It is being accepted more and more and the results are encouraging.

The only limitation seems to be the prohibitive cost of the laser machine.

Lasik procedure for high myopia is now being practised in which a superficial disc of stroma is removed by a special microtome after cutting a flap of epithelium. This is a procedure like the one practised earlier in keratomileusis. The epithelial flap is then reposited.

The laser is also being used for correction of hypermetropia, presbyopia and astigmatism. However, even the new techniques with excimer laser have not yet proven effective and safe for hyperopia (hypermetropia) correction.

### Holmium laser

It is a laser which operates in the infrared zone. Like neodymium, holmium is a rare earth element and utilises YAG crystal (yttrium, aluminium and garnet).

Its use in correction of refractive errors is still in experimental stage.

## NON-CORNEAL INTERVENTIONS

The second group of operation are either on the lens or on the sclera.

### Operations on the lens

#### Lens extraction

In very high myopia several surgeons are removing the clear lens. This operation was fraught with complications when intracapsular extraction was in vogue as it caused vitreous prolapse, retinal detachments and cystoid macular oedema. Vitreous being fluid in most of the cases vitreous prolapse into anterior chamber was quite common. It is based on the optical principle that if in a myopia of 25 D lens is removed the eye becomes emmetropic.

With the advent of intraocular implants and planned extracapsular cataract extraction (ECCE) the operation has become less hazardous.

The operation has the following disadvantages :

1. Loss of accommodation.
2. Increase in size of retinal image.

#### Anterior chamber lens implantation

A concave lens of appropriate lens power is implanted into the anterior chamber without interfering with the patient's own lens. Theoretically it is a good idea but in practice it suffers from all the drawbacks of anterior chamber IOL implantation, particularly the corneal endothelial decompensation and angle changes. Although early visual results are good yet in view of the complications stated above and which are of a severe nature the procedure is not recommended.

### Surgery on the sclera

**Scleral shortening :** In view of the progression of the posterior segment pathology scleral shortening operations have been recommended. The operation helps to restrict the axial length of the eyeball, the tension in the choroidal and retinal vessels is lessened and the nutrition of these membranes is thereby improved, possible haemorrhages are prevented and degenerative changes are checked. The shortening is achieved by an annular scleral resection. However, the end results over a period of time do not justify this procedure.

**Scleral support :** As a preventive support to the sclera by strips of tendons, fascia lata or scleral implants have been resorted to. The results are, however, not encouraging and the procedures are not recommended.

Combined corneal surgery and tension reducing operation

Radial keratotomy along with operations for reduction of intraocular tension are advocated and practised by some. They claim excellent results in growing children to stop the progression of myopia. However, such a procedure is erratic, results are unpredictable and it is hazardous. The same is not recommended.

## Prophylactic laser or cryosurgery

This is a useful method to prevent retinal detachment. For indications and techniques the reader is referred to surgery for detachment of retina.

## Surgery for hypermetropia

The operations for this condition are again grouped into two :
1.  Surgery on the cornea
2.  Non-corneal interventions

**Surgery on cornea :** It is essentially a thermo-keratoplasty on the cornea. A regular hexagon is marked (Fig. 18.7) around the optical zone reaching the mid-periphery. On the angles of the

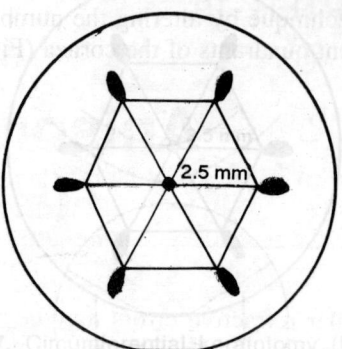

**Fig. 18.7.** Circumferential keratotomy (hexagonal keratotomy).

hexagon burns are made with cautery going to the stroma. When these burns heal, the periphery is flattened and in the central part of the cornea the corneal curvature is increased. In many cases observed by the author over a period of time the corneal opacities are considerably, if not totally, resolved and the visual results are fairly satisfactory particularly in aphakia.

**Non-corneal intervention :** Anterior chamber convex lenses are being implanted in high hypermetropia but as for myopia they produce endothelial damage and angle change.

Piggy back convex lenses on the patient's own lens are being tried but they are too experimental to comment on. The danger of pupillary block glaucoma is real.

Excimer and holmium lasers are being used more frequently and the results are quite encouraging. It will take some time for the procedure to get established.

# CHAPTER 19

# Anisometropia and Aniseikonia (Binocular Optical Defects)

Uniocular refractive errors may be amenable to correction and the patient may have good uniocular vision in each eye after correction. Binocularly he may be uncomfortable in spite of correction. The refractive errors should also be considered in relation to binocular functions. These basically are :

1. A difference in the refraction between the two eyes (anisometropia),

2. A difference in the size of the two images formed on the two retinas (aniseikonia), and

3. A disturbance in the muscular balance particularly the two images not falling on the corresponding retinal areas.

In this chapter it is proposed to discuss the first two and the third one will be described in later chapters.

## Anisometropia

If the refraction in the two eyes is equal the refraction is termed isometropia. An ideal isometropic person is rare. If the total refraction of the two eyes is unequal the refractive state is termed as anisometropia. There is some degree of anisometropia almost always present. In smaller degree of anisometropia binocular vision is not interfered with. Each 0.25 D difference in refractive error causes 0.5% difference in the size of two retinal images. A difference of more than 4.6% is rarely tolerated with ease. With higher degree of anisometropia fusion is not possible. It is this anisometropia which is clinically more troublesome.

1. **Simple :** In which one eye is normal and the other eye is either hypermetropic (simple hypermetropic) or myopic (simple myopic).

2. **Compound :** In which both eyes are ametropic, either hypermetropic (compound hypermetropic) or myopic (compound myopic).

3. **Mixed :** In this both eyes are ametropic. One eye is myopic while the other is hypermetropic. This is also called antimetropia.

4. **Simple astigmatic anisometropia :** When one eye is emmetropic and the other has either simple myopic astigmatism or simple hypermetropic astigmatism.

5. **Compound astigmatic anisometropia :** When both eyes are astigmatic but of unequal degree.

6. **Mixed astigmatic anisometropia :** When both eyes are astigmatic but one eye has myopic astigmatism and the other eye has hypermetropic astigmatism.

**Classification of anisometropia**

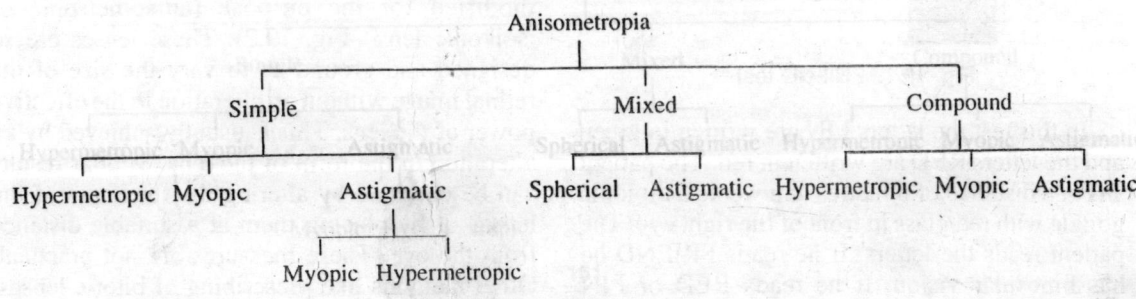

Anisometropia may be congenital or acquired. Acquired type is due to either uniocular disease or injury (operative or traumatic scars). Congenital anisometropia is associated with differential growth of the eyeball either associated with or without the developmental anomalies of the face. It is hereditary in origin but the mode and mechanism of this transmission is not known.

In young anisometrope, whose one eye is emmetropic, the size of the image of an object placed at reading distance or the image of an object at the far point of a myopic eye may be sufficient to interfere with binocular functions.

A difference of more than four dioptres in the refractive power of the two eyes usually interferes with binocular vision and makes fusion almost impossible and tolerance very difficult. Before the glasses are prescribed and after correction is given, one should make sure that the two eyes are functioning simultaneously. FRIEND test (Fig. 19.1) is a simple device by which this can be easily assessed.

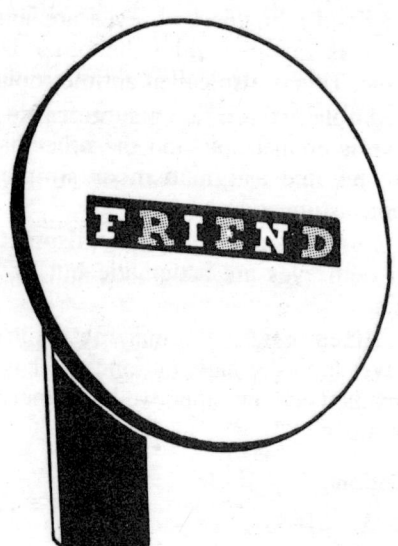

**Fig. 19.1.** FRIEND test.

In this test the letters FIN are written in green and the letters RED are written in red. The patient sits at a distance of 6 metres and wears a diplopia goggle with red glass in front of the right eye. The patient reads the letters. If he reads FRIEND he has binocular vision. If he reads RED or FIN

persistently he has uniocular vision with the eye having the corresponding glass. If he reads FIN at one time and RED at others, he has got alternating vision. Alternating vision is likely to occur when both eyes have good visual acuity. In these cases one eye is usually hypermetropic and the other myopic (antimetropia). In these cases one eye is usually used for distance (hypermetropic eye) and the other for near myopic eye. The patient is so comfortable in this that he seldom seeks any optical aid.

**Treatment**

The refractive error has to be corrected by glasses. It would be easy to settle small differences of refractive power by the prescription of ordinary spectacle lenses. If we can place the lens at the anterior focal plane of the eye to be corrected, there is no change in the size of the image but in practice it is not possible to place lens at this distance. If the lenses are nearer to the eye than this distance, then the size of the retinal image is diminished with convex and enlarged with concave lenses. If the lenses are farther from the anterior focal plane the image is diminished with concave lenses and increased with convex. Difficulties arise from irregularities of peripheral distortion, where ordinary correcting lenses are employed. Artificial heterophoria is created when the pupillary centre does not coincide with the optical centre of the lens. A prismatic effect is produced when the eyes move to either direction from the primary position. The problems are, therefore, many and the solutions are inadequate. No rule of thumb procedure can be laid down for the treatment of these cases and each case may be considered on its own. The anisometropic discomfort can sometimes be reduced or abolished with the use of suitable lenses especially modified for the purpose (anisometropic or isoikonic lens—Fig. 19.2). These lenses are so designed and ground as to vary the size of the retinal image without an alteration in the effective power of the lens. This is usually achieved by an alteration in the form of the lens. Similar results can be obtained by altering the thickness of the lenses or by placing them at a suitable distance from the eye. These measures are not practical. Other methods like prescribing of bitoric lenses,

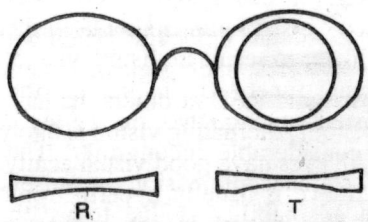

**Fig. 19.2.** Anisometropic lens.

which include air space between the two curves, has been claimed to be useful. These are rather difficult to manufacture and are now seldom in use.

In children under the age of 12 every attempt should be made to induce the full correction to be worn; the younger the child the more persistent should be the attempt, the easier it may prove, the more successful may be the result.

In the experience of the author, however, it is easier said than done. Children seldom use these glasses.

Contact lenses offer the solution to many of the problems of anisometropia and are now being frequently used. Artificial heterophoria and to a great extent aniseikonia are eliminated, myopic anisometropia is no exception. In order to avoid the occurrence of amblyopia and promote the development of binocular vision, extended wear contact lenses are being quite frequently used in children by some even in infancy.

Anisometropia may be treated by any of the operations or combination of operations described in the chapter of refractive surgery (Chapter 18). Excimer laser surgery may be the ultimate answer.

## Aniseikonia

Aniseikonia is defined as the condition wherein the images presented to the cortex from the two retinas are abnormally unequal in size or shape. In general terms aniseikonia includes all the incongruities of the ocular images. The images which are formed in the two eyes are carried to the brain. They are, as stated above, unequal in size and/or shape. The anomaly becomes apparent only in binocular vision. This may not be strictly true as diminution or increase in size and distortion in shape may be uniocularly appreciated. Such a state of uniocular distortion is not included under the generic name of aniseikonia which is essentially a disturbance of binocular function.

### Classification

Aniseikonia may be classified as difference in size (symmetrical) or difference in shape (asymmetrical).

**Symmetrical :** This type of aniseikonia is further classified into :

*Overall :* In this the size of one ocular image is symmetrically larger than the other.

*Meridional :* In this the size of retinal image of one eye is symmetrically larger or smaller than that of the other in one meridian only, i.e., vertical, horizontal or oblique; or the retinal image of one eye is symmetrically larger in one meridian and smaller in another than that of the other eye.

*Compound :* In which a combination of overall and meridional difference is manifest.

**Asymmetrical :** This is of three types :

*General :* There is a progressive increase or decrease in size across the visual field.

*Pincushion or barred type :* In this type there is a progressive increase or decrease in all directions from the visual axis.

*Irregular :* In this warping may occur or may have combination of any of the above.

### Aetiology

The aniseikonia may be

1. **Optical :**

### Classification of aniseikonia

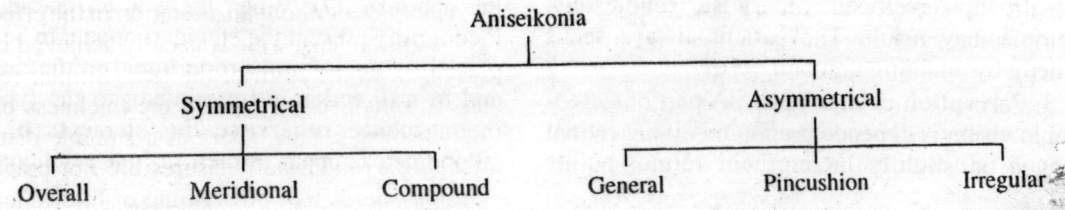

(a) *Inherent* : Due to defects in the dioptric system of the eye and is usually related to anisometropia.

(b) *Acquired* : This depends upon the correction lenses worn, their power, position, thickness and form. Cylinders create aniseikonia by introducing meridional size differences.

2. **Anatomical :** This may be due to :

(a) Displacement of retinal elements towards the nodal point in the eye.

(b) Separation of neuro-epithelial elements of the retina.

(c) Stretching or oedema of the retina.

3. **Central :** The asymmetrical simultaneous perception in spite of equal size of images formed in the retina.

## Symptoms

The symptoms may be :

1. Subjective of eye strain.
2. Disturbance of binocular vision.
3. Disturbances of stereoscopic spatial functions.

1. **Subjective symptoms :** These symptoms are characteristically those of asthenopia. Ocular discomfort, itching, lacrimation, blurred vision, fixation difficulties, heaviness of eye and ocular fatigue and are quite common. Visual fatigue is particularly evident when seeing moving objects, e.g., motion pictures and while concentrating for near work. Frontal and other forms of headache with general fatigue, irritability, lack of concentration, nausea, nervous tension, etc. are common features.

2. **Binocular vision :** The disturbance of binocular vision occurs only if the difference between the two retinal images exceeds 5%. A difference lower than this can be compensated, even though with effort by the adaptability of perceptual visual processes. The disturbance of binocular function adopts the form of suppression in one eye at an early age if binocular vision has not already developed; otherwise troublesome diplopia may result. The patient always seeks remedy by attaining uniocularity.

3. **Perception of the depth :** A part of stereoscopic vision is dependent upon receiving retinal images on slightly incongruent retinal points

which results in physiological aniseikonia. Any disturbance caused by aniseikonia in this incongruity is likely to result in disturbance of stereoscopic visual functions. In practice the stereoscopic visual function has the ability to adapt itself to considerable incongruity. The disturbance of stereoscopic vision in aniseikonia is rare. The adaptability is due to psychological interpretations (based on experience) of the perceptual depth. If the patient is transferred to surroundings in which uniocular perception occurs, as in aviation or in motoring, resulting in diplopia, ocular fatigue and accidents. The condition of instability is comparable to a latent heterophoria which becomes manifest when fusion is lost. In both cases the defect is present all the time but is elicited only in special circumstances.

## Clinical measurement

The degree of aniseikonia can be measured by eikonometer. This instrument is based on the principle of preventing fusion by presenting dissimilar objects of the same size of such a design that discrepancy between them could be easily assessed. Based on this principle a space eikonometer has been developed. Three clinical measurements are taken, i.e.,

1. Image size difference in horizontal meridian,
2. Image size difference in the vertical meridian, and
3. Correction of inclination which is indicative of meridional aniseikonia.

The space eikonometer and its principle are shown in Figs. 19.3 to 19.9. Space eikonometer consists of four vertical lines (A, B, C, D) arranged two in front and two behind a cross consisting of two cords at right angles (F and G) through the centre of which a vertical limb (E) passes at point Q (Fig. 19.4). The whole is viewed through a test lens unit (L) upon a uniform background (T). The patient directs his gaze through the aperture (O). When there is an anomalous incongruity present the elements appear to be displaced by an amount proportional to the degree and in a direction corresponding to the type of incongruence otherwise the elements of the eikonometer appear in their normal relationship.

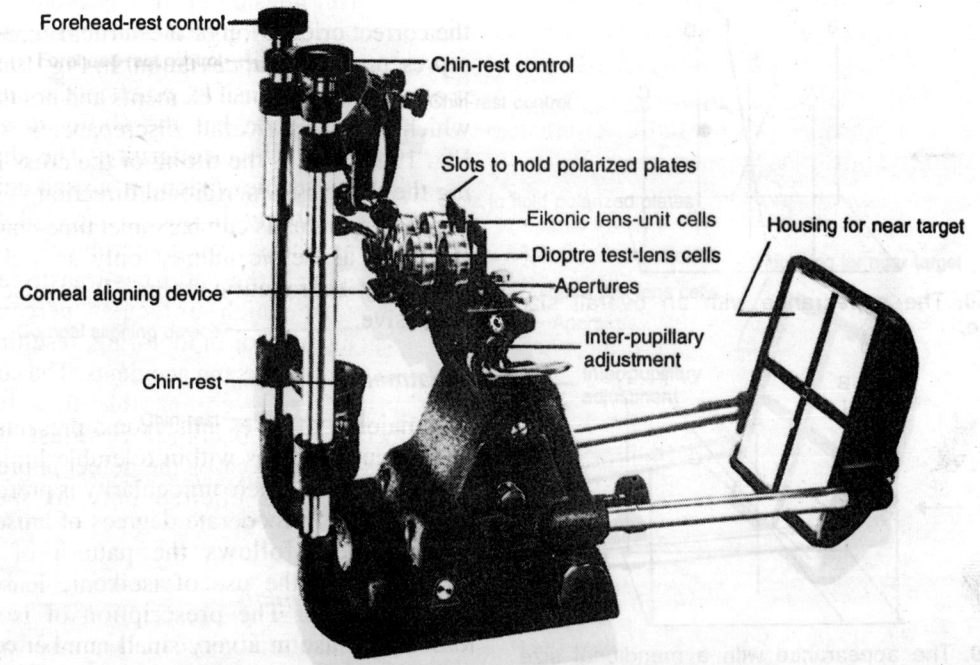

**Fig. 19.3.** The standard eikonometer (American Optical Co.).

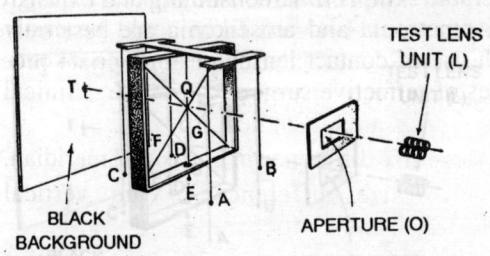

**Fig. 19.4.** The structure of the space eikonometer.

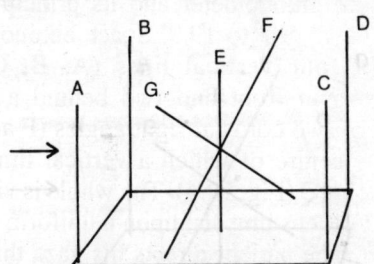

**Fig. 19.5.** The normal appearance.

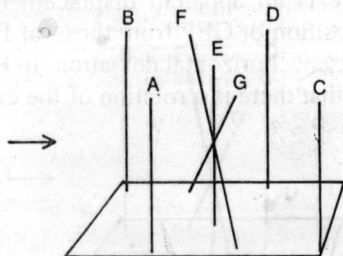

**Fig. 19.6.** The appearance with a horizontal size difference.

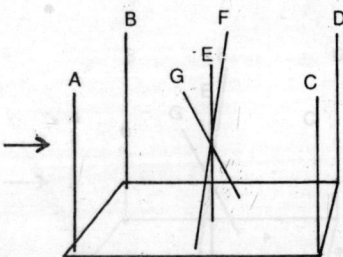

**Fig. 19.7.** Appearance with vertical difference.

The incongruity can be corrected by appropriate isoikonic lenses from a special trial case.

To be able to comprehend the above statement

look at Fig. 19.5. There is no displacement and this represents the normal appearance. In Fig.

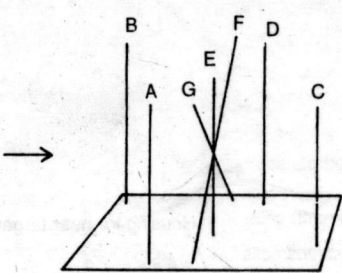

**Fig. 19.8.** The appearance with an overall size difference.

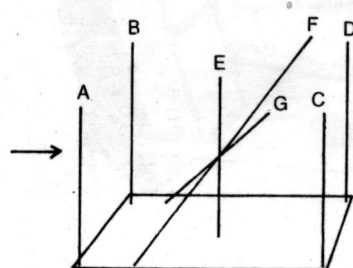

**Fig. 19.9.** The appearance with a meridional size difference.

19.6, there is an apparent displacement of the front in position of GEF from those of Fig. 19.5. This represents horizontal deviation. In Fig. 19.7, one finds that there is a rotation of the cross with the correct orientation of the vertical cords which represents a vertical deviation. In Fig. 19.8, there is a rotation of vertical elements and not the cross which indicates overall discrepancies while in Fig. 19.9, there is the tilting of the cross indicating the defects in meridional direction.

The apparatus is cumbersome, time-consuming and is of academic interest only as it does not have any therapeutic value. It is also fairly expensive.

### Treatment

In a majority of cases aniseikonia presents either no difficulty as it is within tolerable limits or is insurmountable where uniocularity is preferred to binocularity. In moderate degrees of aniseikonia the treatment follows the pattern of aniso-metropia, i.e., the use of isoikonic lenses and contact lenses. The prescription of isoikonic lenses is of use in a very small number of cases and relieves distressing symptoms only of some patients. The method of correction requires considerable skill, is time-consuming and expensive. Anisometropia and aniseikonia are best treated with use of contact lenses or appropriate procedures of refractive surgery.

# SECTION V

# Accommodation and Convergence

# CHAPTER 20

# Accommodation

The refractive indices of various ocular media, curvature of refractive surfaces and position of retina in normal eyes are such that when the eyes are at rest the parallel rays coming from the infinity (6 metres are considered as the same) are focused on to the retina in an emmetropic eye. The objects may be moved within a short range and yet remain in focus without any change in the refractive power of the eye. This distance range is depth of focus. If the object is brought nearer to the eye the image will be formed behind the retina (Fig. 20.1) there are large diffusion circles. The image is out of focus and blurred. There are only two ways by which this image can be seen properly, i.e.,

1. either the axial length of the eyeball should increase so that image now falls on the retina which is not possible; or

2. it should increase its dioptric power to cause greater convergence of rays so that the image is formed at the retina (Fig. 20.2). This is what actually happens in real life.

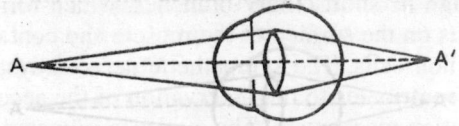

**Fig. 20.1.** Eye not accommodating for A.

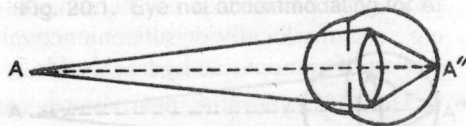

**Fig. 20.2.** Eye accommodating for A.

There are, thus, two processes by which the clarity of retinal images is maintained in spite of change in distance. The first is the inherent char-acter in which the object remains in focus without any change in the refractive power of the eye (depth of focus) and the second is the process by which an individual by his effort increases dioptric power of eye brings about the image of a near object to focus on the retina and this is termed as accommodation.

## Depth of focus

The depth of focus is defined as the distance through which an object may be moved closer to or farther away from the eye and still the object remains in focus, i.e., probably the blur circles overlap a single cone. Depth of focus is considerably increased with the narrowing of the pupils and decreased with dilatation of the same. An emmetropic eye with a pupil of 2 mm has a depth of field from infinity to approximately 15 metres but if the pupil enlarges to 4 mm the depth of field is shortened from infinity to 30 metres. The depth of focus also varies with the distance of the original fixation point from the eye. It is more with a fixation point at a distance while it is less if the fixation distance is less.

## Anatomy of parts of eye concerned with accommodation

Accommodation is brought about by a change in the form of lens due to contraction of ciliary muscle and relaxation of zonule of Zinn. There is a thickening of the lens, a decrease in its diameter (vertically and horizontally), with protrusion forwards of the centre and relative flattening of the periphery at the same time.

The lens is composed of two layers, i.e., the zonular lamellae and the capsule proper (Fig. 20.3) which can be shown by appropriate staining methods. The lens capsule is elastic though no

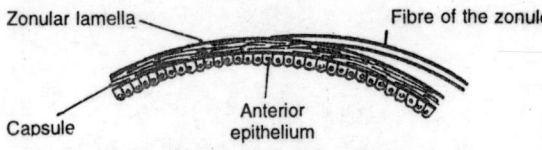

**Fig. 20.3.** Lens capsule.

quantitative measurements have been made. The anterior capsule is much thicker than the posterior capsule and it varies in thickness in different parts (Fig. 20.4). The lens substance has plasticity, the cortex can be easily deformed; the posterior cortex has more malleability than the anterior. The

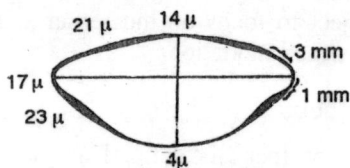

**Fig. 20.4.** Thickness of lens capsule.

nucleus does not modify the refractive power until the age of 30 years when it becomes large and dense. At this age it interferes with deformation of the lens during accommodation. There is thickening of cortex with advancing age which further modifies accommodation. The lens is held by fibres from ciliary body to all around the equator of the lens which are called zonules of Zinn.

The ciliary muscle is classically described as consisting of three kinds of fibres (Fig. 20.5)—meridional, radial and circular (Müller's muscle).

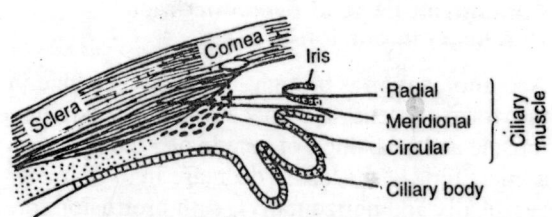

**Fig. 20.5.** Fibres of ciliary muscle.

Meridional fibres are attached to the scleral spur anteriorly and mix up with fine trabeculae in the suprachoroidal space up to the equator, or even beyond this, ending in branched stellate figures (muscle stars). Radial fibres have no definite origin or insertion but extend in between

the meridional and circular fibres (oblique junctional fibres). Circular fibres form a bundle round free edge of the ciliary body just behind the root of the iris. The form of ciliary muscle is determined largely by the grade of development of this portion. It is highly developed in hypermetropic and poorly developed in myopic eyes. On contraction the circular fibres decrease the radius of the circle which they constitute thus relaxing the zonule (Fig. 20.6) which in turn decreases the tension on the lens capsule. The lens then moulds into a more strongly curved system. This also

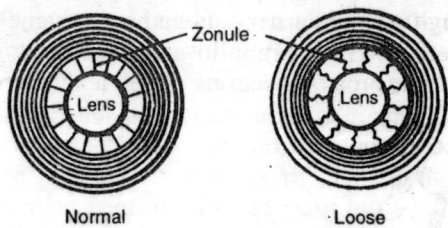

**Fig. 20.6.** Looseness of zonule on contraction of ciliary muscle.

applies to the radial fibres. The longitudinal fibres thicken on contraction and increase the cross-sectional diameter of the whole muscle. Thus the whole muscle acts as a sphincter. It is important to note that the muscle is thickest opposite the equator of the lens so that it bulges first where one would expect it to have the greatest slackening effect on the zonular fibres. The ciliary muscle is supplied by oculomotor (III cranial) nerve through its short ciliary branches, which form a plexus on the surface of the muscle and contains ganglion cells. The sympathetic nervous system also contributes to the innervation of the accommodation mechanism. The evidence is as under :

- Drugs having sympathomimetic action produce a partial loss of accommodation, e.g., cocaine locally or subconjunctival injection of epinephrine hydrochloride.

- In Horner's syndrome, near point is closer to the eye on the affected side. Some people attribute this to miosis and increase in depth of focus.

- In the dark, the state of human lens corresponds to about +0.8 D of accommodation. To focus infinity there must be an active flattening of lens from this state of partial accommodation and sympathetic innervation helps in this flattening.

- In dogs and rabbits stimulation of the sympathetic nerves causes flattening of the lens.
- Sympathetic and parasympathetic nerves probably act antagonistically. Section of the III cranial nerve, which allows uninhibited action of the sympathetic, increases the negative accommodation.

## Pathway of accommodation

The mechanism of accommodation is mediated through a definite nervous pathway (Fig. 20.7). The efferent pathway follows the visual fibres to the striate area of calcarine cortex and is re yed

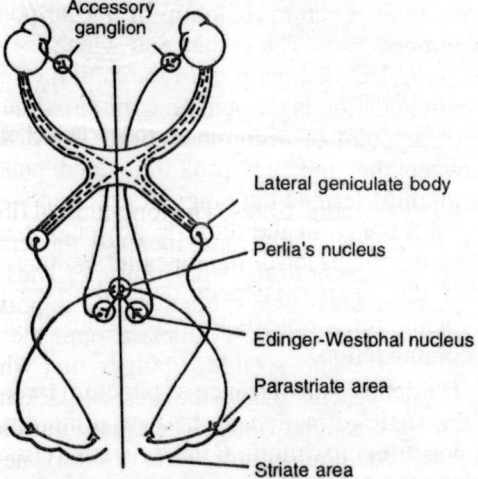

**Fig. 20.7. Pathway for accommodation.**

to the parastriate area. The efferents travel to Perlia's nucleus via occipito-mesencephalic tract. From Perlia's nucleus fibres go to Edinger-Westphal nucleus from where they are carried to the sphincter through the third nerve via an accessory ganglion. The path from Perlia's nucleus to the sphincter is common both for accommodation and convergence.

## Changes in eye during accommodation

Essentially the following changes occur in the process of accommodation.

- Increase in the curvature of anterior surface of lens.
- Moving forwards of the anterior pole of the lens without any change in the position of the posterior pole.
- Consequent increase in the thickness of the lens in the centre.
- The anterior capsule becomes slack and separates more from the posterior pole.
- Contraction of pupil.

That during accommodation changes take place in the lens, this is supported by the following evidence :

- Lens becomes tremulous as if its all suspension has been relaxed.
- Wrinkles usually seen at the equator of the unaccommodated lens disappear.
- Purkinje image as formed by the anterior surface of the lens becomes smaller indicating an increase in the curvature of this surface (Fig. 20.8).
- Studies in congenital aniridia show that the lens becomes smaller and thicker during accommodation.
- The central zone of the anterior surface becomes more convex in relation to peripheral parts.
- Mobile opacities in the lens, on accommodation, move as an axial flow from the periphery. This is easily revealed under slit-lamp microscopy.
- Extracted lens is in a state of complete relaxation and has an increased dioptric power which shows that increase in dioptric power of the lens in accommodation is due to a relaxation of the capsule and consequent change in the sphericity of the lens.
- Photographic and gonioscopic evidence shows that in accommodation the anterior surface of the lens approaches the cornea, making the anterior chamber shallower, while its posterior surface remains comparatively stationary.

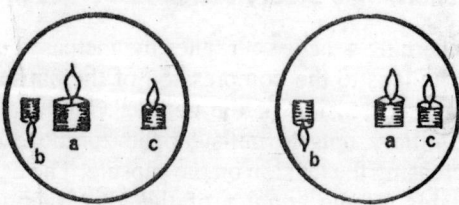

**Fig. 20.8. Purkinje images in accommodation.**

## THEORIES OF ACCOMMODATION

Various theories have been advanced to explain the mechanism of accommodation. According to some of these theories there is alteration in the length of the eyeball, increase in the curvature of the cornea or the pushing of the lens forwards but none of these theories have been found to be accurate. There are two important theories which account for the changes in the lens. The first is the Young-Helmholtz relaxation theory and second is Tscherning's theory of increased tension. Most of the people adhere to the relaxation theory and believe that the two factors—mouldability of the lens and power of ciliary muscle—contribute to the efficiency of the mechanism of accommodation.

### Young-Helmholtz theory

When the eye is at rest and not accommodating, the lens is compressed on the capsule by the stretched zonule. When the ciliary muscle contracts the choroid is pulled forwards and the ring formed by the ciliary processes is narrowed mostly by the circular fibres of the ciliary muscles which now release the tension on the zonule and make it lax. With the relaxation of the zonule the anterior capsule of the lens is also relaxed. The lens has plasticity and, therefore, it moulds itself. The posterior pole rests on the vitreous and cannot mould itself. The moulding occurs in the anterior pole and is determined by the thickness of the capsule. The anterior pole lies opposite the thinnest part of the anterior capsule. In the pupillary area, there occurs a nipple-like bulging of the anterior pole of the lens. All the processes increase the dioptric power of the eye and thus focus the near object on the retina.

### Tscherning's theory of increased tension

Tscherning's theory attributes the increased power of the lens to the compression of the capsule by increased tension of the zonule. Contraction of the ciliary muscle pulls on the zonule directly increasing the tension on the capsule. The capsule presses on the equator of the lens making the poles bulge. The posterior pole cannot bulge due to its resting on the vitreous. Therefore, it is the anterior pole of the lens which shows a nipple-like bulging in the pupillary area.

The weight of evidence is in favour of the relaxation theory coupled with the evidence that the substance of the lens in its relaxed state assumes the form determined by its own elasticity. During accommodation this is overcome by the greater elasticity of the capsule which moulds it in its accommodation form.

## RANGE AND AMPLITUDE OF ACCOMMODATION

The maximum distance at which the eye can see an object without any accommodative effort is termed the punctum remotum or the far point of accommodation. The distance at which they can see an object distinctly with maximum effort of accommodation is termed punctum proximum or the near point of accommodation. The distance between the punctum proximum and punctum remotum is termed the range of accommodation. The difference in the dioptric power of the eye when it is focused for the far point (static refraction) and when it is focused for the near point (dynamic refraction) is termed the amplitude of accommodation.

If $r$ denotes the distance of punctum remotum, $R$ the static refraction of the eye, $p$ the distance of punctum proximum, $P$ the dynamic refraction, $a$ the range of accommodation, and $A$ the amplitude of accommodation, then the range and amplitude of accommodation can be expressed by the following equations :

$$a = r - p$$
$$A = P - R$$

In emmetropic eye (Fig. 20.9) the distance of far point from the eye ($r$) is infinity and for an average adult the distance of near point from the eye ($p$) is at 10 cm, R = 0, and P = +10 D. Range of accommodation ($a$) is infinity – 10 = infinity,

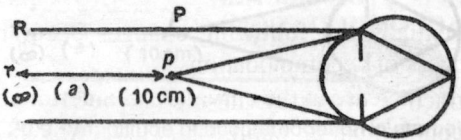

Fig. 20.9. Amplitude of accommodation in emmetropic eye.

while amplitude of accommodation (A) is 10 – 0 = 10 D.

In myopia (Fig. 20.10) the distance of far point from the eye (r) is at a fixed distance say 20 cm (myopia of –5 D), the near point is at 10 cm. Hence R = 5 D, and P = 10 D.

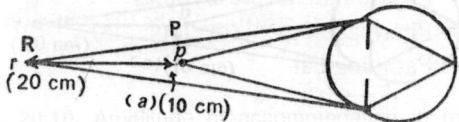

**Fig. 20.10.** Amplitude of accommodation in myopic eye.

Range of accommodation (a) = 20 cm – 10 cm = 10 cm, while amplitude of accommodation (A) = 10 D – 5 D = 5 D.

In hypermetropia (Fig. 20.11) far point is a hypothetical point beyond infinity and in order to see objects clearly at infinity the subject has to exert an accommodative effort equivalent to

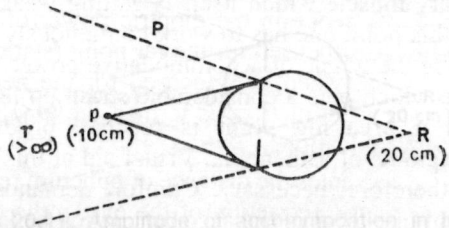

**Fig. 20.11.** Amplitude of accommodation in hypermetropic eye.

hypermetropia. The distance of far point from the eye (r) is more than infinity. All the distances behind the eye are taken as negative. In case of hypermetropia of +5 D, the hypothetical point will be 20 cm behind the eye and the static refraction R will be +5 D. The near point P is 10 cm in front of the eye. Hence P = +10 D. The range of accommodation (a) shall be infinity and amplitude of accommodation is 10 D – (–5 D) = 15 D.

## EFFECTOR MECHANISM AND BINOCULAR ACCOMMODATION

The essential factor in accommodation is a contraction of ciliary muscle, convergence and the contraction of pupil. This associated action is called synkinesis. The convergence and accommodation are closely related physiologically as both are used together in binocular vision. However, the two can be independent of each other and also exhibit a certain degree of elasticity. Hypermetrope exerts more accommodation and less convergence while myope has less accommodation and more convergence and this dissociation in itself causes a breakdown and may result in strabismus. It may be stated that maximum efficiency can be attained by accommodation and convergence supplementing each other in synkinetic action when both eyes are being used together, the initial stimulus being the act of convergence. The elasticity of the relationship is determined largely by accommodation. The pupillary contraction which accompanies this synkinetic action occurs independently. This synkinetic action is also not influenced by fusion of the two images from the two eyes, for an increase in binocular accommodation is also seen in amblyopic patients with divergent squint.

Of the various factors stimulating accommodation, accommodative convergence is of great importance. It is certain that an increase in accommodation normally brings about an increase in convergence. The relationship between change in convergence expressed in prism dioptres brought about by an increase in accommodation expressed in dioptres is termed accommodative convergence/accommodation ratio (AC/A). In a given individual this ratio is remarkably constant so that it can be safely said that accommodative convergence varies with accommodative stimulus. If, however, there is greater miosis (size less than 1.5 mm) this linear relationship is disturbed because of the additional factor of the depth of focus.

The ratio is upset by a change in the tone of ciliary muscle or in presbyopia. It can thus be increased when cycloplegics are used and decreased in miosis.

In presbyopia there are two opposing views expressed to explain the decrease in accommodative power :

1. Change in the power of the ciliary muscle which means that greater amount of change of accommodation. Amount of contraction of ciliary muscle is constant for 1 D change of accommodation but the sclerosis of lens does not allow this to be effective.

2. There is a view that since when accommodative stimulus is increased accommodative convergence can increase without any dioptric change suggests that there exists an inflexible relationship between the two. It seems that though ageing process has an effect on the ciliary muscle yet major role in producing presbyopia is played by the change in the mouldability of the lens through a sclerotic process.

The excess of binocular over uniocular accommodation averages about half dioptre although individual variations are large. It may be as high as 1.5 D.

### Variations with age

The power of accommodation varies with age. The punctum proximum in a child is situated at about 7 cm from the eye and the accommodative power is about +14 D. As the age advances the near point recedes and the power of accommodation decreases. At about puberty the near point is at 10 cm and the power of accommodation is +10 D. At about 30 years of age the near point is situated at about 14 cm and the power of accommodation is +7 D. In this modern civilisation most of the work is done at 28 to 30 cm and, therefore, the recession of near point with age goes unnoticed. In India the recession of near point is more rapid than is seen in many western countries where at about 45 years of age the accommodation is 3.5 to 4 D. In our country the figure is reached at about 40 years of age and the near point recedes to 25 cm. At the age of 60 only 1 D accommodation remains but at this age cataract usually starts to form in this country. When near point reaches 25 to 30 cm it would entail working at the near point continuously

which is extremely fatiguing and not possible. It follows that when the near point is at a distance of some 30 cm presbyopia is said to have to have set in.

## ANOMALIES OF ACCOMMODATION

1. Insufficiency of accommodation
   - Physiological (presbyopia)
   - Pharmacological (cycloplegia)
   - Pathological
     - Insufficiency
     - Ill-sustained
     - Inertia
     - Paralysis
2. Excess and spasm of accommodation

### Presbyopia or physiological insufficiency

We have seen that the punctum proximum usually recedes to about 25 cm at the age of 40 years in this country due to lens becoming hard and sclerosed and less mouldable by action of the ciliary muscle which itself is getting weakened. At this point one has to work continuously exercising the whole of accommodative power available which puts a considerable strain on the eye and a breaking point is reached producing symptoms of asthenopia. Visual aid at this point is, therefore, necessary. Comfort demands that about one-third of the accommodation be kept in reserve, so that aid becomes necessary even earlier in professions needing working at small distances, e.g., in goldsmiths, engravers, darners, compositors, etc.

Presbyopia is considered to have set in when the diminution in the power of accommodation has reached a stage needing aid for near work. In myopes of 3 to 4 dioptres this stage never reaches

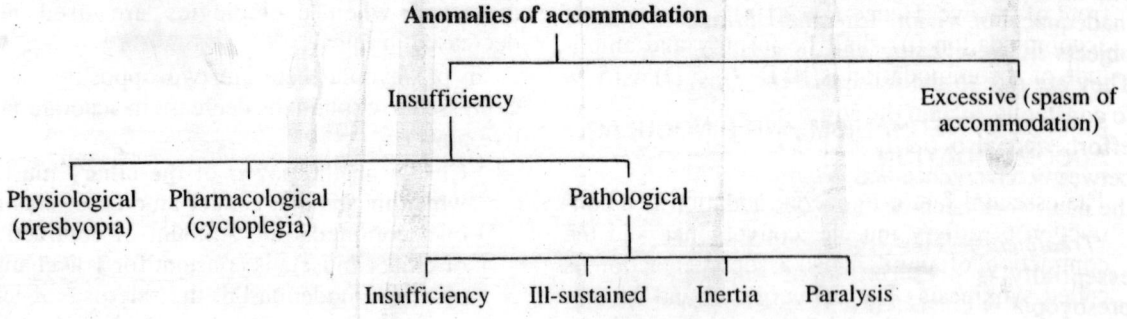

as the punctum remotum of these persons corresponds with the comfortable working distance. In uncorrected hypermetropes this stage is reached earlier as part of the hypermetropic error needs to be corrected by the patient's own voluntary effort. The premature onset of presbyopia, due regard having been paid to refractive error, should always excite suspicion that factors other than physiological are involved. An early failure of accommodation may indicate premature sclerosis of the lens, development of cataract, premature senility affecting musculature, i.e., ciliary body, chronic simple glaucoma or suppression of ovarian function in elderly females. The early appearance of presbyopia in India particularly in poorer class of persons and farmers can probably be correlated with early lenticular changes which in turn may be due to poor nutrition and greater exposure to sunlight. It may be recalled that cataract is quite common in India and it is not uncommon to see it in patients between 45 and 60 years of age. There are two main factors in the production of presbyopia, i.e., the tone of ciliary muscle and plasticity of lens apart from secondary factors as state of refraction and profession of the person.

*Symptoms :* The small print becomes indistinct at the usual reading distance; especially so if the illumination is inadequate. The patient begins to hold the head back and the book slightly at a greater distance. The difficulty is increased in the evening partly due to slight dilatation of pupil and less of illumination and partly due to fatigue of the whole day work. The patient prefers bright light for near work. Fortunately at this time senile miosis also begins to set in which offers some help in compensating the evening mydriasis. The symptoms of eye strain appear after a time but in the beginning the patient complains of inadequacy of vision for small print and finer objects in the evening and in dim illumination. They are due to the failure of the ciliary muscle to constantly sustain the strain of accommodative effort, and also partly due to the dissociation between convergence and accommodation. Finally the near work becomes an impossibility.

*Treatment :* The treatment of presbyopia essentially is prescription of glasses. Before presbyopia is corrected it is essential to correct the static refraction. To do this, an objective and subjective assessment of the static refraction should be done under cycloplegia and mydriasis. At the postmydriatic test the glasses for distant vision should be worn and then the presbyopic error corrected. The correction should be such that the accommodation is reinforced and the near point is brought within a useful working distance. It may differ with the profession of the individual. About one-third of the accommodation should be kept in reserve. The correction should be made on individual basis as limits of accommodation and the working distance vary with individuals. It is always advisable to prescribe weakest glasses which are compatible with good vision, rather than to over correct the error as stronger glasses may disturb the accommodation convergence equilibrium and give rise to headache. In such cases either the power of the convex glass prescribed should be reduced, compatible with good vision, or asthenopia can be relieved by prescribing glasses with base-in-prisms. The same effects can be obtained by decentring of the lenses by a corresponding amount. In our experience the condition can be relieved by suitable orthoptic exercises.

As a general rule it is found that an individual requires +1 D for every five years of age over 40 years but this should only be taken as a rough guide. Individual testing should be resorted to. Usually both eyes are prescribed equal addition but different correction for each eye can be given if individual eye testing gives different results. The other method is to find out the punctum proximum of the individual by a near point rule (Fig. 20.12) or Livingston's binocular gauge, from which can also be found the amplitude of accommodation. The latter can be measured by dynamic retinoscopy, which is a procedure employed to assess the refractive state of the eyes

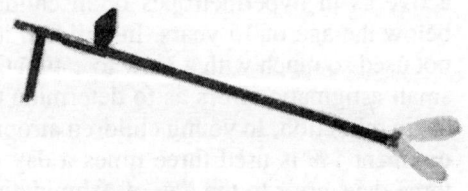

**Fig. 20.12.** Near point rule.

while they are fully accommodating or converging. The value of this test is equivocal as there is not complete agreement as to the interpretation of results.

Let us suppose that in an emmetrope the near point has receded to 33 cm, i.e., the amplitude of accommodation is 3 D. As pointed out earlier, one third of this amplitude should be left in reserve, therefore, utilisable amplitude is two-thirds of 3 D or 2 D. If the patient's working distance is 25 cm, he requires a total of 4 D of accommodation. He has an available accom-modation of 2 D, of utilisable amplitude, so he needs 2 D as an aid, i.e., difference between required accommodation and utilisable accom-modation should be prescribed.

## Cycloplegia or pharmacological insufficiency

The ciliary muscle is supplied mainly by the para-sympathetic nerves. Instillation of parasympathico-lytics in the conjunctival sac causes paralysis of the ciliary muscle. It is called cycloplegia. As the supply of the sphincter pupillae is the same as of ciliary muscle the pupil also dilates (mydriasis). The drugs causing this are called cycloplegics and mydriatics, respectively. Most of the drugs, e.g., atropine sulphate, homatropine hydrobromide, hyoscine hydrobromide, are both cycloplegics and mydriatics. The cocaine and neosynephrine group of drugs, which are sympathomimetics, are only mydriatics and not cycloplegics. These drugs if given with atropine augment the effects of the latter and probably help to produce quicker cycloplegia.

### Indications of cycloplegia and mydriasis

The use of cycloplegia and mydriasis is of utmost value in the evaluation of refractive errors. It is recommended in the following cases :

- Where accommodation is abnormally active as in hypermetropes or in children below the age of 15 years. In children it is not used so much with a view to estimating small astigmatic errors as to determine the static refraction. In young children atropine ointment 1% is used three times a day for three days prior to the day of examination. In hypermetropes, by the paralysis of the

ciliary muscle, nearly all accommodation for near is abolished and latent hyper-metropia is rendered manifest.

- Where definite symptoms of accommoda-tive asthenopia are present and where refractive error is not sufficient to explain this asthenopia. This is due to spasm of accommodation. In these cases homa-tropine may be advised for some time which may force a rest upon the eye. The eye is enabled to recover from its state of fatigue and is prevented from further over-action of accommodation until the correcting glasses are prescribed.

- Where convergence and accommodation are not within the range for the age of the patient. It is especially applicable to hyper-metropes.

- Above the age of 40 years where excessive accommodation may occur at the commence-ment of presbyopia.

- Where dilatation of the pupil is helpful in examination of the fundus.

- Where the pupil is small and presents tech-nical difficulties in estimating error of refraction.

### Disadvantages of cycloplegics

The use of these drugs is not without disad-vantage. They are :

- The dilatation of the pupil considerably alters the optical properties of its refractive apparatus and intensifies the physical error due to aberration through the peripheral parts of the refractive media. The periphery of the pupillary aperture has a refraction different from the central part. With a mydriatic the refraction of the peripheral part of the lens is often estimated leading to inaccuracies in the prescription. Besides this technical difficulties of disturbing shadows due to dilated pupil exist. It may be very different from the refraction of the central part which is used in normal circumstances of life. Some people even consider refraction under cycloplegia as pathological because the shape of lens has been altered and ordinarily after the lens has assumed its normal shape, minute errors cannot be reasonably transposed to the dioptric system.

- In the routine use of mydriatics the danger of producing glaucoma in the eye with a shallow anterior chamber is by no means negligible. The possibility of such a serious complication should always be avoided especially in patients over 40 years of age, by taking the tension before instilling a cycloplegic. When in doubt the patient should be kept under observation until the pupil is fully contracted by the subsequent instillation of pilocarpine.

- Cycloplegia involves certain economic disadvantages as during the period of its activity near work is impossible apart from annoying and incapacitating glare. The patient may not be willing or be able to put up with cycloplegics unless he is assured that it is essential for his well being.

As a rule, patients under 15 years of age should be refracted under atropine. Homatropine can be relied upon in hypermetropes above the age of 15 years. Neo-synephrine group of drugs are also useful as mydriatics where cycloplegia is not essential. Over 40 years of age it is not necessary to do refraction under cycloplegia. Some people recommend cycloplegia in all cases below the age of 40 years and where considerable accommodative activity may be assumed to exist. They suggest that smallest astigmatic error should be forced on the patient which does not seem to be a healthy practice considering the fact that small astigmatic error is not uncommonly found in majority of people. To correct a minute error, which is not associated with definite asthenopic symptoms especially when it is measured in pathological condition of cycloplegia, and transpose it to the eye in its normal dynamic state even when it is further complicated by optical defects inseparably associated with the fitting of glasses is to misinterpret completely the whole economy of living organisms.

The quantity and type of cycloplegia should not be the same for every individual. There is considerable variation in dosage in which cycloplegics produce a satisfactory degree of paralysis. Even anisocycloplegia, i.e., different amount of cycloplegia in two eyes of the same individual by the same dosage of the cycloplegic is known to occur. Some people, therefore, recommend that depth of cycloplegia should be tested before the refractive examination is done. It can be easily done by testing it on the accommodation cards. If the patient can read at 1 metre further cycloplegia is needed if the patient is not myopic.

The effect of some of these drugs is counteracted by pilocarpine 2%. Effect of atropine is not usually counteracted by miotics so the post-mydriatic test after atropine should be done at least after 10 days.

DFP is employed in some clinics to counteract the action of atropine but it should not be used as it is not without its hazards. Accommodation comes to normal within 4 to 5 days after homatropine instillation. Although pupillary reaction is obtained normally in 48 hours, it is better to do a post-mydriatic test after 5 to 7 days when homatropine has been used as a cycloplegic.

## Pathological insufficiency of accommodation

It is a common condition in which the accommodative power is consistently poor and below the lower limit than what may be considered as normal for the patient.

In dynamic form it is due to weakness of ciliary muscle. Ciliary muscle fatigue may be due to general debility, malnutrition, and anaemia, general toxaemia due to chronic infections or due to chronic alcoholism. Excessive use of the eye especially for close work in unfavourable conditions in the presence of ciliary fatigue may break down accommodation to produce asthenopia. Among local causes onset of cyclitis in sympathetic ophthalmia may give rise to insufficiency. Glaucoma needs special mention because many a time there is a gradual paresis of accommodation manifesting either as rapid change of presbyopic correction or too high a correction for the age of the patient. It is also seen in neurosis, neurasthenia and hysteria.

The insufficiency may be due to sclerosis of the lens, frequently referred to as premature presbyopia which is stable.

The patient complains of incapacity to do near work which brings asthenopic symptoms. He remains comfortable if near work is not attempted. If the local or general causes are attended to, the condition improves considerably to recur again if the same conditions prevail again. It may be accompanied by insufficiency of convergence. Excessive convergence may occur if the patient exerts to overcome accommodation insufficiency.

### Treatment

When the accommodative failure is associated with general debility the cause is reasonably clear and should be treated. When it is not, as is often the case, the treatment is on symptomatic lines. Optical treatment should be the first consideration. Any static refractive error should be corrected and if the symptoms persist, additional convex glasses should be prescribed. If it is associated with convergence insufficiency, base-in-prisms add to patient's comfort. Weakest glasses should be prescribed to exercise the accommodation, if convergence is weak. Full correction can be unhesitatingly given in cases with convergence excess. Additional correction for reading should be made progressively weaker with recovery if presbyopia is dynamic. Accommodation exercises in presbyopia, given at short periods throughout the day to intelligent patients who can appreciate the physiological limits of their powers, prove very useful. These are not useful in cases with general debility or lenticular sclerosis. The exercises are taken wearing distance correction, using each eye separately if there is convergence excess and both eyes simultaneously if there is convergence deficiency.

### Ill-sustained accommodation

The accommodation is normal initially but cannot be maintained over any length of time. On doing near work for a prolonged period near point gradually recedes and vision becomes blurred. It is an initial stage of true insufficiency. It is characteristic of convalescence from debilitating illness or in a state of general tiredness or general relaxation. The treatment consists of curtailing near work during convalescence. Give better instructions for visual hygiene to the patients pointing out conditions of illumination and posture during study.

### Inertia of accommodation

Difficulty is experienced in altering the range of accommodation. Normally the focus is altered readily and accurately within one second. Difficulty may be experienced in bringing the focus on to a near object after looking at a distant one. Most cases are functional and probably depend on insufficiency of accommodation. Check-up of refractive error and accommodation exercises do help in real cases.

### Paralysis of accommodation

The paralysis of accommodation may be due to diseases affecting the ciliary muscles or the oculomotor nerve. It is usually associated with paralytic mydriasis. It may or may not be associated with paralysis of any extraocular muscle. It may be unilateral or bilateral, insidious or sudden. If the loss of accommodation occurs as an isolated event, it is nuclear or peripheral in origin. In other lesions paralysis of accommodation is associated with other cranial nerve palsies.

Congenital defects like aniridia or gross abnormalities of the ciliary body or zonule may cause lack of accommodation. It may be of central origin, i.e., in acute or sub-acute infections of the central nervous system, epidemic encephalitis, rarely in anterior poliomyelitis, nervous involvement in acute exanthemata and infective diseases. It is not uncommon in herpes zoster and chronic infections like tuberculosis, syphilis and leprosy. Diphtheritic paralysis of accommodation is common. It usually occurs two to three weeks after faucial infection but may rarely occur as early as 2nd to 5th day of the illness or as late as 8 weeks after diphtheria. It comes on suddenly and appears to be invariably bilateral. It is almost always incomplete. The power of accommodation slowly returns. The mechanism of palsy is little understood. It is toxic and either the nerve trunk or the nucleus or both are affected. There is no action on the musculature as the pupil contracts on instillation of miotics. Probably the toxin is firmly and rapidly fixed in the nerve tissue by the time palsy appears. Schick's test is negative and there is usually no effect of anti-diphtheritic serum in the treatment of diphtheritic paralysis of accommodation. It is also found in chronic alcoholism, food poisoning, botulism and in poisoning from belladonna, lead, ergot or even arsenicals.

Uncommonly paralysis may occur in hereditary degenerative conditions of the brain stem. Metabolic toxaemias like diabetes, Wernicke's encephalopathy and lactation may cause paralysis of accommodation. The onset in diabetes is usually sudden and the palsy is seen in young individuals. It is bilateral. The pupils are normal. Oculomotor nerve palsy, trauma, local conditions (cyclitis and glaucoma) and hysteria may also account for a few cases of accommodation palsy.

*Treatment*

The treatment of the condition, as is seen from its varied etiology, is directed against the cause. Local drugs like pilocarpine may be of some help. In cases of partial paralysis their value lies not only in ciliary stimulation but also in optical improvement due to small pupil. In cases where either recovery is incomplete or not at all, suitable correction with glasses is the treatment of choice although under-correction rather than over-correction should be the rule.

**Excessive accommodation**

In this the tone of the ciliary muscle is increased inducing a condition of pseudomyopia, i.e., an emmetrope becomes myopic, the myope more short-sighted and the hypermetrope may become less hypermetropic, emmetropic, or even myopic. It may be functional or organic. Functional accommodative spasm occurs in fatigue of accommodation. The irritability in asthenopia is precipitated by overwork in bad hygienic conditions; optical or muscular anomalies in the eye, especially myopia and heterophoria and constitutional make-up of the individual, i.e., ténseness, anxiety and emotional upset may result in over-accommodation. The organic excessive accommodation is usually due to the following causes :

- Use of strong miotics, e.g., D.F.P.
- Lesions of brain stem in their irritative phase, e.g., tabetic crisis, epidemic encephalitis and meningitis.
- Local inflammatory conditions, e.g., iridocyclitis and inflammatory conditions of the orbit.
- Toxic reaction to exogenous poisons, e.g., sulphonamides, arsenic, or even smoking.
- Trauma.
- Trigeminal neuralgia.
- Refractive errors like hypermetropia and astigmatism.
- Sympathetic underactivity or excessive parasympathetic activity.

*Symptoms :* The distant vision is blurred because of pseudomyopia and accommodative astigmatism but the near vision usually remains unimpaired. The patient may complain of macropsia which is due to optical illusion. Symptoms of ocular asthenopia are marked especially when near work is attempted. Sometimes gastric disturbances occur due to this accommodative spasm and these are reflex in origin. The condition is many a time missed and pseudomyopia is corrected. Once the glasses are given a vicious circle starts increasing the spasm of muscle requiring increasing correction. In such cases full examination under complete cycloplegia reveals the true state of affairs.

*Treatment :* All contributory factors should be taken into account and visual rest for 3 to 4 weeks may sometimes be necessary. Proper correction of refractive error especially under cycloplegia is very essential. Homatropine instillation may be advised in the beginning only if full correction cannot be worn. Stronger lenses for near work and orthoptic stereoscopic exercises may bring some relief.

# CHAPTER 21

# Convergence (Binocular Muscular Coordination)

When the eyes are looking at a distant object the visual axes are parallel to each other. To see a near object the eyes must not only accommodate so that the object is brought into focus but the visual axes should also be rotated inwards so that both are directed at the object. The inward rotation of visual axes is termed convergence or sometimes it is called positive convergence. Similarly both eyes can be turned outside and the movement is called divergence or sometimes as negative convergence. Convergence can be voluntary or involuntary.

The voluntary rotation of the two eyes to fix the object of regard at a near distance is initiated in the frontal lobe of the cerebrum and is the only disjunctive movement which can be initiated at will. Involuntary convergence is a psycho-optical reflex based on fixation and refixation reflexes. It is also a part of near reflex (reflex convergence).

Normally, when at rest, the eyes are in a state of slight divergence. To retain parallelism of eyes in primary position convergence is required. It is known as tonic convergence. It is separate from accommodative and fusional convergence, which is convergence employed synergistically with accommodation for fusion. The reflex is centred in the peristriate area of the central cortex.

## Pathway for convergence (Fig. 21.1)

The precise path for convergence is not known. The centre for voluntary convergence lies in the frontal oculogyric area (area 8) and the centre for reflex convergence which is initiated by visual stimuli from the retina is situated in the peristriate area of occipital cortex along with the centre for fixation reflex. The two are connected by occipito-frontal tract and are also connected with the lower convergence centre (Perlia's nucleus)

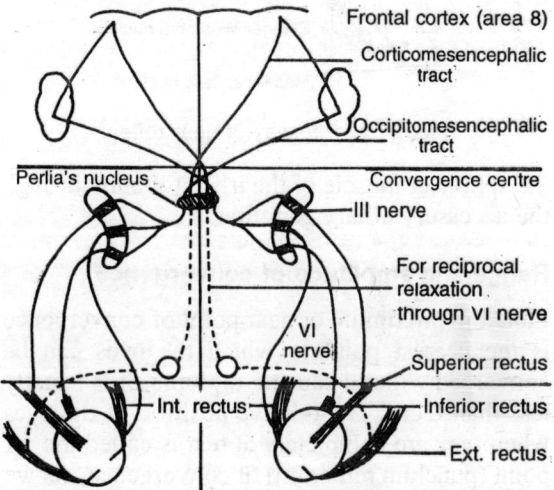

**Fig. 21.1.** Pathway of convergence.

by the occipito-mesencephalic and corticomesencephalic tracts, respectively. The precise path of fibres is not very clear. The fibres probably travel down the internal sagittal stratum through the posterior part of the internal capsule to reach the oculomotor nuclei. From the oculomotor nuclei the path runs to the internal recti and the associated vertical recti while reciprocal relaxation is conveyed to external recti and the obliques. There is pupillary constriction along with convergence (near reflex—Fig. 21.2) which is controlled by a definite pathway. The near reflex starts in the fibres of the internal rectus muscles which contract on convergence. From the muscles the afferent fibres probably run through the III cranial nerve towards the Perlia's nucleus, passing through the mesencephalic roof of the V nerve or they are mediated all along through the V nerve. From the Perlia's nucleus, they are connected to the Edinger-Westphal nucleus from which they are relayed to

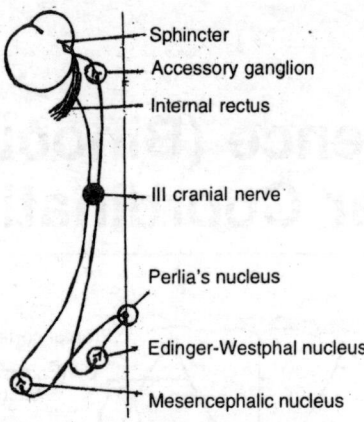

**Fig. 21.2.** Pathway of near reflex.

the sphincter muscle of the iris, probably through the accessory ciliary ganglion.

### Range and amplitude of convergence

Punctum proximum or near point of convergence is the nearest point to which the eyes can be converged without causing diplopia. It is usually less than 8 cm. The relative position of the eyes when they are completely at rest is called the far point (punctum remotum) of convergence. As we have seen that at rest the eyes are in a position of slight divergence, the far point instead of being at infinity is situated beyond infinity. It can be mathematically found by producing the axis backwards so as to meet at a point behind the eyes. It would be situated in front of the eyes if there is no divergence or if there is slight convergence, when the eyes are at rest. Range of convergence is defined as the distance between the far point and the near point. It is described as positive when it is between the eye and infinity. Difference in converging power required to maintain the eyes in a position of rest and in a position of maximum convergence is the amplitude of convergence. The part of the range of convergence between the eye and infinity is described as positive; that part beyond infinity, that is behind the eye and which in reality is divergence, is termed the negative convergence.

### Measurement of convergence

Convergence is measured either in metre angles or in prism dioptres. When the eyes are at rest,

the visual axes are practically parallel to each other and the eyes are directed straight ahead. When the eyes are now directed to an object at a distance of one metre of the median line between the two eyes the visual axes make an angle with this line (Fig. 21.3). This angle is called the metre angle (ma) which is inversely proportional to the

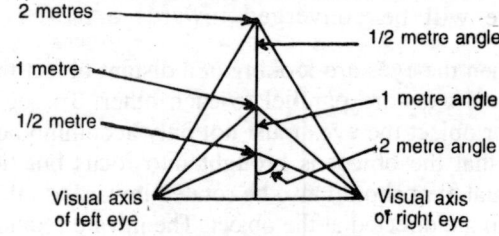

**Fig. 21.3.** Metre angle.

distance in metres, i.e., it would be 0.5 ma at 2 metres, and 2 ma at half metre. The angle also varies, to an extent, with the distance between the two eyes but this variation is negligible. The normal amplitude of convergence is 10.5 ma which has 9.5 ma of positive and 1 ma of negative convergence. The amount of accommodation expressed in dioptres is the same as the amount of convergence expressed in metre angles in normal accommodation convergence relationship. The convergence can also be measured in prism dioptres. If an adducting prism is placed before the eye (base out—Fig. 21.4) the rays of light entering the eye will be deviated outwards through a degree depending on the strength of the prism and diplopia will tend to be produced, but

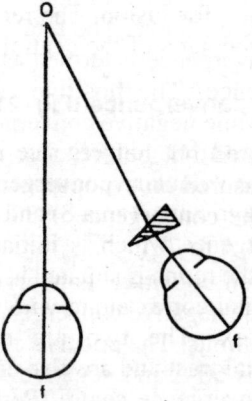

**Fig. 21.4.** Action of abducting prism.

to maintain the binocular vision the eye is turned inwards, through a corresponding degree. The strongest converging prism through which the binocular vision can still be maintained is the measure of power of convergence. This component is called the positive convergence. If now an abducting prism (base in—Fig. 21.5) is placed in front of one eye the rays of light entering the eye will be converged inwards and tend to

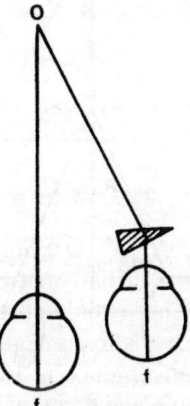

**Fig. 21.5.** Action of abduction prism.

produce diplopia but if binocular vision is to be maintained the eye must move outwards through a corresponding degree. The strongest abducting prism which can be tolerated without producing diplopia gives the degree of measurement of divergence or negative convergence. In all these the degree of convergence or divergence is shared equally between the two eyes so that the effect is the same whether one prism is placed before one eye or two prisms, each of half the strength, one placed before each eye. The total of positive and negative convergence is termed as the amplitude of convergence. The positive convergence is about 30 $\Delta$ while negative convergence is 4 $\Delta$. As already pointed out before, fusion and convergence is measured on synoptophore as the range of fusion. The convergence is 30 $\Delta$ to 60 $\Delta$ and divergence 3 $\Delta$ to 7 $\Delta$.

As is seen, positive convergence is much larger than the negative convergence. Each varies within wide limits. The positive convergence can be as large as 60 $\Delta$ and negative convergence as much as 7 $\Delta$

3 $\Delta$ corresponds to one metre angle on con-

vergence scale. It is, therefore, not difficult to convert readings in $\Delta$ to the ones in metre angles; 60 $\Delta$ is 20 ma and 6 $\Delta$ is 2 ma.

**Relation of accommodation and convergence**

The functions of accommodation and convergence are synkinetic and are closely interrelated.

The relationship between accommodation and convergence has already been briefly described. In convergence a large component is that of accommodative convergence. This type of convergence is induced by a stimulus to accommodation. The accommodation effort and the nature of the convergence response which it evokes forms an important part of the linkage between accommodation and convergence in each individual and which is surprisingly quite firm and quite constant. The amount of accommodative convergence measured by prism dioptres induced by each dioptre of accommodation is called the accommodative convergence/accommodation (AC/A) ratio. The average normal numerical value of this ratio is said to be 3 : 1 to 5 : 1 or 3 to 5 times because it is taken for granted that the convergence measurement is related to one dioptre of accommodation. There are several methods by which this can be measured.

There are two important situations which lead to a breakdown of accommodative convergence/accommodation ratio.

1. Excessive convergence is brought about by uncorrected hypermetropia with its excessive accommodative requirement as against emmetropia for the same distance at which the object of regard is placed.
2. There is a high AC/A ratio so that there is an excessively high response of the convergence mechanism to any accommodative effort.

There may also be dissociation in other refractive errors, in cycloplegia and in advancing years. However, the amount of dissociation possible is limited. It can be increased by practice through an increase in fusional response. It varies in different individuals under certain conditions. Convergence may be required without accommodation, e.g., under cycloplegia and moderate myopia when the object is placed at punctum remotum. Accommodation is similarly not fully associated with convergence in hypermetropia or artificially created hypermetropia by placing weak concave lens in front of the eye. The effort to dissociate the two may be the cause of considerable distress. It gives rise to symptoms of asthenopia in refractive errors. Necessary degree of dissociation may on occasions be impossible of attainment. Since a clear image is of more immediate advantage than retention of binocular vision, one eye may eventually deviate to produce a squint.

Convergence is made up of four components :

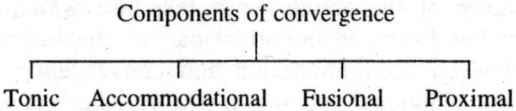

1. *Tonic convergence* : It is the convergence which determines the position of visual axes in relation to each other and is primarily responsible for maintaining parallelism of the eye in the primary position.
2. *Accommodational convergence* : As stated above, it is employed synergistically with accommodation.
3. *Fusional convergence* : It works in unison with accommodation augmenting it with a view to direct the eyes to the object of attention and interest and the eyes are maintained in such a position relative to each other so that the images of the object of fixation fall on the fovea of each eye simultaneously. The fusion mechanism compensates for any errors in ocular alignment induced either by dioptric power of the eye, the accommodative convergence and accommodation relationship or by excessive tonic or proximal convergence.
4. *Proximal convergence* : It is stimulated by the perception of the position of an object of attention and is independent of accommodation.

**Relative convergence**

The relative accommodation, i.e., accommoda-

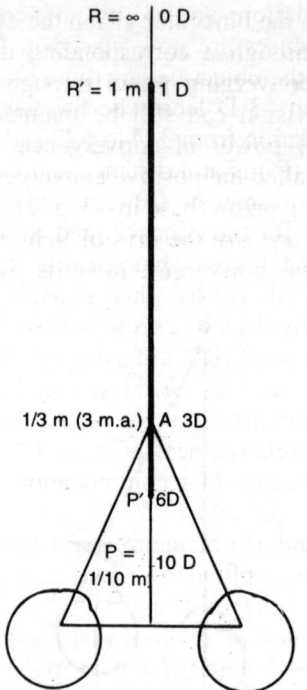

**Fig. 21.6.** Relative accommodation.

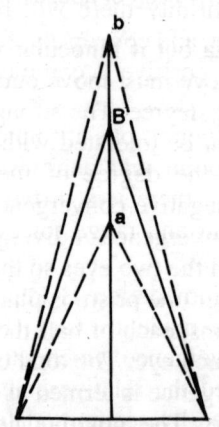

**Fig. 21.7.** Relative convergence.

tion for a given point of convergence is given in Fig. 21.6.

Similarly, convergence for a given point of accommodation is termed relative convergence and is given in Fig. 21.7.

In Fig. 21.6, the subject is an emmetrope and has his far point (R) at infinity and his near point P at 10 cm. Suppose he looks at object A situated 1/3 metre away, he will then be exercising 3 D of accommodation and 3 ma of convergence. Concave lenses are now placed in front of his eyes until the object begins to be blurred; if this occurs with –3 D lenses he has augmented his accommodation from 3 D to 6 D and his relative near point (P′) is at a distance equivalent to 6 D or 1/6 of a metre. Convex lenses are now substituted for the concave, and it is found that the image begins to be blurred when lenses of 2 D are presented. He has thus relaxed his accommodation by 2 D, i.e., from 3 D to 1 D and his relative far point (R′) is at a distance from the eye equivalent to 1 D, i.e., 1 metre. For 3 ma of convergence, therefore, the relative far point is 1 metre, the relative near point is 1/6 of a metre, the relative range of accommodation (R′P′) is 5/6 of a metre, of which 2/3 of a metre (R′A) is negative and 1/6 of metre (AP′) is positive and the relative amplitude is 5 D (i.e., 6 D – 1 D) of which 2 D is negative and 3 D is positive.

It is, therefore, obvious that nearer the object is to the eye, smaller will be the positive and larger the negative range of accommodation.

If the eyes are emmetropic and the object of fixation is at infinity there will be no negative accommodation, and conversely if the object is at near point, the positive accommodation will be nil.

Thus while there is one absolute far point, one absolute near point and one absolute range of accommodation, there is a different relative far point, near point and range for every degree of accommodation.

If the accommodation is kept constant and convergence is made to vary (Fig. 21.7), the amount of convergence which can be exerted or relaxed is called the relative convergence. This can be measured by accommodating for a fixed object and varying the convergence by prisms. The strongest prism, base outwards, which can be tolerated without producing diplopia is a measure of positive portion of convergence (Ba) of the relative convergence (ab) or the amount by which the normal convergence can be augmented. Similarly, the strongest prism, base inwards, which can be tolerated is a measure of the negative portion of convergence (Bb) of the relative convergence and is the amount by which the convergence can be relaxed.

**Binocular accommodation :** Not only are convergence and accommodation closely related, they also have a mutual effect of the one upon the other. Binocular accommodation is usually seen to be higher than uniocular accommodation (the range is 0.5 to 1.5 D).

**Binocular convergence :** It is no doubt influenced by accommodation but several factors influence it as under :

- basic tonus
- accommodative convergence
- fusional convergence
- proximal convergence

The term relative convergence thus is applied to the convergence which is the amount that can be exerted (positive relative convergence) or relaxed (negative relative convergence) while the accommodation is kept constant (Fig. 21.8). If accommodation is maintained for a fixed object (Q) at the reading distance or working distance

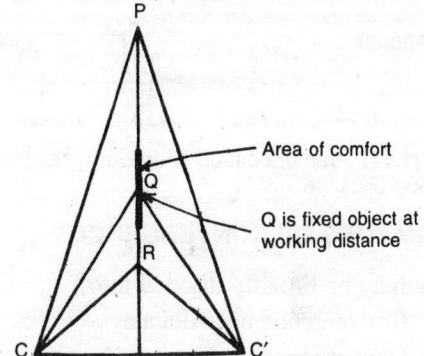

**Fig. 21.8.** Relative convergence when accommodation is constant.

the strongest adducting prism, base out, which can be tolerated without producing diplopia is the positive portion (QR) of relative convergence (RP) or the degree by which the normal convergence can be augmented. The strongest abducing prism, base in, which can be tolerated is the negative portion (QP) of the relative convergence. If comfort is to be maintained in close work the positive portion of the relative convergence should be larger than the negative so that ample convergence is in reserve otherwise it is advisable to prescribe prisms (base in) or convergence exercises to assist those who do continuous near work. Middle third of the range of relative convergence is called the area of comfort. If the convergence is reduced beyond this aids should be given. If at 33 cm a patient can tolerate abducting prisms of 4 dioptres and adducting prisms of 8 dioptres (Fig. 21.9), the convergence at working distance (D) falls just within the area of comfort. If he can tolerate abducting prisms of 2 dioptres and abducting prisms of 10 dioptres though the relative convergence is the same, i.e., 12 dioptres yet the area of comfort falls between 2 to 6 dioptres (Fig. 21.10), i.e., the working distance (D) is outside the area of comfort hence he will be uncomfortable and requires either relief by prisms or reduction in working distance.

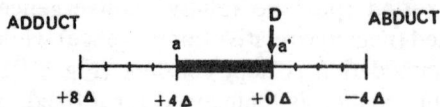

**Fig. 21.9.** Area of comfort in convergence for a given working distance.

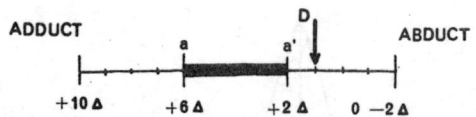

**Fig. 21.10.** Area of comfort in convergence for a given working distance.

## ANOMALIES OF CONVERGENCE

They may be broadly divided into :
- Convergence insufficiency
- Convergence excess

### Convergence insufficiency

It is the condition is which parallel movements of the eyes are normal but the associated process of simultaneous contraction of medial recti muscle is reduced in its power. A condition of insufficiency is said to exist if the near point of convergence is more than 11 cm away from the interocular baseline which is about 10 mm from the cornea (or 10 mm from the apex of the cornea). If measured on synoptophore the insufficiency of convergence is said to exist if there is difficulty in attaining 30° of convergence. Dissociation of accommodation and convergence or working outside the area of comfort is more

productive of symptoms, hence more important clinically. We may also consider this as fusional range deficiency.

Convergence insufficiency may exist as a separate clinical entity, unassociated with exo- or esophoria, or it may exist in association with esophoria, or exophoria, or even with hyperphoria.

Convergence insufficiency may be classified as under :

**Classification of convergence insufficiency**

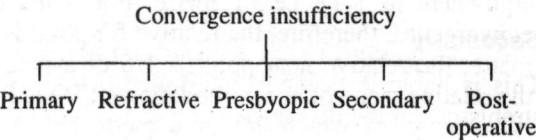

- Primary or idiopathic
- Refractive
- Presbyopic
- Secondary
- Postoperative

### Primary or idiopathic

*Anatomical factors :* Wide inter-pupillary distance and delayed and inadequate functional development are the usual aetiological factors in this type of insufficiency.

*Systemic :* General diseases or debility due to toxic conditions, e.g., illness, metabolic or endocrinal disorders, may cause convergence insufficiency. Overwork, worry and psychological instability are undoubtedly important factors in several cases. In this country it has been quite commonly seen in girls at puberty, persons with nutritional deficiency, and as the presbyopic age is approaching.

### Refractive

This involves the question of formation of a sharply and clearly defined image upon each foveal region. It is also a question of accommodation convergence relationship. Convergence tends to suffer if accommodation is not normally employed. Insufficiency is frequently seen in uncorrected myopes and hypermetropes. It is also deficient in those who do not call upon it as in high hypermetropes, anisometropes or amblyopes. Convergence insufficiency is also evident in patients who have habitually worn too full a plus spherical correction. These cases, specially children, need to be periodically reviewed for the refraction at suitable intervals.

### Presbyopic

The near point of convergence recedes as accommodation decreases with age and there tends to develop exophoria for near fixation. Neglect of presbyopia may lead to fixation of this anomaly.

### Secondary

This is liable to occur in intermittent divergent strabismus of the divergence excess type if treatment has been neglected until later in life. In cases of vertical muscle imbalance, convergence tends to become weakened apparently as a result of the effort required to overcome the vertical deviation to maintain binocular single vision. This results in exophoria for near with a gradually receding near point of convergence.

### Postoperative insufficiency

It occurs as a result of symptoms of an over-liberal recession of one or both medial recti or of an over-liberal resection of both lateral recti.

### Symptoms of convergence insufficiency

The presence of symptoms largely depends upon patient's visual requirements. These symptoms are, therefore, seen more commonly in desk workers and precision workers rather than in farm or manual labour.

The most usual story is unsuitability of glasses in those wearing spectacles. The patient roams about from one place to another in search of glasses which will give him comfort but seems to be dissatisfied with every pair he gets. The common complaint, however, is of ocular fatigue associated with headaches and pain in the eyeballs, especially so after near work. A mild constant headache is not unusual although some patients show migrainous tendencies and the pain is not relieved by analgesics. Soreness of the eye and redness of conjunctiva especially of the nasal half, commonly occur after prolonged close work. The author has seen several cases where recurrent marginal corneal ulcers have been produced by this deficiency. They disappeared after the deficiency was corrected by exercises. Blurred vision and sometimes horizontal diplopia for near vision is not uncommon. The absolute range of convergence may be satisfactory. It may be working outside the area of comfort or convergence accommodation dissociation which may be responsible for symptoms.

### Diagnosis

There is no limitation of uniocular adduction movement of each eye yet the eyes fail to converge fully. The diagnosis is based on the presence of orthophoria in the distance and the increase of divergence as the near point is reached. There is remoteness of the near point, the low prism convergence and the normal prism divergence. There may or may not be an associated exophoria of the convergence weakness type.

### Treatment

As the aetiology of the condition is varied, the main treatment should be directed against causative factors. The prognosis is good with treatment provided general causes, physical and psychological, are adequately rectified. Working under strain and poor visual hygienic conditions should be eliminated.

The treatment essentially consists in orthoptic training with convergence exercises by stereoscopic slides of increasing complexities on the stereoscope and then on the synoptophore for about 2 to 6 weeks, to start with daily and then on alternate days. It is more practical and perhaps more fruitful to give these exercises on fusion slides as the main aim is to increase the fusional convergence which has a corrective influence on other forms of convergence.

These are supplemented by simple exercises of convergence carried out at home whereby the patient attempts to approximate the near point by fixing the object as it approaches his eyes until it appears double.

Training of voluntary convergence is very helpful if the patient is intelligent and cooperative. It aims at developing the control of the position of eyes. The patient is made to understand physiological diplopia which he practices. If a finger is brought in the field of vision while the patient is fixing a distant light, there appear to be two fingers, and now if he fixes at the finger then there appear to be two lights at the distance. While the finger is moved to and fro, the distance between the lights increases or decreases. The patient tries to maintain the two lights apart as long as possible. The finger may again be brought in if the two lights become single as soon as the finger is removed. The exercise is completed by doubling the lights without the aid of the finger. Development of voluntary convergence goes a long way in relieving symptoms. In the beginning the exercises may have a fatiguing influence on the patient, of which he may be forewarned, and there is exacerbation of symptoms but as the practice continues remarkable relief is obtained.

Duction exercises are given by placing prisms of gradually increasing strength, base out, in front of one or both eyes in order to produce convergence in the distance. The patient is asked to look at an object and while the gaze is still fixed at the object, prisms of gradually increasing strength are placed, base out, before the eyes at an interval of 5 seconds or so, the patient being encouraged to fuse the two images into one. The exercise can be continued at home. The patient is given 2 D prism with which to exercise, practice for one week which may be increased by 1 D at weekly intervals. If all these exercises fail then relieving prisms, base in, are incorporated in spectacles for near work in which sufficient correction is given to bring convergence just within the area of comfort for a particular distance required. These are mostly required for presbyopes who have insufficient converging power for near work. Hypermetropes are given under correction and myopes full correction to stimulate their accommodation which will simultaneously stimulate convergence thus increasing the content of accommodative convergence required for comfortable work. Relieving prisms and bifocals in young age should be avoided as far as possible. Relieving prisms sometimes aggravate the condition and prisms of increasing power are required.

If the patient's intelligence and temperament do not hamper cooperation and since the reflexes concerned are usually plastic, fusion amplitude of some 70° can be developed with relief of symptoms. Orthoptic training, which consists of developing adequate convergence including fusional amplitude by convergence exercises in stereoscopes or synoptophore (amblyoscope), duction reserve by prism exercises and simple exercises at home give beneficial results. Voluntary effort is enlisted to aid development of fusion amplitude.

Operation of advancement or resection of internal recti in absence of divergent squint is not advisable since the deficiency at near point is corrected at the cost of equally serious esophoria for distance. In such cases external recti should be recessed as it does not produce the same degree of esophoria.

### Convergence excess

It can occur only when associated with related orthophoria for distant vision and normal horizontal movement of either eye. It is due to innervational influences of hyperkinetic type. It can be of the following types :

- Primary
- Secondary
- Accommodative (associated with excessive accommodation)

**Primary :** It is of spasmodic nature and is associated with spasm of accommodation and contraction of pupil. It occurs in irritative lesions of the central nervous system, e.g., meningeal irritation, increased labyrinthine pressure and lesions near the aqueduct of Sylvius giving rise to nystagmus retractorius. Hypersensitivity of nervous system and unstable neurotic temperament may augment reflex irritability from dental or paranasal sinus disease which produce hyperkinesia. Traumatic neurosis or hysterical spasm of convergence with miosis and accommodative spasm is not uncommon.

**Secondary :** Secondary convergence excess may follow an insufficiency of divergence.

**Accommodative :** Increase in accommodation in refractive conditions with miosis and increase in convergence excess are responsible for most of the cases as these functions are synergic and usually vary in consonance with each other.

It may, therefore, be termed as a spasm of near reflex. It is typically seen in uncorrected hypermetropes, recently fully corrected myopes and in early presbyopes. It is due either to excessive accommodation becoming a habit as in hypermetropes or to the use of accommodation for the first time as in fully corrected myopes and presbyopes who are making persistent efforts to mobilize their failing accommodation. It also occurs when desire for clear vision, in spite of difficulties, calls for unusually accentuated effort of accommodation as in those whose vision is embarrassed by poor illumination, opacities in ocular media or going to work early in convalescence. It may also occur in child starting near work for the first time or a conscientious young desk worker starting his work life.

## Symptoms

Reading and close work are difficult. The print rapidly becomes blurred. Ocular fatigue and headache come on any effort at concentration, particularly so if the patient is ill. These may be merely annoying or may be completely incapacitating. Sometimes convergence may go into spasm, near-work becoming impossible, and homonymous diplopia may occur. In worst cases, especially of traumatic neurosis or hysteria, the spasm may result in fixed position of extreme convergence resembling bilateral abducens palsy. There is a concomitant spasm of accommodation and the pupil is smaller and fixed. The condition is sometimes accompanied by intermittent horizontal and rapid nystagmus.

## Treatment

The first principle is elimination of the causative factor. Refractive errors are corrected judiciously. Near work for all patients is curtailed. Treatment for any significant heterophoria should be instituted. Physical and mental health is attended to particularly during convalescence. Visual hygiene is ensured. Orthoptic exercises, except for the heterophoria, are usually unhelpful. Divergence exercises on diploscope or synoptophore are difficult to do but may prove to be helpful. Exercise for relaxation of accommodation and convergence may be tried but are difficult and many a time abandoned by the patient.

# SECTION VI

# Orthoptics and Squint

This section in brief presents some basic factors and guidelines. For detailed study, the reader is referred to Clinical Ophthalmology in India, Volume VII, edited by the same author and published by the same publishers. The co-editor of this volume is Prof. O.P. Kulshreshta.

# CHAPTER 22

# Anatomy and Physiology of Binocular Functions

## ANATOMY AND PHYSIOLOGY OF BINOCULAR FUNCTIONS

For the understanding of the binocular functions, it is of paramount importance to go into the fundamentals of ocular anatomy and physiology specially dealing with the structure of the extrinsic ocular muscles, their related fascial membranes and their neural control.

### Extrinsic ocular muscles (Fig. 22.1A)

The movements of the eyeball are controlled by six extrinsic ocular muscles—four recti (superior, inferior, lateral and medial) and two obliques (superior and inferior). These muscles can rotate the eyes on three axes, viz.,

1. horizontal axis,
2. vertical axis, and
3. anteroposterior axis.

Both uniocular and binocular movements are executed on these axes with fine neuromuscular

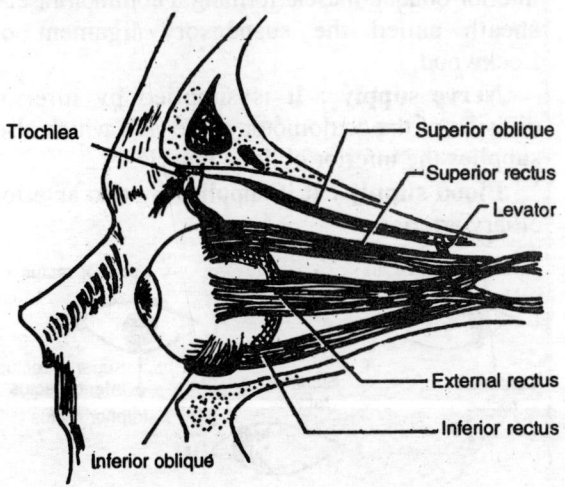

**Fig. 22.1A.** Muscles of the eyeball.

coordination between the muscles of the same eye as well as among those of the two eyes.

### Medial rectus

It arises near the apex of the orbit from the medial aspect of the annulus of Zinn with fascial connections with optic nerve and superior and inferior rectus muscles. It is 40.8 mm long, runs forwards almost parallel to the medial wall of the orbit and is inserted by a tendon 3.7 mm long, 10.3 mm broad and 5.5 mm away from the limbus of the medial aspect of the globe (Fig. 22.1B).

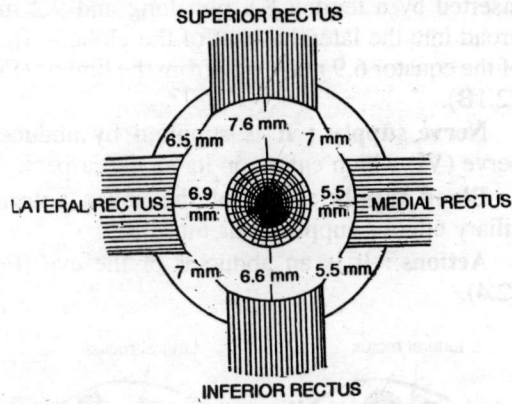

**Fig. 22.1B.** Insertion of recti on anterior surface of the globe.

**Nerve supply** : It is supplied by the oculomotor nerve (III).

**Blood supply** : It is supplied by two anterior ciliary arteries.

**Actions** : It is an adductor of the eye (Figs. 22.2 and 22.3).

### Lateral rectus

It arises from the lateral aspect of the annulus of

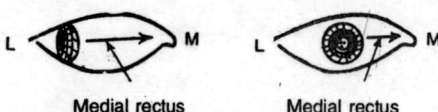

**Fig. 22.2.** Actions of medial rectus.

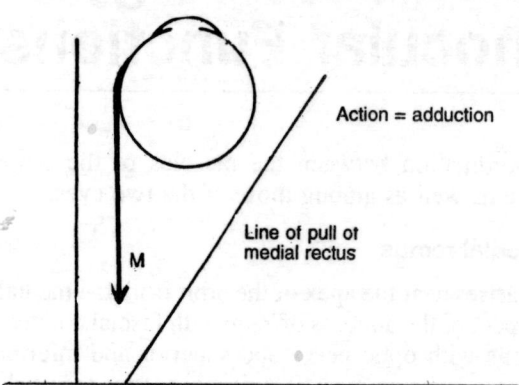

**Fig. 22.3.** Adduction by medial rectus.

Zinn and from the spina recti lateralis. It is 40.6 mm long and passes forwards between the eyeball and the lateral wall of the orbit. It is inserted by a tendon 8.8 mm long and 9.2 mm broad into the lateral aspect of the globe in front of the equator 6.9 mm away from the limbus (Fig. 22.1B).

**Nerve supply :** It is supplied by abducent nerve (VI) which enters on its medial aspect.

**Blood supply :** One of the seven anterior ciliary arteries supplies this muscle.

**Actions :** It is an abductor of the eye (Fig. 22.4).

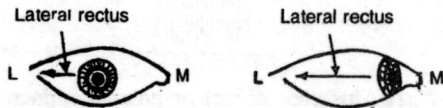

**Fig. 22.4.** Actions of the lateral rectus.

### Inferior rectus

This muscle arises from the lower aspect of the annulus of Zinn in common with the tendon of the medial rectus. It is 40 mm long and runs along the floor of the orbit underneath the eyeball in a plane inclined at 23° to the nasal side of the vertical meridian of the eyeball. It is inserted by a 5.5 mm long and 9.8 mm broad tendon on the inferior aspect of the sclera in front of the equator

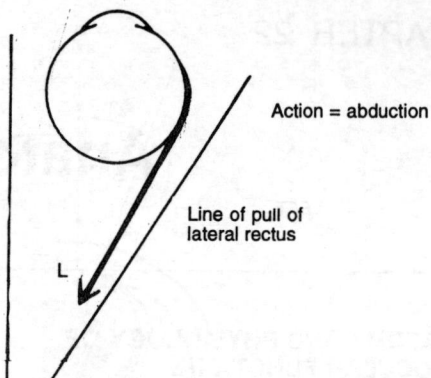

**Fig. 22.5.** Abduction by lateral rectus.

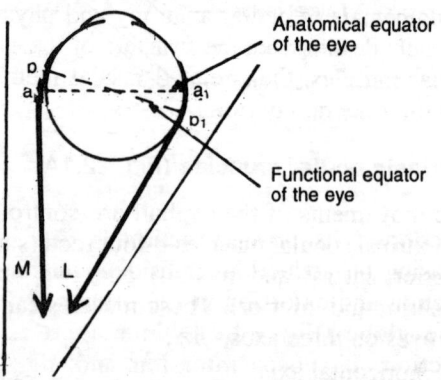

**Fig. 22.6.** Action of medial and lateral recti.

and about 6.6 mm away from the limbus (Fig. 22.1B). During its course it is crossed by the inferior oblique muscle forming a common fascial sheath called the suspensory ligament of Lockwood.

**Nerve supply :** It is supplied by inferior division of the oculomotor nerve (III) which also supplies the inferior oblique muscle.

**Blood supply :** It is supplied by two anterior ciliary arteries.

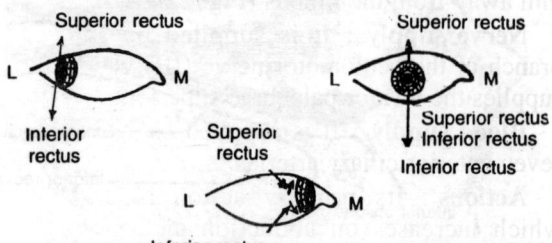

**Fig. 22.7.** Actions of superior and inferior recti.

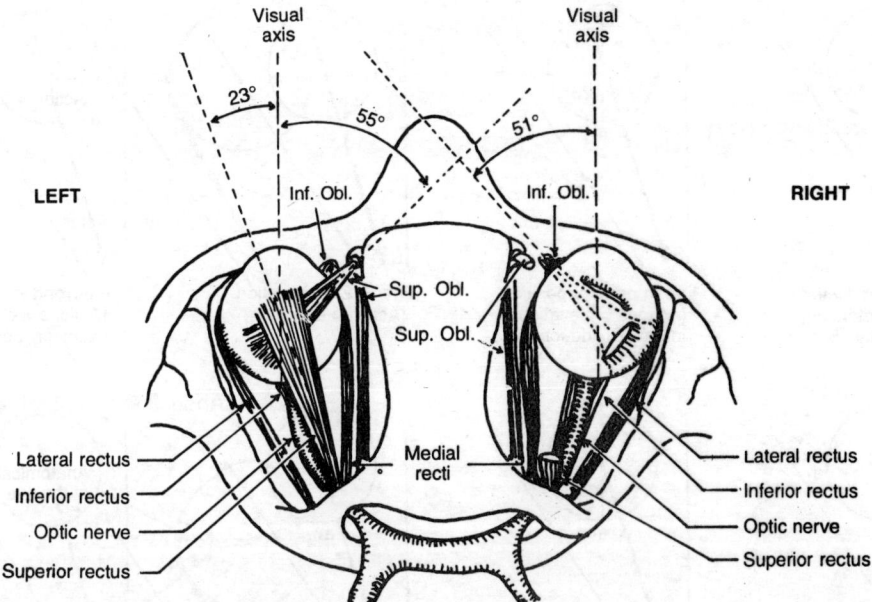

**Fig. 22.8.** Position of extrinsic ocular muscles.

**Actions :** Its primary action is depression, increasing on abduction. Subsidiary actions are adduction and extorsion in the primary position of the globe (Fig. 22.7) which increases on adduction. It causes intorsion and abduction beyond 23° of abduction.

### Superior rectus

It arises from the superior margin of the annulus of Zinn. It is 41.8 mm long and passes forwards through the orbit between the eyeball and the levator palpebrae superioris. With the latter it has a close relationship at its origin. It runs in a plane inclined at 23° to the nasal side of the vertical meridian of the eyeball. It is inserted by a tendon 5.8 mm long and 10.8 mm broad into the superior aspect of the sclera in front of the equator and 7.7 mm away from the limbus (Fig. 22.1B).

**Nerve supply :** It is supplied by superior branch of the oculomotor nerve (III) which also supplies the levator palpebrae superioris.

**Blood supply :** It is supplied by two of the seven anterior ciliary arteries.

**Actions :** Its primary action is elevation which increases on abduction and subsidiary actions are adduction and intorsion in the primary position of the globe (Fig. 22.10) which increases

on adduction. Beyond 23° of abduction it causes extorsion and abduction.

### Superior oblique

It arises from the apex of the orbit from the superior and the medial aspect of the optic foramen. It is the longest muscle of the eyeball (40 mm muscular part and 20 mm tendinous part and runs forwards in the upper and the medial aspect of the orbit between superior and medial rectus muscles till it reaches the superomedial angle of the orbit where it passes through the cartilaginous pulley to become rounded tendon. Then it is reflected backwards, downwards and laterally and after passing under the superior rectus, it is inserted into the posterolateral aspect of the eyeball behind the equator. The reflected tendinous portion of the muscle makes an angle of 54° to the nasal side of the vertical meridian of the eyeball. Its functional origin is from the trochlea (Fig. 22.11).

**Nerve supply :** It is supplied by the trochlear nerve (IV).

**Blood supply :** It is supplied by the muscular branch of the ophthalmic artery.

**Actions :** The primary action is depression

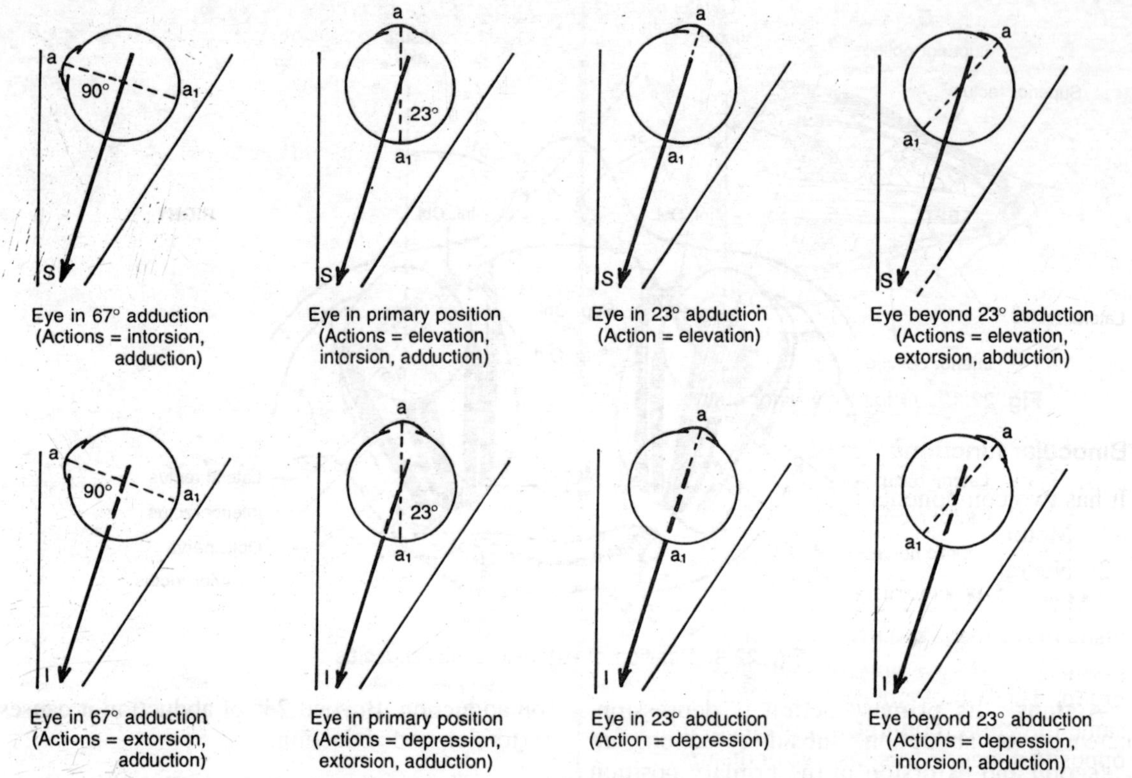

Eye in 67° adduction
(Actions = intorsion,
adduction)

Eye in primary position
(Actions = elevation,
intorsion, adduction)

Eye in 23° abduction
(Action = elevation)

Eye beyond 23° abduction
(Actions = elevation,
extorsion, abduction)

Eye in 67° adduction
(Actions = extorsion,
adduction)

Eye in primary position
(Actions = depression,
extorsion, adduction)

Eye in 23° abduction
(Action = depression)

Eye beyond 23° abduction
(Actions = depression,
intorsion, abduction)

**Figs. 22.9 and 22.10.** Actions of right superior and inferior recti in various positions and right orbit in horizontal section viewed from above. S = line of pull of the superior rectus; I = line of pull of the inferior rectus; aa₁ = direction of the vertical meridian of the eye.

increasing on adduction. Its subsidiary actions are abduction and intorsion increasing on abduction.

### Inferior oblique

It arises from the shallow fossa in the orbital portion of the maxillary bone immediately behind the lower orbital margin and the lateral side of the lacrimal fossa. It is 37 mm long and runs laterally and backwards at an angle of 51° to the nasal side of the vertical meridian of the eyeball. It passes underneath and in close association with the inferior rectus muscle making a common sheath (ligament of Lockwood) to be inserted at the lower temporal quadrant of the eyeball behind the equator (Figs. 22.11 and 22.12).

**Nerve supply :** It is supplied by a branch from the inferior division of the oculomotor nerve (III). The branch to the muscle sends the motor root to the ciliary ganglion.

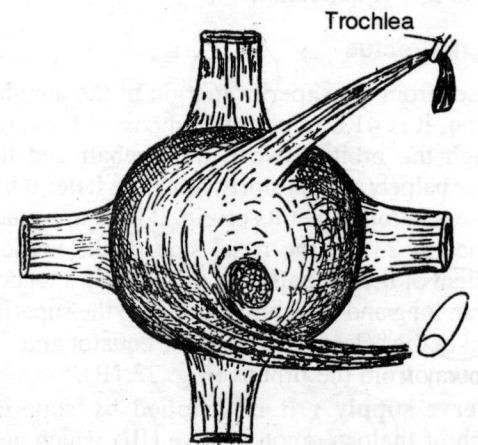

Trochlea

**Fig. 22.11.** Insertion of superior and inferior oblique.

**Blood supply :** It is supplied by muscular branches of the ophthalmic artery.

**Actions :** Its primary action is elevation increasing on adduction. Its subsidiary actions are abduction and extorsion increasing on abduction

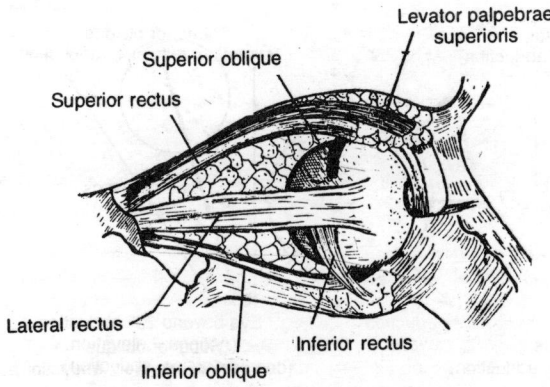

**Fig. 22.12.** Origin of inferior oblique.

## Binocular functions

It has two components :

1. Motor
2. Neural

**Motor :** The binocular movements are synergistic movements requiring the contraction of one group of muscles and relaxation of the other group. These movements may take place in the same direction (conjugate movements) or in the opposite direction (disjunctive or disjugate movements). The rotatory movements of the eye from the primary position are shown in Figs. 22.13, 22.14, 22.15 and 22.16.

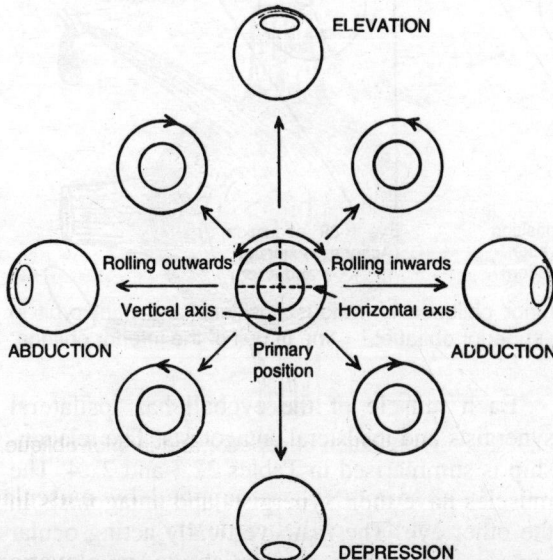

**Fig. 22.13.** Rotating movements of the right eye as viewed from in front.

**Table 22.1. Muscles involved in various ocular movements from the primary position of the globe**

| Movement | Muscles | Axis on which performed |
|---|---|---|
| 1. Intorsion | Superior rectus<br>Superior oblique | Anteroposterior axis |
| 2. Extorsion | Inferior rectus<br>Inferior oblique | |
| 3. Elevation | Superior rectus<br>Inferior oblique | Horizontal axis |
| 4. Depression | Inferior rectus<br>Superior oblique | |
| 5. Abduction | Lateral rectus<br>Inferior oblique<br>Superior oblique | Vertical axis |
| 6. Adduction | Medial rectus<br>Superior rectus<br>Inferior rectus | |

The synergistic actions of the ocular muscles from the primary position are given below and individual actions in Tables 22.1 to 22.6.

The muscles performing the movements depend upon the position of the eyeball. The eyeballs can be moved on an anteroposterior axis (intorsion and extorsion) or on a horizontal axis (elevation and depression) or on a vertical axis (abduction and adduction). When the eyeballs are in a primary position the muscles perform the movement as shown in Table 22.1 and Figs. 22.13 to 22.16.

If the eyeballs are looking to the right, the muscles taking part in elevation and depression differ in the two eyes. In the right eye, the anatomical axis of the eyeball corresponds to the long axis of the inferior and superior recti while in the left eye the anatomical axis of the eyeball coincides with the long axis of the superior and inferior obliques. The muscles whose long axis corresponds with the anatomical axis of the eyeball perform the movements of elevation and depression. The action of the muscles when the eyes are looking to the right are summarised in Table 22.2 and Fig. 22.17.

When the eyes are looking towards the left, the anatomical axis of the left eyeball coincides with the long axis of the left superior and left inferior recti and the anatomical axis of the right

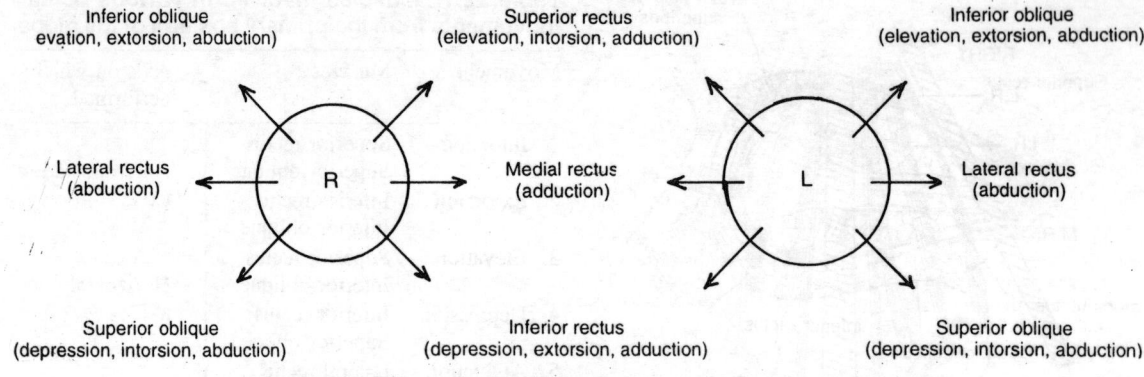

Inferior oblique
evation, extorsion, abduction)

Superior rectus
(elevation, intorsion, adduction)

Inferior oblique
(elevation, extorsion, abduction)

Lateral rectus
(abduction)

Medial rectus
(adduction)

Lateral rectus
(abduction)

Superior oblique
(depression, intorsion, abduction)

Inferior rectus
(depression, extorsion, adduction)

Superior oblique
(depression, intorsion, abduction)

**Fig. 22.14.** Action of extraocular muscles from primary position.

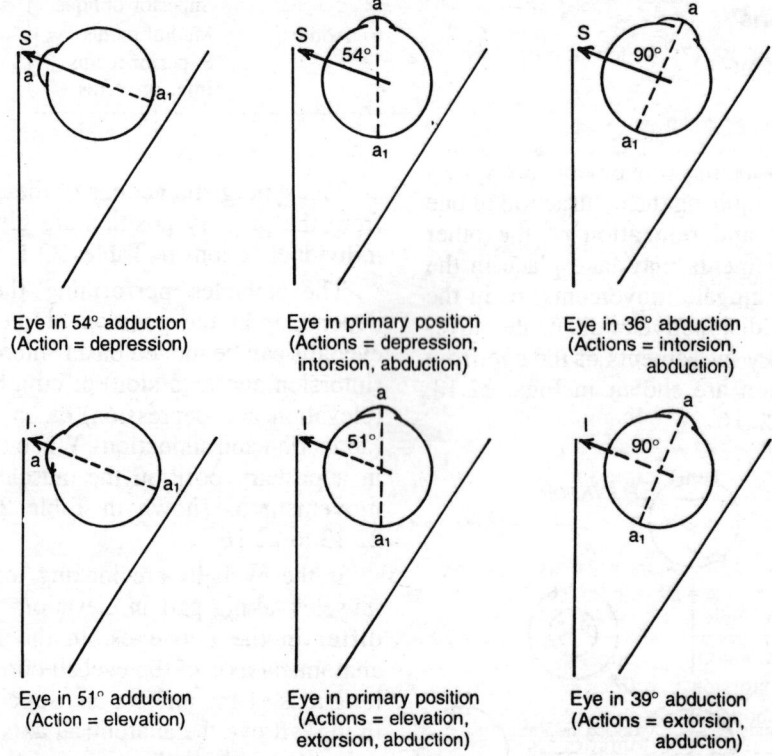

Eye in 54° adduction
(Action = depression)

Eye in primary position
(Actions = depression,
intorsion, abduction)

Eye in 36° abduction
(Actions = intorsion,
abduction)

Eye in 51° adduction
(Action = elevation)

Eye in primary position
(Actions = elevation,
extorsion, abduction)

Eye in 39° abduction
(Actions = extorsion,
abduction)

**Figs. 22.15 and 22.16.** Actions of right superior and inferior obliques in various positions and right orbit in horizontal section viewed from above. S = line of pull of the superior oblique; I = line of pull of the inferior oblique; $aa_1$ = direction of the vertical meridian of the eye.

eyeball coincides with the long axis of the right inferior and superior obliques. The left eyeball is elevated or depressed by the left superior or left inferior rectus and the right eyeball is elevated or depressed by right inferior or right superior obliques. The actions of muscles when the eyes are looking to the left are summarised in Table 22.3 and Fig. 22.18.

Each muscle of the eyeball has ipsilateral synergists and ipsilateral antagonists. The relationship is summarised in Tables 22.3 and 22.4. The muscles have their synergists and antagonists in the other eye. The main vertically acting ocular muscles have their antagonists and synergists. These are given in Tables 22.5, 22.6 and 22.7 and Figs. 22.1 to 22.6.

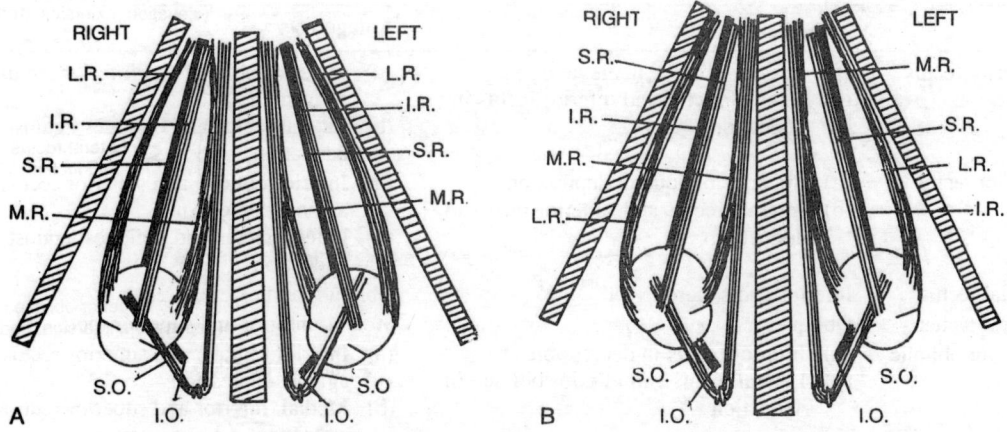

**Fig. 22.17.** Action of muscles in dextroversion (A) and in laevoversion (B).

**Table 22.2.  Action of muscles in dextroverted position of eyeballs**

| Movement | Right eye | Left eye | Axis of movement |
|---|---|---|---|
| 1. Intorsion | Superior oblique | Superior rectus | Anteroposterior axis |
| 2. Extorsion | Inferior oblique | Inferior rectus | |
| 3. Abduction | — | Lateral rectus Superior rectus Inferior rectus | Vertical axis |
| 4. Adduction | Medial rectus Superior oblique Inferior oblique | — | — |
| 5. Elevation | Superior rectus | Inferior oblique | Horizontal axis |
| 6. Depression | Inferior rectus | Superior oblique | |

**Table 22.3.  Action of muscles in laevoverted position of eyeballs**

| Movement | Right eye | Left eye | Axis of movement |
|---|---|---|---|
| 1. Intorsion | Superior rectus | Superior oblique | Anteroposterior axis |
| 2. Extorsion | Inferior rectus | Inferior oblique | |
| 3. Abduction | Superior rectus Inferior rectus Lateral rectus | — | — |
| 4. Adduction | — | Medial rectus Superior oblique Inferior oblique | Vertical axis |
| 5. Elevation | Inferior oblique | Superior rectus | Horizontal axis |
| 6. Depression | Superior oblique | Inferior rectus | |

**Neural :** The above mentioned synergistic and antagonistic actions of the muscles are governed by certain innervational factors controlled by the central nervous system. There are two important laws governing these actions :

·1.  Law of reciprocal innervation

**Table 22.4. Ipsilateral synergists and antagonists**

| Muscle | Synergists | Antagonists |
|---|---|---|
| 1. Superior rectus | (a) Inferior oblique in elevation<br>(b) Internal rectus and inferior rectus in adduction | (a) Superior oblique and inferior rectus against elevation<br>(b) Lateral rectus and obliques against adduction |
| 2. Inferior rectus | (a) Superior oblique in depression<br>(b) Internal rectus and superior rectus in adduction | (a) Inferior oblique and superior rectus against depression<br>(b) Lateral rectus and obliques against adduction |
| 3. Medial rectus | Inferior and superior recti | Obliques and external rectus |
| 4. Lateral rectus | Obliques | Medial, inferior and superior recti |
| 5. Superior oblique | (a) Inferior rectus in depression<br>(b) Lateral rectus and inferior oblique in abduction | (a) Inferior oblique and superior rectus against depression<br>(b) Medial, inferior and superior recti against abduction |
| 6. Inferior oblique | (a) Superior rectus in elevation<br>(b) Lateral rectus and superior oblique in abduction | (a) Superior oblique and inferior rectus against elevation<br>(b) Medial, superior and inferior recti against abduction |

**Table 22.5. Synergists and antagonists of vertically acting muscles**

| Muscle | Superior rectus | Inferior rectus | Superior oblique | Inferior oblique |
|---|---|---|---|---|
| *Synergists* | | | | |
| Ipsilateral (indirect) | Inferior oblique | Superior oblique | Inferior rectus | Superior rectus |
| Contralateral (direct) | Inferior oblique | Superior oblique | Inferior rectus | Superior rectus |
| *Antagonists* | | | | |
| Ipsilateral (direct) | Inferior rectus | Superior rectus | Inferior oblique | Superior oblique |
| Contralateral (indirect) | Superior oblique | Inferior oblique | Superior rectus | Inferior rectus |

## 2. Hering's law

The law of reciprocal innervation ensures that the contraction of each muscle is accompanied by a simultaneous and proportional relaxation of its antagonist.

Hering's law postulates equal and simultaneous innervation to the yoke muscles of the eye.

In binocular coordination movements of the eye the reciprocal innervation is controlled at three levels (Fig. 22.18). There is a level of binocular control (I level) which determines the direction of the two visual axes with regard to each other; the second level is the level of monocular coordinating areas which distribute the final contractile impulses to the individual

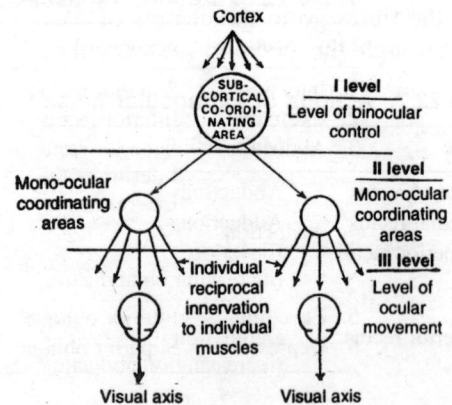

**Fig. 22.18.** Reciprocal innervation.

extraocular muscle; the third level is the peripheral level or the ocular movements. The

**Table 22.6.**

|  | | Elevation | | |
|---|---|---|---|---|
| Dextro-elevation | R.S.R.\nL.I.O. | R.S.R.\nL.S.R. | L.S.R.\nR.I.O. | Laevo-elevation |
| Dextro-version | L.M.R.\nR.L.R. | Primary position | R.M.R.\nL.L.R. | Laevo-version |
| Dextro-depression | L.S.O.\nR.I.R. | R.I.R.\nL.I.R. | R.S.O.\nL.I.R. | Laevo-depression |
|  | | Depression | | |

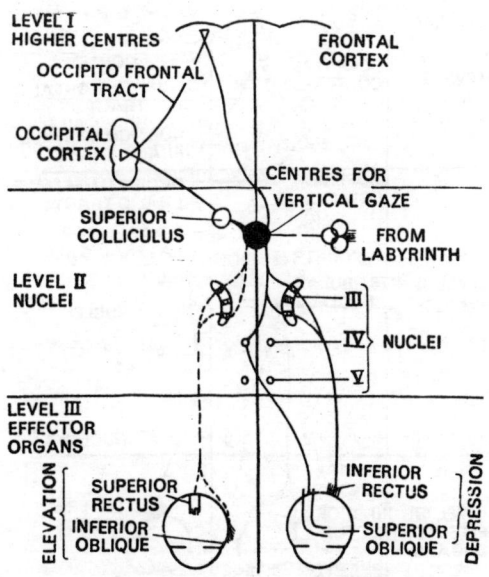

**Fig. 22.19.** Pathway for vertical gaze.

highest control is in a centre in the second frontal gyrus in the posterior part of the frontal convolutions where movements and not individual ocular muscles are represented except the muscles of the lid.

The pathway of voluntary movements starts from the second frontal convolutions in the frontal lobe. The fibres pass into the corona radiata of the white matter and enter the knee of the internal capsule as a part of the pyramidal tract. The fibres run in the internal capsule and proceed downwards into the pons. The fibres of the vertical and other conjugate movements are given off in the superior colliculus where they probably go to a centre for vertical gaze (Fig. 22.19). From this centre the fibres pass on to the nuclei of III and IV nerves in the mid-brain to be ultimately distributed to the respective muscles. There is a relay between the frontal and the occipital cortex and when the fibres go to the centres of the vertical gaze through the occipito-mesencephalic tract

passing through the superior colliculus on their way.

The contingents of the lateral gaze (Fig. 22.20) leave as two bundles of fibres. One passes to the mid-brain and the other to the upper pons. They descend for a short distance in the mesial fillet and then pass to the centre of lateral movements in the tegmentum. There is a relay between the frontal and the occipital cortex via the occipito-frontal tract. The fibres from the occipital cortex go to the centre for lateral gaze via the occipito-mesencephalic tract passing through substance of superior colliculus. Fibres from the vestibular nucleus enter the centre for the lateral

**Table 22.7. Actions of extraocular muscles**

| Muscle | Main action | Subsidiary | Actions |
|---|---|---|---|
| 1. Lateral rectus | Abduction |  | Retraction of globe |
| 2. Medial rectus | Adduction |  | Retraction of globe |
| 3. Superior rectus | Elevation (increasing on abduction) | Intorsion and adduction increasing on adduction; or extorsion and adduction beyond 23° abduction | Retraction of globe |
| 4. Inferior rectus | Depression (increasing on abduction) | Extorsion and adduction increasing on adduction; or intorsion and abduction beyond 23° abduction | Retraction of globe |
| 5. Superior oblique | Depression (increasing on adduction) | Intorsion and abduction increasing on abduction | Protraction of globe |
| 6. Inferior oblique | Elevation (increasing on adduction) | Extorsion and abduction increasing on abduction | Protraction of globe |

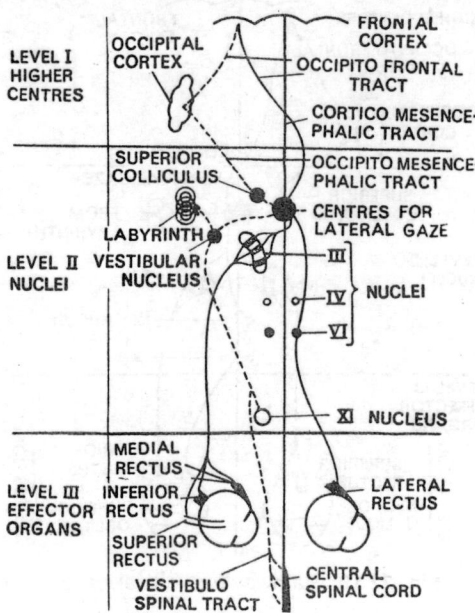

**Fig. 22.20.** Pathway for lateral gaze.

gaze via the posterior longitudinal bundle. Similar is the neural control of disjunctive movements, viz., convergence and divergence which have been described earlier (see convergence).

## Binocular vision

Binocular vision has been classically described to have the following components :

- Simultaneous macular perception
- Fusion
- Stereopsis

The function of binocular vision is to produce a single mental impression of the same object by the coordination of two separate eyes of an individual. Achievement of good binocular vision is dependent upon :

- Proper receipt of sensory stimuli (normal sensory apparatus and normal dioptric mechanism).
- Proper muscular coordination.
- Correct psychological (cortical) interpretation.

The advantages of binocular vision are :

- The field of vision is enlarged.
- Blind spot and other defects of each eye are compensated by the other.

- Binocular acuity is higher than uniocular.
- Stereopsis (depth perception).

### Simultaneous macular perception

This is the most primitive binocular function from evolutionary point of view and is the first to develop in a child. For the proper development of the function both the maculae should be efficient. The prerequisite is that two clear and almost equally distinct images should be formed. To do this aid is necessary from the physiologically fully functioning extraocular muscles as it is only then that the eyes can be readily, precisely and efficiently directed towards the object whose image is to be formed on the two maculae. Once these images are formed an efficiently working nervous mechanism will be able to receive the two impressions and psychologically interpret them into one image. It is an ability to interpret two sets of impulses coming from the maculae of the two eyes as one by the visual cortex. It is the first concept towards the development of fusion. Slight dioptric differences of the two eyes and little muscular incoordination can be compensated in a normal healthy person. Clinically it can be tested on a synoptophore by placing two dissimilar pictures which do not require fusion but which do not antagonise each other, e.g., lion and cage (Fig. 22.21). A normal individual usually sees these two dissimilar images as one, i.e., the lion in the cage. Inability to see them simultaneously shows the absence of the faculty of simultaneous perception. If only one image is seen at one time simultaneous perception is absent. The eye which sees the image most of the time has the macular dominance. If they are seen alternately there is an equal macular function in both eyes. Thus it might be noted in such a case uniocular or alternate suppression. The size of the

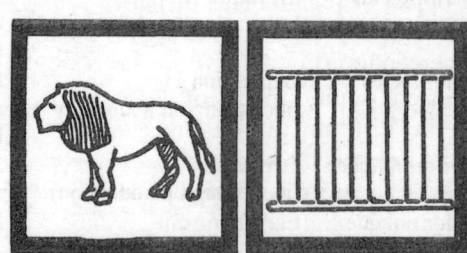

**Fig. 22.21.** Simultaneous macular perception.

slides should always be mentioned, i.e.,. whether foveal, macular or paramacular slides have been used.

## Fusion

This is the second faculty to be acquired in the evolution of binocular vision. This is a process by which visual cortex combines two almost similar objects into a single perception. There is also a faculty of fusing two dissimilar colours (colour fusion) when presented simultaneously to the two eyes, the resulting mixture being different from the original colours. Thus fusion can be achieved in spite of limited amount of difference in size, shape and colours. It can be tested on synoptophore with appropriate similar slides with some control to check the participation of both the eyes (Fig. 22.22). Fusion is present in a particular amplitude of ocular deviation which measures the amplitude of fusion. The presence of the fusion faculty in a case of squint carries a better prognosis in its functional cure.

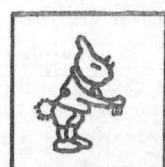 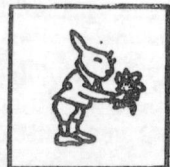

**Fig. 22.22.** Fusion slide.

## Stereopsis

It is the third and last step in the development of binocular vision which enables the person to develop depth perception (tridimensional vision). Because of the linear distance between the two eyes, an object in space forms slightly different angles in the two eyes. This results in slight but perceptible difference in the two retinal images of the object of regard. This disparity in the two images is interpreted at the higher centres as depth perception (Fig. 22.23).

The stereoacuity (extent of depth perception) varies in different individuals and can be measured by special slides on a synoptophore. These slides are so constructed as to project their images at the slightly disparate points on the retina, i.e., the right eye sees more on the right and the left eye sees more on the left. So long as

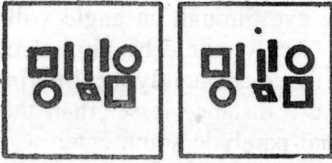

**Fig. 22.23.** Stereoscopic vision.

the disparate images fall on the Panum's area, no diplopia is experienced and fusion of such images produce stereopsis.

Actually a small degree of diplopia which should be produced by this projection is suppressed. At the same time impressions from both the eyes reach the brain and their integration results in an appreciation of a third dimension, i.e., stereoscopic vision.

A quicker and simpler method of testing stereopsis and stereoacuity is Titums fly test in which the use of polaroid glasses is made to see two disparate images on a small booklet. Stereopsis no doubt is a binocular function but certain monocular clues also help perceiving depth to a limited degree.

The monocular depth perception is limited to a degree but it is achieved by a process of rapid monocular movement to obtain two dissimilar images reproducing the conditions of binocular function.

## Judgement of distance

On this depends the process of projection and orientation of the subject in space and their relation to each other. In a normal individual it seems that the process is achieved and appreciated by the angular movements of the eyeball. This is an erroneous impression. The distance is interpreted not on the angular movement alone but in terms of the muscular force applied to move the eye through a particular angle. Thus, projection in space is computed graphically against the quantum of muscular force applied. This distance varies directly as the quantity of force. The relationship of force and distance is fixed as an impression on the basis of the past experiences. If the muscle is congenitally weak, the dissociation between force and angular deviation may not be appreciated. If some muscle becomes weaker in later life then the amount of force required to move the eye through an angle will be greater than the force required by normal muscle. The object will consequently be interpreted to be situated at a distance lesser than the actual. In paretic and paralytic squint such a condition is well manifested. In phorias also the judgement of distances and faculty of stereopsis may be impaired. This leads to false projection and false orientation.

## Development of binocular vision

Because of lack of structural development of the eye at birth, the binocular vision of eye is very poor which is attained fully by the age of 5-6 years.

At birth the eyes are linked only by unconditioned compensatory fixation reflex of an object to be maintained in spite of movement of the head and neck.

At 2-3 months the orientation reflex (enabling conjugate movements of the eye to maintain fixation of a moving object across the field of vision), refixation reflex and vergence reflex are developed. The vergence reflex is well developed at the age of 6 months. At 2-3 years, the accommodation reflexes are well developed. By 5-6 years binocular reflexes are well grounded.

# CHAPTER 23

# Methods of Examination and Diagnosis of Muscular Imbalance

For orthoptic investigations and treatment, several instruments are required. Some of the important ones are listed below :

- Synoptophore
- Stereoscope
- Diploscope
- Worth's four-dot test
- Livingston's binocular gauge
- Maddox tangent scale
- Maddox wing
- Bishop-Harman diaphragm test
- Hess screen
- Lees screen
- Cheiroscope
- Myoscope
- Remy separator
- Bar reader
- Bagolini striated glasses

### Synoptophore (Fig. 23.1)

It is an instrument which is utilised for

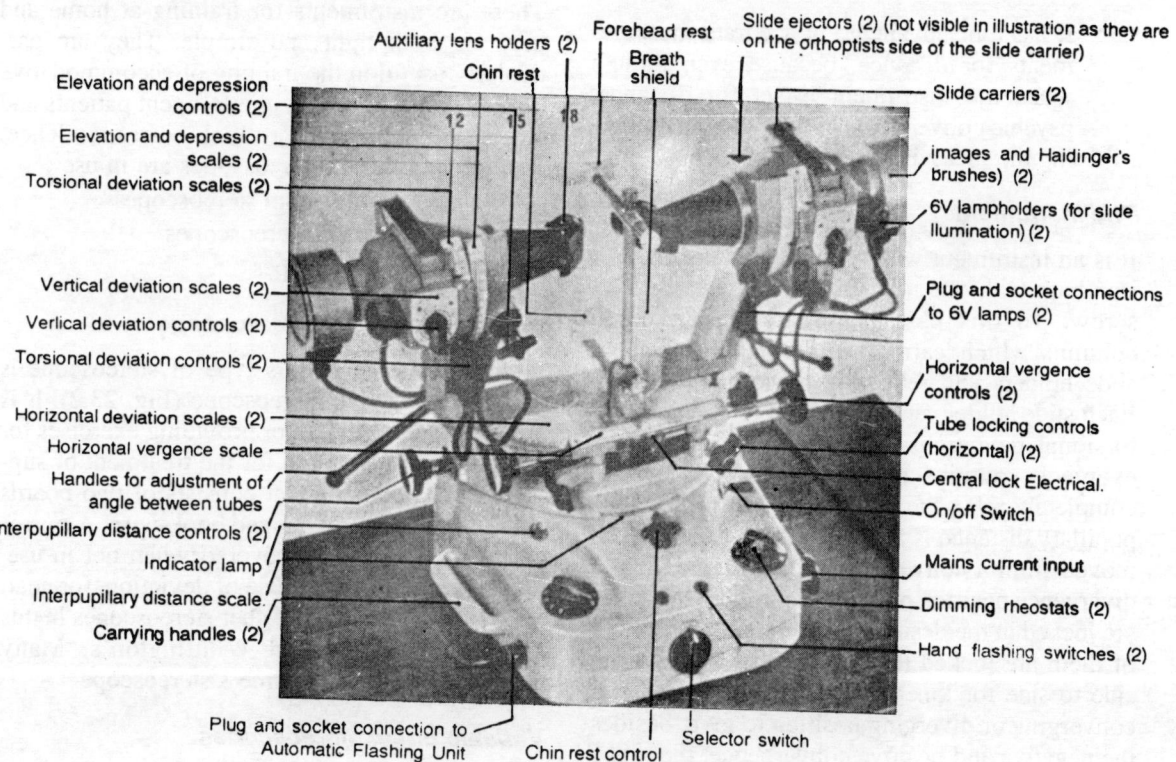

**Fig. 23.1.** Synoptophore.

195

- the measurement of the subjective and objective angles of squint;
- the diagnosis of a latent or manifest squint;
- the assessment of the degree of binocular functions; and
- the orthoptic exercises to develop the binocular functions in defective individuals.

### Advantages

- Over the instruments utilised for these purposes synoptophore presents certain advantages :
- It is more accurate in measuring the imbalance and in detecting the incomitance.
- The images can be moved both sideways and up and down by tapping the finger lever. It helps in stimulating the suppressing eye.
- An objective check can be maintained by an orthoptist on the patient's doing.

### Disadvantage

- It has a disadvantage in accurate measurements for distance, because even though when the instrument is set for distance, psychic convergence comes into play vitiating the measurements for distance.

### The instrument

It is an instrument which stands on a heavy cast iron base with one movable foot adjustable by a screw. To this base are attached gun metal columns which carry the illuminating system, slide holders and reflecting mirrors and lenses. Each slide holder can be adjusted for vertical and torsional deviations by separate screws. Each eyepiece contains a lens of +6.5 D sph. to completely relax the accommodation. The interpupillary distance is adjustable. The tubes can be moved from a convergence position of 70° to a divergence position of 40°. One or both the tubes are locked in the desired positions and when both of them are locked the two can be rocked from side to side for kinetic exercises or moved in a converging or diverging position to give, besides the negative and positive convergence, the range of fusion. The illuminating system is so constructed as to avoid any intense reflection. The intensity of the light can be regulated by rheostat. An arrangement of extinguishing the light in front of any one of the slide carriers also exists. This arrangement results in the rapid flashing of light and stimulates the underfunctioning macula.

The transparencies are inserted at the ends of each limb and are seen with the two eyes by reflection and the amblyopia with eccentric fixation and abnormal retinal correspondence.

The synoptophores are useful instruments. Mirrors are placed at 45° to the direction of the tubes. The pictures are thus fused. Synoptophore is an excellent instrument as it is adjustable for several measurements. Horizontal, vertical, rotatory movements are controlled and measured in scales. Centrally there is a chin and forehead rest. Recently Haidinger's brushes and after-image devices in the two arms of synoptophores have been incorporated which are very useful for diagnosis and treatment.

### Stereoscopes

These are instruments for training at home and they are both light and simple. They are particularly useful in the training of accommodative type of young children, unintelligent patients and cases with abnormal retinal correspondence. Several varieties of stereoscopes are in use :

- Non-variable prism stereoscopes
- Variable prism stereoscopes
- Kinetic stereoscopes

### Non-variable prism stereoscope

A good example of this type of stereoscope is Pigeon-Cantonnent stereoscope (Fig. 23.2). It is an inexpensive device for providing exercises for encouraging fusion and for the treatment of suppression. The instrument consists of two boards and a central septum, hinged book-wise. A mirror on the septum can be covered when not in use. The scale permits the angle of deviation, for near, to be readily measured. Other stereoscopes in this type are Holme's and Whittington's. Many people prefer to use Holme's stereoscope.

### Variable prism stereoscopes

A good example of this variety is Cruise's home training stereoscope (Fig. 23.3). It is small and

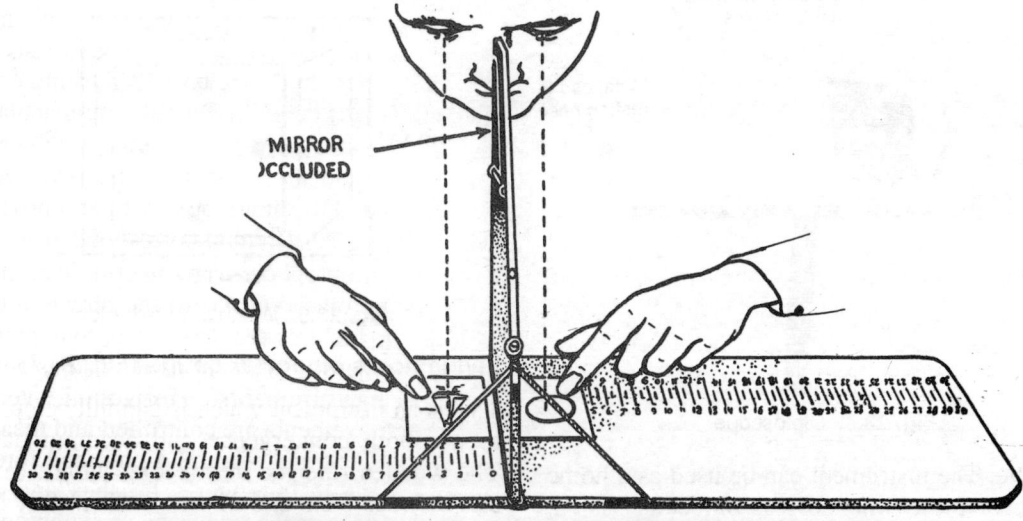

**Fig. 23.2.** Pigeon-Cantonnent stereoscope.

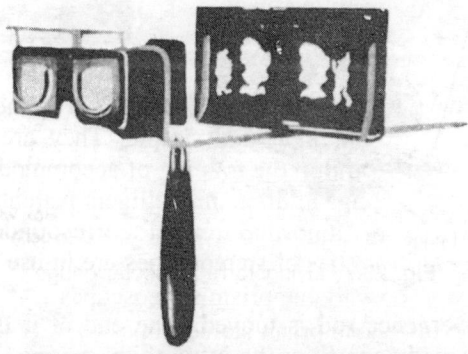

**Fig. 23.3.** Cruise's home training stereoscope.

convenient model for teaching amplitude of fusion in small degrees of squint. The prisms can be varied up to 20 dioptres. Additional prisms may be added for convergence. One of the prisms is detachable for vertical adjustments. It is a clinical instrument which may be used for both testing and training.

### Kinetic stereoscopes (Fig. 23.4)

This is a useful instrument for home exercises in small degrees of incomitance as it provides a swinging movement in all directions. It is the only stereoscope which can be adjusted for cyclo- and hyperphoria. It is used for fusion and stereopsis. The instrument is unsuitable for small children and for those in whom fusion has not developed.

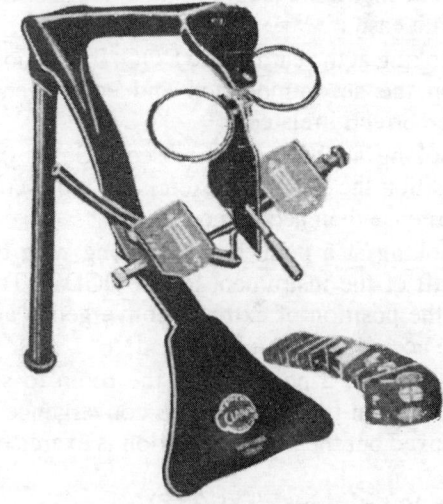

**Fig. 23.4.** Kinetic stereoscope.

### Diploscope (Fig. 23.5)

This is a simple instrument which is used for diagnosis and treatment of ocular deviations. The patient looks through a four-holed septum at a card bearing three letters, DOG. If binocular vision is present the patient sees the letters in their true arrangement. If there is exophoria or relative divergence, the patient sees the letters as DOOG. While if there is relative convergence or eso-phoria, the letters will be seen as OGDO. If there is left suppression, the letters are seen as DO while OG are seen if there is suppression of the

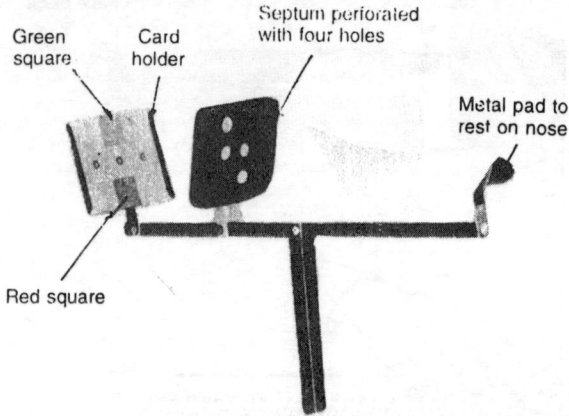

**Fig. 23.5.** Diploscope.

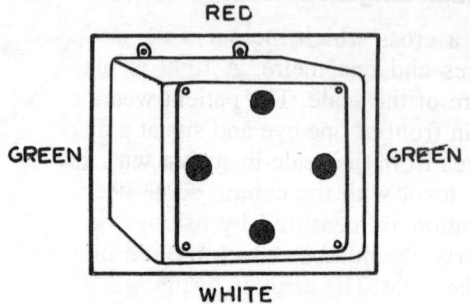

**Fig. 23.6.** Worth's four-dot test.

right eye. The instrument can be used as a home trainer for those who possess binocular vision. The following are the four possible positions and the patient should be taught to obtain any one of them with ease :

1. Looking at the card to see DOG. In this position the accommodation and convergence are correctly related.

2. Looking at the septum to see DG. At this position the patient is exercising more convergence than accommodation.

3. Looking at a point halfway along with the shaft of the instrument to see OGDO. This is the position of extreme convergence and the accommodation is relaxed.

4. Looking at a point across the room to see DOOG. In this position the convergence is relaxed but the accommodation is exercised.

### Worth's four-dot test (Fig. 23.6)

The instrument consists of an illuminated box with four apertures. Coloured glasses are placed before each aperture (one red, two green and one yellow or ground glass). The patient wears a diplopia goggle, with red glass in front of the right eye. If the patient sees three green spots he uses the left eye only. If he sees two red spots he is using the right eye only. If he sees sometimes two red and sometimes three green spots he uses the eyes alternately. If he sees five spots he has diplopia, but if he sees four spots both eyes work in harmony.

### Livingston's binocular gauge (Fig. 23.7)

This is an instrument which is gainfully employed to use both convergence and accommodation. The wooden ruler is 36 cm long with a central slot between 6 cm and 21 cm marks in which the

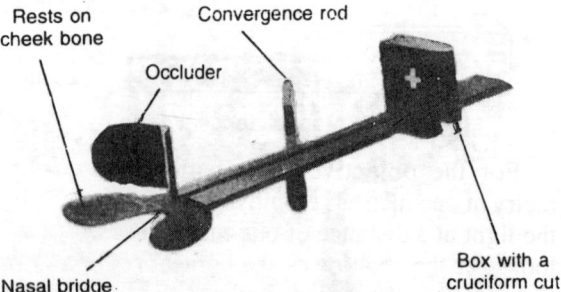

**Fig. 23.7.** Livingston's binocular gauge.

convergence rod is moved. One end of it is so designed as to fit at the infraorbital margin. The wooden rule is marked in centimetres from the anterior corneal surface. There is a shield provided to cover one eye in case uniocular accommodation is to be tested. There is a slot in the rule and in this a central rod is slid towards the eyes until the limit of convergence is reached, i.e., when one eye diverges. There is a box-like attachment with a cross opening at the other end of the rule which can be slid towards the eye. A card with a vertical line is placed in it opposite the vertical line of the cross. The box is slid towards the eye till the line diverges either to the left or to the right indicating the divergence of the corresponding eye. When accommodation is measured, the card, with the line, is replaced by a card with the print and the near point is the point at which the print becomes blurred.

## Maddox tangent scale (Fig. 23.8)

It is a cross which measures the deviation at 5 metres and one metre. A light is placed at the centre of the scale. The patient wears a Maddox rod in front of one eye and sits at a distance of 5 metres from the scale in such a way that the eye is at level with the central spot. The amount of deviation is measured by asking the patient to observe the number which the red line traverses on the scale. The position of the Maddox rod can be so adjusted as to obtain readings both for vertical and horizontal deviations. This gives a subjective assessment of deviation at 5 metres in degrees.

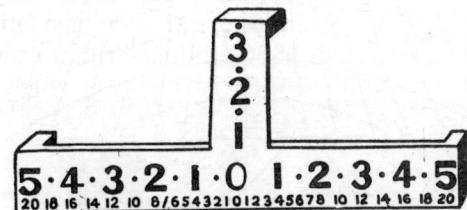

**Fig. 23.8.** Maddox tangent scale.

For the objective examination, strabismometry at one metre is employed. The patient faces the light at a distance of one metre. The observer looks for the position of the corneal reflex in the fixing eye as the patient looks at the light. If the corneal reflex is in the centre of the fixing as well as the deviating eye, there is no squint. If the reflex is not central in the deviating eye, the patient then looks along the scale until the reflex in the deviating eye occupies a position similar to one occupied by the fixing eye and the number at this point represents the angle of squint in degrees.

## Maddox wing (Fig. 23.9)

This instrument makes use of mechanical dissociation of the fields of the two eyes.

It is an extremely valuable test for vision at near distance. It is a rapid means of detecting the presence of and measuring the degrees of heterophoria.

The field of the two eyes are separated by a diaphragm. The right eye sees the scale and the left eye sees the arrow. The patient is asked to point out the number at which the arrow points,

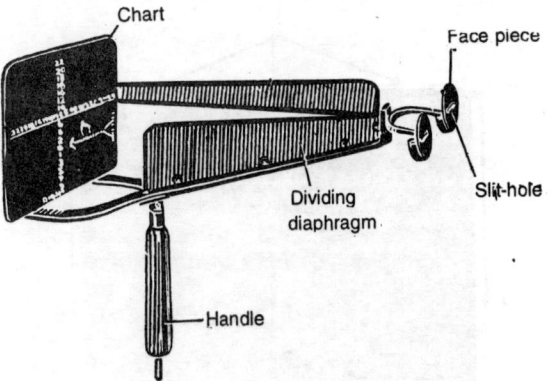

**Fig. 23.9.** Maddox wing

which gives the measure of the degree of heterophoria. It can measure horizontal, vertical and cyclophorias. If he sees the arrow at 0 he is orthophoric for near.

## Bishop-Harman diaphragm test (Fig. 23.10)

It is an instrument for detecting heterophoria and the capacity for fusion. This instrument does not measure the degree of heterophoria. The patient's inter-pupillary distance is first measured. The pointer on the scale of the diaphragm is set at the patient's inter-pupillary distance. The handle is held by the patient who holds the metal end of the instrument firmly against his upper lip just below the nose. The diaphragm of the instrument is fully opened and the patient is asked to read the letters or the numbers on the charts from left to right. As the diaphragmatic opening is gradually

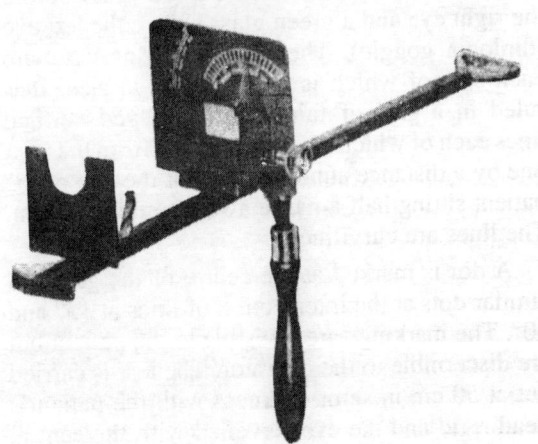

**Fig. 23.10.** Bishop-Harman diaphragm.

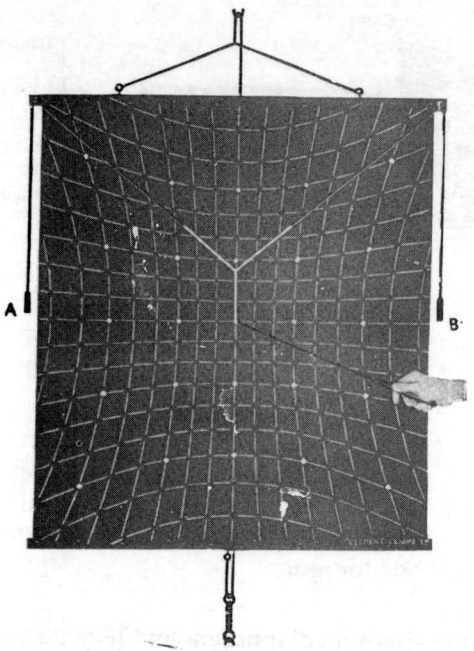

**Fig. 23.11.** Hess screen.

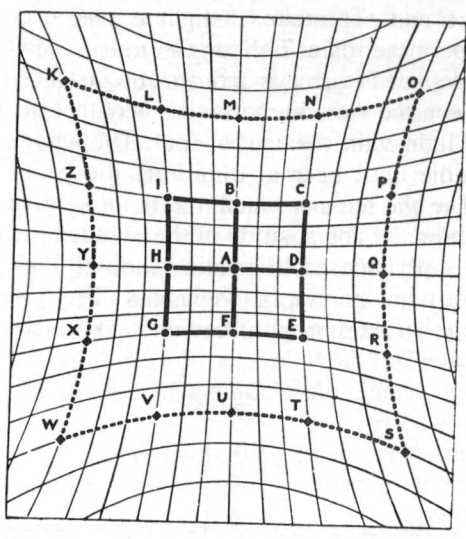

**Fig. 23.12.** Diagram of the Hess screen.

narrowed in, the numbers may be evident. The letters may be crowded in the centre (esophoria) or may be separated into two groups with a dividing line or bar in the centre (exophoria). One group of letters may be higher or lower than the other (hyperphoria) or the number at one end may disappear (indicating a uniocular response). This instrument is used for measuring the ocular poise.

### Hess screen (Fig. 23.11)

The test is based on the mutual exclusion of fields by colour. The patient wears a red glass before the right eye and a green glass before the left eye (diplopia goggle). The screen is a grey square each side of which is about 3 feet in size. It is ruled in a grid of faint horizontal and vertical lines each of which line is separated from the next one by a distance subtending 5° at the eye of the patient sitting half a metre away from the screen. The lines are curvilinear.

A dot is marked at the centre of the grid and similar dots at the intersection of lines at 15° and 30°. The markings are invisible to the patient but are discernible to the operator. The test is carried out at 50 cm in semi-darkness with the patient's head rigid and the eyes levelled with the central dot.

One torch (red) is flashed by the observer on the point to be examined and the patient is asked to cross the light by the other torch (green). The test is carried on each spot one by one. The results are charted on a special chart. Electrically operated Hess screens are available.

### Lees screen (Fig. 23.13)

This apparatus is also based on the principle of

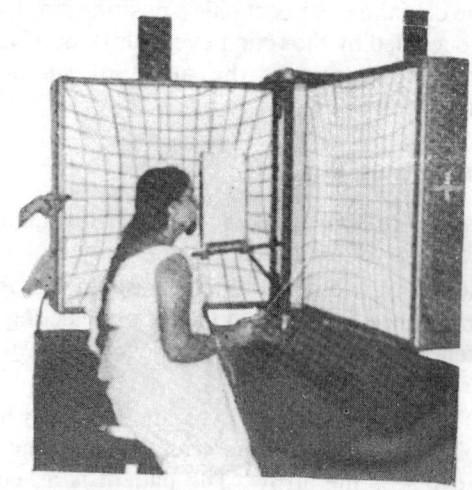

**Fig. 23.13.** Lees screen.

providing dissociation but does not utilise coloured filters for the purpose. It is essentially a twin screen. The two screens are placed rigidly and permanently at right angles to each other. A double-sided mirror is fixed to bisect the angle between the two. Each screen, which is backed by a light-tight casing, bears a tangent marking invisible until internal illumination is switched on. The two screens which may be independently lit, under the control of the foot-switch, are optically superimposed. The patient looks through the mirror with one eye and views the screen immediately before him with the other. The examiner indicates, on the indirectly observed illuminated tangent screen, those points which he wishes the patient to fix with a hand on the other blank screen. A momentary illumination of the blank screen demonstrates displacement and this is recorded on the chart similar to that of Hess.

### Cheiroscope

This apparatus was first designed by Maddox. It is a useful instrument (Fig. 23.14) for anti-suppression exercise. The instrument has a working base, an upright picture carrier, a headrest in which are contained a pair of +8 dioptre spherical lenses and an obliquely placed septum extending from a point midway between the lenses to the base of the picture carrier. The working base of

the cheiroscope is at a distance of 12.5 cm (i.e., the focal distance of the lenses) from the lenses. The patient uses both hand and eye. It provides a stimulus to the suppressing eye. Permits direction, observation and guidance of the hand by one eye only. The other eye sees an image in the mirror. This image controls the task set to the hands. Adequate and even illumination is provided by a mains lamp fitted to the instrument. Exercises for the development of binocular vision on this instrument can be given only in the presence of normal retinal correspondence.

### Myoscope (Fig. 23.15)

This instrument is based on the principle of mutual exclusion of field by colours. Two slides of complementary colours are fitted in front of

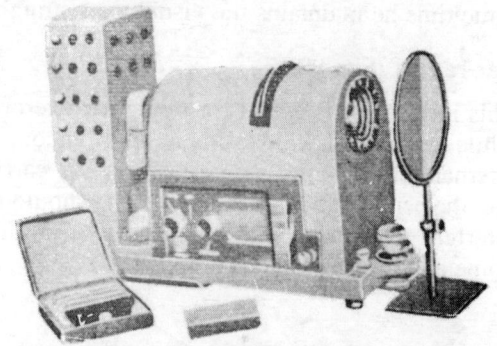

**Fig. 23.15.** Myoscope.

the lamp and their images are projected upon a screen. These images travel at various speeds over the screen in any meridian in a circle of varying diameter. The instrument provides for kinetic type of orthoptic exercises to more than one person at a time. It has the disadvantage that the orthoptist has no control over the patient. It can also be used for cases of slight incomitance and in cases of recent paralysis due to trauma where other instruments are not useful.

### Remy separator (Fig. 23.16)

It is a simple and inexpensive instrument which helps in the restoration of parallelism of the visual axis. It consists of a septum to one end of which is fitted a carrier for transparencies. Without the maintenance of parallelism of the visual axis the

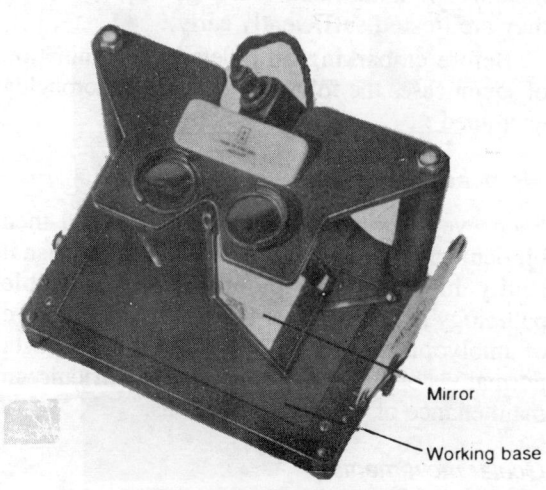

Mirror

Working base

**Fig. 23.14.** Cheiroscope.

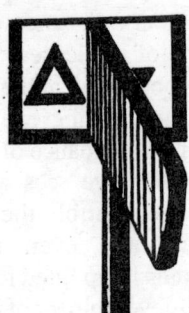

Fig. 23.16. Remy separator.

paired pictures held at either side of the septum cannot be observed as a single unit. By relaxing the convergence, the two pictures become super-imposed. With practice the patient learns to accommodate till the pictures are clear and at the same time he maintains the visual axes straight.

**Bar-reader** (Fig. 23.17)

This instrument is useful for binocular exercises while reading. The instrument may encourage alternation. When the exercise is properly carried out, the bar should be seen double and should not interfere with the point. It can be used both at home and in the hospital.

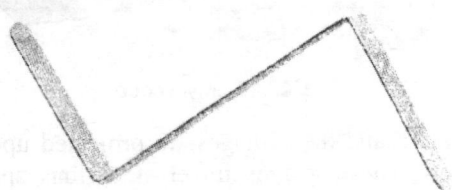

Fig. 23.17. Bar-reader.

**Bagolini's striated glasses**

Each glass consists of cylinders which convert a source of light into a line in the same way as in a Maddox rod. Both the glasses are kept in front of each eye with the axes of cylinders at right angles to each other, which results in the forma-tion of a cross when a spot of light is observed. The peculiarity of these glasses is that there is minimal dissociation of the eyes and the objects are viewed under the most natural conditions pos-sible. These glasses help in the detection of the presence or absence of binocular functions in space or the type of correspondence present.

## METHODS OF DIAGNOSIS

In the diagnosis, management and prognosis of muscular imbalance a careful history-taking is essential particularly with reference to :

- The age of onset of squint and its duration.
- Whether the squint was of sudden or gradual onset.
- Whether the squint is intermittent or constant and if it is intermittent under what circumstances does it manifest.
- Whether the squint is unilateral or alternating and whether the degree of the squint is con-stant or variable. If it is variable under what circumstances it increases. It should also be enquired whether the deviation is horizontal or vertical.

Information should also be elicited with regard to the precipitating causes of the disease :

- Family history : A strong family history of the squint makes the prognosis unfavour-able.
- General illness preceding squint.
- Trauma or infections
- Shock
- Ocular disorder interfering with the passage of light.

Squints dating from birth usually indicate some degree of amblyopia and the prognosis is usually not good. Squints of gradual onset from the age of three years or so are usually accom-modative in nature and bear a good prognosis if they are treated sufficiently early.

Before embarking on a detailed examination of squint cases the following should be thoroughly examined :

*Visual acuity*

Each eye should be tested separately and then binocularly. Considerable lowering of visual acuity in one eye without any demonstrable pathology in the media or the fundus is indicative of amblyopia. Lowering of binocular vision with normal vision in each eye indicates a difficulty in maintenance of binocular functions.

*Ocular movements*

Ocular movements should be tested for each eye

separately and then for both eyes. Six movements should be tested in each eye separately :

- Down and in
- Down and out
- Up and in
- Up and out
- In
- Out

These movements indicate the actions of various extraocular muscles. Binocular movements should be similarly tested to give an idea of binocular synergism and antagonism :

- Left
- Right
- Right and up
- Right and down
- Left and up
- Left and down

Besides this, the movements of elevation and depression should also be tested from the primary position of the eyeball. This examination may reveal the presence of weakness or paralysis, if any, of the extrinsic ocular muscles.

### Pupillary reactions

The reactions to light and convergence serve to distinguish a secondary deviation from primary deviation, due to the disease of retina or optic nerve.

### Media and fundi

This helps to eliminate a secondary deviation due to a local cause, i.e., defect in the media, retina or optic nerve.

### Refraction

This should be done under full cycloplegic effect.

After having obtained preliminary information from the history and the above-mentioned examinations, a detailed examination of the cases of squint is carried out. The examination may be grouped as under :

- Tests for fixation
- Tests for binocular dissociation
- Measurement of deviation
- Tests for binocular projection
- Ocular movements

## Test for fixation

One eye is covered and the other eye fixes the object. Fixation may be present, absent, or eccentric. In case of small children the object to be shown must be of interest. Though one can get an idea whether the fixation is present or absent yet it is difficult by this simple test to be sure about eccentric fixation.

A more complicated instrument like the visuoscope should be used for the determination of eccentric fixation.

## Visuoscope

This instrument is used to detect amblyopia with eccentric fixation. The visuoscope (Fig. 23.18) is a type of modified ophthalmoscope provided with a disc which can be brought in front of the lighting beam so that a star can be focused on the retina. The patient is asked to fix the projected star. If the patient fixes the star and the observer finds that the patient has fixed it foveally the case is

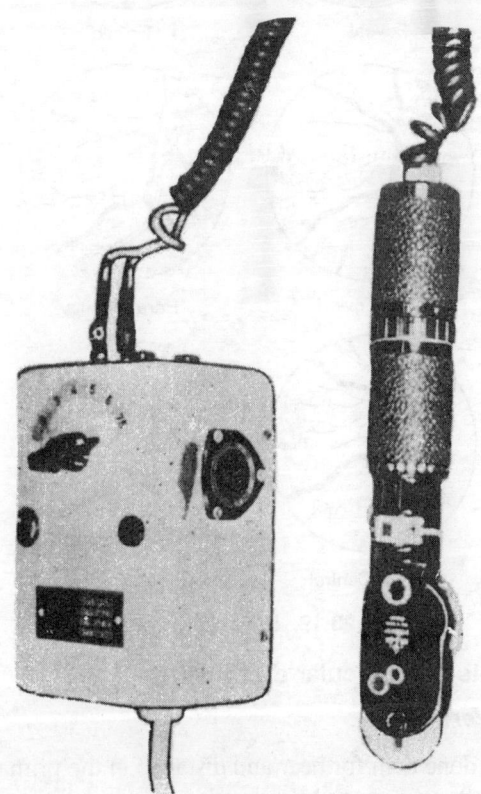

**Fig. 23.18.** Visuoscope.

then of amblyopia with central fixation. If the observer notices that the fixation star is extra-foveal the case is of eccentric fixation. At the same time it may be ascertained whether principal visual direction of the fovea is straight or not.

The eccentric fixation (Fig. 23.19) may be :

- Erratic
- Para-foveal
- Para-macular
- Centro-caecal
- Paracaecal
- Temporal
- Non-fixation

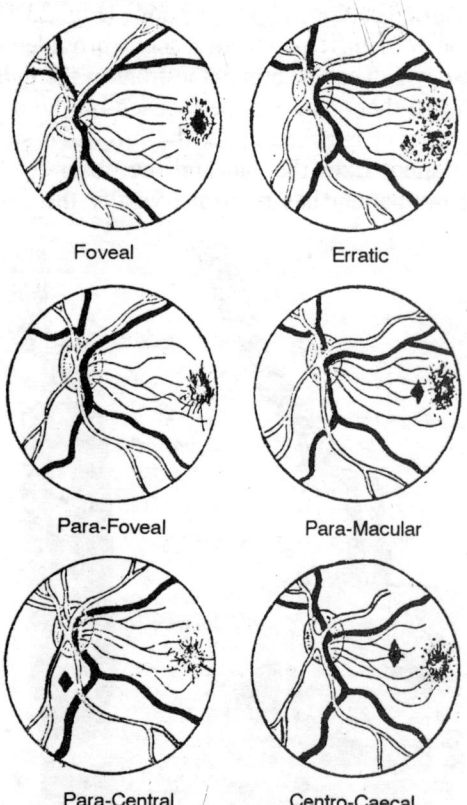

**Fig. 23.19.** Eccentric fixation.

## Tests for binocular dissociation

### Cover test

It is done both for near and distance in the primary position of gaze and also in other cardinal directions of the gaze.

### Alternate cover test (binocular)

In this test the examiner covers the eyes alternately, and any movement of the eye would show the presence of squint. On removal of the cover from the eye, it has to be observed whether the covered eye comes to take over fixation with the loss of fixation in the already fixing eye or remains deviated. In case it remains deviated, it shows the presence of a manifest squint of the eye. On repeating the test with the other eye, it would be possible to know whether it remains as a uniocular squint or alternating squint depending upon whether it can maintain fixation on uncovering the other eye or not. The direction of the movement would tell us whether it is convergent, divergent or vertical squint.

### Cover and uncover test (uniocular)

In case it has been detected that there is a movement of the eyes with alternate cover test, one can easily detect whether it is phoria or not by the cover and uncover test. In this test the examiner covers one eye and lets the other fix. On removal of the cover it is noted whether the covered eye comes to take up fixation without any loss of fixation of the other eye. In case it can do so, it shows the presence of phoria.

The amount of movement would let us judge the degree of deviation and in case of phoria, would also tell us the rate of recovery.

The change in the amount of deviation with alternate fixation by the eye would let us know whether there is any difference in the primary angle of deviation and the secondary angle of deviation (Fig. 23.20).

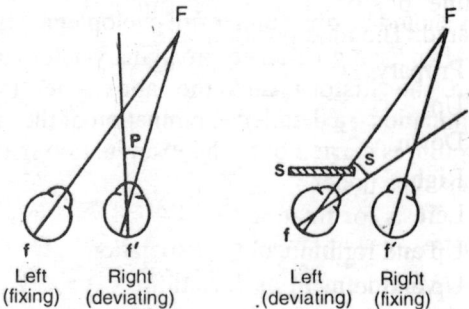

**Fig. 23.20.** Primary angle of deviation (primary angle equal to secondary angle).

- Primary angle of deviation is the angle which is measured when the normal eye is the fixing eye.
- Secondary angle of deviation is the angle which is measured when the affected eye is the fixing eye.

In concomitant squints the angle of primary deviation is equal to the angle of secondary deviation (Fig. 23.20) whereas in the incomitant squint, secondary angle is greater than the primary (Fig. 23.21).

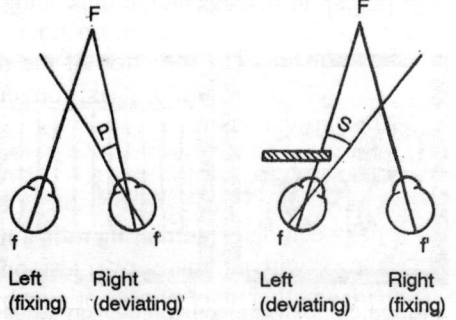

**Fig. 23.21.** Secondary angle of deviation (primary angle less than secondary angle).

The cover test may be done in various positions of gaze.

*Diplopia test*

If incomitance is suspected a simple diplopia test may be helpful in diagnosing the group of muscles involved. The patient wears a diplopia goggle in the darkroom with the red glass in front of the right eye and the green glass in front of the left eye.

The patient is shown the flame of the candle in nine positions and the diplopia chart is prepared. The nine positions are :

1. Primary
2. Up
3. Down
4. Right
5. Left
6. Up and right
7. Up and left
8. Down and right
9. Down and left

The diplopia chart is then interpreted (Fig. 23.22), e.g.

- If there is no diplopia there is orthophoria.
- If diplopia is present in right and up position the muscles involved are either right superior rectus (RSR) or left inferior oblique (LIO).
- The farther image belongs to the paralysed muscle. If the green image is farther the paralysed muscle is of the left eye but if the red image is farther the paralysed muscle is of the right eye.
- In heterophorias the distance of the images would remain constant in all directions of gaze.

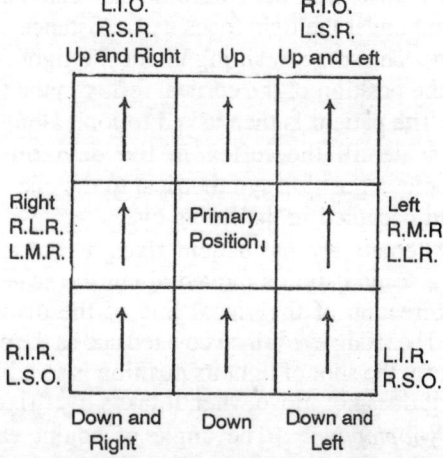

**Fig. 23.22.** Diplopia chart. LIO, left inferior oblique; LSR, left superior rectus; LLR, left lateral rectus; LMR, left medial rectus; LIR, left inferior rectus; LSO, left superior oblique; RIO, right inferior oblique; RSR, right superior rectus; RLR, right lateral rectus; RMR, right medial rectus; RIR, right inferior rectus; RSO, right superior oblique.

**Measurement of deviation**

The patient is seated on a stool and the examiner sits at a distance of at least one foot from him. He holds a lighted ophthalmoscope or a lighted candle in front of him and notes the position of the corneal reflex from behind the candle. Normally the corneal reflex of the light is in the central position. In either case it may be displaced. Its position in relation to the pupil is noted. If the image is at the pupillary margin the squint is about 15°; if it is between the pupillary margin and the limbus the squint is about 30°; if it is at the limbus the squint is about 45°. Beyond this a higher degree of squint is present. The method gives a rough indication only.

*The angle of squint may be measured on an arc perimeter :* The squinting eye of the patient occupies the centre of the perimeter while the other eye fixes an object 6 metres away and directly in front. A candle is lit on the central spot. The corneal reflex is noted and the candle is moved till the reflex is in the centre of the squinting eye. The angular deviation is read off on the arc of the perimeter.

*Maddox tangent scale :* This can be used both for objective and subjective strabismometry. A light is placed in the centre of the scale and the patient under the light faces it at a distance of one metre. The surgeon sitting under the light observes the position of the corneal reflex in the fixing eye. The patient is then asked to look along with the scale till the reflex in the deviating eye occupies a position symmetrical to the one which it had occupied in the fixing eye.

Alternatively the patient fixes a central spot and a second spot is moved along the scale near the direction of the visual line of the diverging eye. The fixing eye is then covered and as the patient looks at the spot of light its position is so adjusted that it does not move when it takes over fixation.

*Synoptophore :* The angle of squint can be more accurately measured on the synoptophore. If the patient wears glasses he would retain them on the face. Angle alpha interferes with an accurate measurement of the angle of the squint, particularly so if the angle alpha is large. Angle alpha should always be measured by the method described earlier. To measure the objective angle, slides of small lion and small cage are used (Fig. 23.23). The cage is in front of the right eye. The patient looks steadily at the picture in front of his right eye, and the position of the corneal reflex in this eye is noted. The tube, containing the picture, in front of the left eye is moved till the corneal reflex is identical in position to that in the right eye. The right eye does not move if the measurement has been correct.

**Measurement of binocular functions**

Three grades of binocular functions should be tested :

*Simultaneous perception* (Fig. 23.23)

Before the patient is tested his objective angle of squint is determined. A slide containing a cage is placed in front of the left eye and a lion in front of the right eye. The patient is now asked to put the lion in the cage. This gives the subjective angle of the squint. If he can do it at the objective angle of the squint, he has simultaneous perception with normal correspondence. The difference between the two angles is the angle of anomaly. If he cannot put the lion in the cage, simultaneous macular perception is absent.

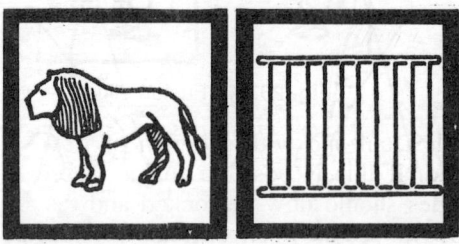

**Fig. 23.23.** Simultaneous perception slides.

In many apparent concomitant squints the angle of primary deviation is less than the angle of secondary deviation revealing a true state of incomitance, which is due to a long-standing paresis. In apparent concomitant squint, incomitance should therefore be tested as follows :

*When simultaneous perception is present :* The patient's subjective angle of squint should be determined at 0° position, at 15° position to the right and then at 15° position to the left. The angle is almost equal in all these three positions in concomitant squint but varies in incomitant ones.

*When simultaneous perception is absent :* The patient's objective angle is measured first with the lion in front of the right eye then with the lion in front of the left eye. There should be no difference in the objective angle if comitance is present. With the lion in front of the right eye the objective angle may be determined with the right tube 15° to the right and then 15° to the left. Similarly the angles are determined with the lion in front of the left eye and the left tube placed at 15° to the right and then 15° to the left. In cases of comitance the angle is the same in all positions. Similarly angle of squint can be measured in other positions of gaze.

## Fusion

Fusion is tested with a pair of similar slides with controls (Fig. 23.24). A slide of Mickey Mouse with flower but no tail and the other Mickey Mouse with no flower in the hand and with tail. The tubes of the synoptophore are so set that the two pictures are seen separately. The patient is instructed to move the handles of the synoptophore till he sees that there is a Mickey Mouse

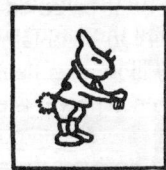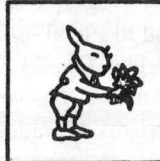

**Fig. 23.24.** Fusion slide.

with a tail and with a bunch of flowers in his hand. If this is possible fusion is present. The angles should now be locked and the tubes are now moved slowly from side to side while the eyes follow the picture. Suppression is present if there is jerking of the eyes when the controls, i.e., the tail and the bunch of flowers come and go.

## Stereoscopic vision

The slides consist of a number of dissimilar figures and these are numbered (Fig. 23.25). The figures are such that their images fall on disparate points of the retina. An attempt to fuse them produces the sensation of depth. The patient sees the numbers in regular order. From that nearest point to the most distant they are either 13572468 or 86427531. If the numbers are not seen one behind the other or if the figures are not in the regular order indicated above stereopsis is defective.

Besides the binocular vision, binocular projection also requires careful assessment. The angle of binocular projection can be measured by the angle of anomaly on the two eyes. A simple method is to deter-

mine the angle of anomaly on the synoptophore as described earlier. Other common methods are :
- By excluding field of one eye from the other.
- By distorting or displacing one image.

### Mechanical dissociation tests

**Maddox wing test :** It is an extremely valuable test for vision at near distance. The method of testing has been described earlier.

**Bishop-Harman diaphragm test :** This instrument detects heterophoria and estimates capacities for fusion. The test has been described earlier.

**Hess screen test :** The principles of this test have already been described. Two positions at which the indicator appears to coincide with the spots are recorded on a chart. The chart is made for each eye by reversing the goggles. A record of primary and secondary deviation is thus made. The area of the field is equal in the two eyes if the squint is comitant. On the paretic side the area is smaller and on the spastic side the area is larger than at the normal. The site of the greatest deviation indicates the involved muscle.

**Diploscope test :** It also utilises the principle of divided fields.

**Synoptophore test :** It is the most reliable amongst these tests.

### Distortion or displacement of image test

**Maddox rods** (Fig. 23.26) : The test is based on the principle of converting the image of a point into a line by utilising a combination of cylinders. The image formed is a focal line perpendicular to the axis of the cylinders. One eye, in front of which the Maddox rod is placed, sees a focal line and the other eye sees the white spot. The line should pass through the spot light; if it does not, suitable prisms can be used to bring the light in

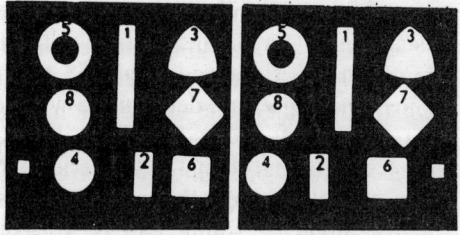

**Fig. 23.25.** Stereoscopic slides.

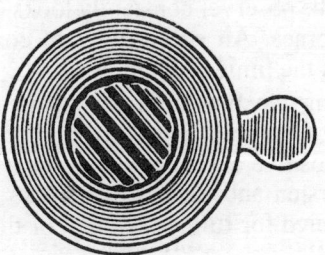

**Fig. 23.26.** Maddox rod.

the centre. The power of the prism is the measure of the displacement. If the line is vertical it measures horizontal deviation and if it is horizontal it measures vertical deviation (Fig. 23.27).

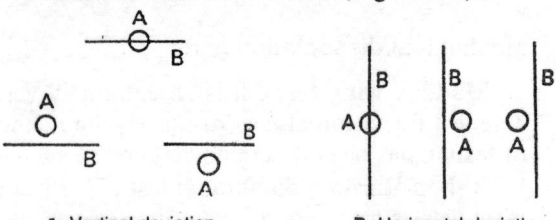

**A.** Vertical deviation          **B.** Horizontal deviation.

**Fig. 23.27.**  Lines formed by Maddox rod. A, horizontal lines; B, vertical lines.

**Prism diplopia test :** This is easily tested by Maddox double prism (Fig. 23.28). Two weak prisms are placed base to base. If they are so placed that the base line between the two cuts the visual axis of one eye a double image is seen while the image of the other eye lies between the two. Any displacement is corrected by placing the prism in front of the other eye. This gives a measure of deviation.

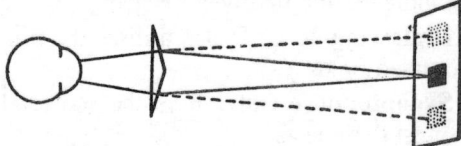

**Fig. 23.28.**  Maddox double prism.

### Tests for ocular movements

**Ocular movements :** Each eye is separately tested for the degree of movement in all the eight directions : up, in, out, down, up and in, up and out, down and in, and down and out. The equality in movement in either eye is noted to determine whether the squint, if any, is concomitant or inconcomitant.

The limits of uniocular movements can be measured readily on the perimeter or a campimeter. The observer constantly looks to the reflex in the cornea. An eccentricity of corneal reflex indicates the limit of fixation.

Among the binocular conjugate movements the most important are convergence and divergence. Positive and negative vertical divergence and intorsion and extorsion are also required to be measured for full assessment of the case.

They may be measured by one of the following instruments : By synoptophore the amplitude of convergence, divergence, positive and negative vertical divergence and amplitude of torsion can be easily measured. Amplitude for fusion with stereoscopic pictures is greater than with other pictures. Some people, therefore, advocate the use of stereoscopic pictures for this purpose but fusion pictures give true measure.

**Prism vergence test :** It is based on similar principles and identical results can be obtained. Maddox prism verger (Fig. 23.29) is an excellent instrument for this purpose. The vergence power is estimated by putting prisms of gradually increasing power in front of the eyes in the desired position depending upon the type of vergence to be assessed, until fusion is broken and diplopia is produced.

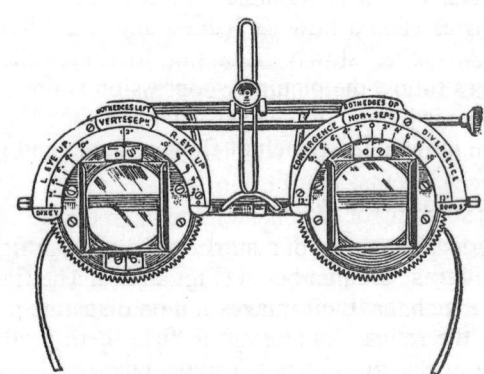

**Fig. 23.29.**  Maddox prism verger.

**Livingston's binocular gauge :** As described earlier the instrument helps in measuring both amplitude of convergence and accommodation.

**Prism divergence :** The measurement of the angle of divergence, i.e., the angle through which the eye can be turned outside (abduction) is tested by putting the base in prism in front of the observed eyes while they maintain parallelism of the visual axes. The maximum power of the base in prisms tolerated without breaking this visual parallelism gives the value of abduction. Similarly the maximum power of the base out prisms tolerated without breaking the parallelism of visual axes gives the value of adduction.

# CHAPTER 24

# Heterophoria

Maintenance of oculomotor apparatus in a perfect equilibrium, so that both the visual axes remain either parallel or remain directed upon the fixation point even when their activity is dissociated by the withdrawal of the controlling influence of fusion and only under the influences of tonic innervation, is called orthophoria. It, like emmetropia contrary to expectations, is uncommon.

Heterophoria is a condition in which the visual axes of the two eyes depart from parallelism when the controlling influence of fusion is removed and the muscles are only under tonic innervation. The faculty of fusion is thus able to maintain parallelism of the two eyes which otherwise are not in perfect muscular equilibrium. A heterophoria of some standing or of considerable degree may put considerable fatiguing strain and as in some debilitating conditions, the ocular musculature cannot cope with this strain, a heterophoria may be converted into a heterotropia. There is thus no fundamental distinction between latent (heterophoria) and manifest (heterotropia) squint.

## Aetiology

There are several factors which are responsible for the causation of heterophoria :

**Faulty muscle origin or insertion :** Faulty insertion, in particular, has been blamed for the development of heterophoria. This view was very widely held few years ago which later was replaced by the recognised innervational changes. In general they are rarely the cause of heterophoria.

**Refractive error :** This is a very frequent cause of heterophoria. In fact most of the anomalies in muscular equilibrium are influenced by the refractive condition and associated accommodation convergence relationship.

Hypermetropia would predispose an individual to esophoria and myopia to exophoria. Some degree of exo-tendency may develop in acquired myopia and presbyopia because of relatively decreased amount of convergence available for near.

**Defective innervation :** It may, to a large extent, be responsible for phorias and is probably the anomalous central distribution of the individual tonic innervation to the muscles of the two eyes.

**Macula :** There may be an anatomical variation in the position of the macula in relation to the optic axis of the eye resulting in heterophoria.

**Systemic causes :** Weakness of muscles may result from illness or general weakness, anaemia or general debility.

**Psychic :** Hysterical or psychic manifestations are usually tropic in nature but may sometimes manifest as heterophoria.

**Toxins :** Various endogenous or exogenous toxins may produce heterophoria commonly exophoria.

**Intracranial structures :** Damage to these may result in phoria although usually tropia is manifested.

**Age :** The tendency for the eyes to move in or out may be dependent upon age, e.g., at birth if one eye is blinded, it tends to deviate outwards. In infancy and childhood, because of the influence of the increased convergence the eye tends to deviate inwards. Above 40 years, the tendency is for outwards deviation.

## Type of phorias

**Esophoria :** There is a tendency for the visual axis of one eye to turn inwards relative to the other under tonic impulses to the muscle without any controlling influences of fusion.

**Exophoria :** There is a tendency for one eye to turn outwards relative to the other under a lack of tonic impulses. Both these conditions are due to the imbalance of horizontal muscles.

**Hyperphoria :** There is tendency for the visual axes to deviate vertically in opposite directions. Usually the terminology used is left or right hyperphoria depending upon whether the right or left visual axis tends to deviate upwards. Hyperphoric eye is not necessarily the faulty eye. The condition is caused due to imbalance of vertical muscles.

**Cyclophoria :** A torsional movement around the anteroposterior axis due to fusional dissociation is known as cyclophoria. When the 12 o'clock meridian of cornea rotates nasally it is called incyclophoria and when it rotates temporally, excyclophoria. The situation is as a result of the imbalance of oblique muscles.

If inferior oblique is overactive or if there is a relative deficiency of superior oblique muscle, an excyclophoria occurs. If there is relative deficiency of the inferior oblique or an overaction of the superior oblique muscle incyclophoria occurs.

### Symptoms of phoria

To overcome the muscular imbalance two factors are very important :

1. Reserve neuromuscular power to overcome muscular imbalance.
2. Individual desire for maintenance of binocular vision.

Small degree of heterophoria are usually overcome by these two factors. Sometimes even larger degrees of heterophoria are overcome without giving rise to symptoms. Such cases, known as fully compensated, are symptomless and need no treatment. If these two factors are weak, the heterophoria is not overcome without symptoms and such cases are known as decompensated cases.

The symptoms of heterophoria closely resemble that of refractive error, viz.,

• Blurring of vision
• Headache
• Asthenopia

• Itching and burning
• Intermittent diplopia

As a rule horizontal phoria causes the least distress and the vertical one causes symptoms and the torsional one is the most troublesome. In severe form the symptoms may assume the form of dizziness, vertigo, nausea and vomiting due to labyrinthine disturbances produced by torticollis.

The severity of symptoms is very variable in different individuals. Similar amount of phoria may result in symptoms of different severity depending upon the individual fusion reserves. The symptoms are usually more marked after the day's work. The symptoms may also occur in the form of faulty judgement of locating objects in space such as in certain games like tennis, cricket etc. Similarly pilots may find it difficult to judge the distance of the ground while landing.

The factors predisposing decompensation are :

• Inadequacy of fusional reserve
• Precision of job
• General debility and lowered vitality
• Psychosis and neurosis
• Advancing age

The objective signs of phoria may be in the form of watering, congestion or hyperaemia of the conjunctiva and lids. There may be head tilt and obvious ocular deviation on cover test.

## Esophoria

In this condition, the eyes tend to deviate nasally when the fusion impulse is withdrawn. There is relative hypertonicity of the internal recti and hypotonicity of the external recti. The symptoms are worse than in exophoria as it is more difficult to surmount.

A deviation of 1-2 dioptres may be taken as within normal limits.

### Aetiology

The causative factors have already been listed under general description. However, few points are stressed again which commonly cause an esophoria.

• Bilateral superable hypermetropia, i.e., hypermetropia which can be overcome by sustainable accommodation in order to give clear image.

- Excessive accommodative convergence.
- Increased convergence in bilateral congenital myopia.
- Innervational.

Presence of hypermetropia may result in esophoria for distance and near in proportion to the accommodation used in presence of excessive convergence esophoria is more in proportion to the accommodation. Esophoria due to these factors is known as accommodative esophoria and it is quite common in children. Esophoria may also be a manifestation of generalised hypertonus of body muscles. Majority of cases which are not accommodative in origin are due to the muscles and is known as tonic esophoria.

### Symptoms

Hypermetropia when present, the symptoms of heterophoria are accentuated on near work. In some cases it may be present for distance also. The condition tends to excite the nervous system as a whole. The psychotic state itself can accentuate esophoria and thus a vicious circle may be established.

### Treatment

It depends primarily upon aetiology. A full correction of the refractive error under complete cycloplegia is advisable. In a purely accommodative esophoria, correction of the refractive error results in a dramatic cure of symptoms. Orthoptic exercises to increase the fusional divergence may be helpful but in general are usually disappointing. Prisms base out may in certain cases prove useful but are not universally advocated. If all these measures fail, surgery may be judiciously employed.

## Exophoria

In this condition the visual axes tend to deviate outwards when the fusional impulse is withdrawn. It is essentially an exaggerated position from the normal specially for near, where up to 6-8 $\Delta$ may be taken as normal.

### Aetiology

- Decreased convergence in myopia because of lesser usage of accommodation.

- Decreased convergence in presbyopia.
- Prolonged uniocular activity.
- Innervational.

### Symptoms

If the fusional convergence amplitude is good, no symptoms may be present. When present the symptoms are typically those of heterophoria in general. Increasing difficulty is felt in close work till it becomes almost impossible to fuse. These are symptoms of asthenopia for near work. Greater effort is required to overcome the convergence deficiency. The accommodation is also, therefore, exercised which itself may go in spasm. There may be intermittent diplopia and it may become difficult to fuse the images from the two eyes. Usually, there is a tendency to develop suppression to overcome diplopia and later after passing the stage of intermittent exotropia it may change into constant exotropia. Headache may become very severe and resemble migraine. There may be generalised muscular hypotonus. With normal fusional convergence amplitude of exophoria of less than 8 $\Delta$ is usually perfectly comfortable.

### Treatment

Firstly, refractive error must be adequately corrected. Full correction in myopes is advisable and hypermetropes may be a little under-corrected. Orthoptic exercises to increase the total range of fusion, both positive and negative, are useful and quite helpful. Anti-suppression exercises are indicated in those who have developed suppression. If exercises fail to give relief, relieving prisms, base in, may be quite useful for near work. If this treatment fails then surgery should be undertaken.

## Hyperphoria

In this condition, the visual axis tends to deviate in a vertical direction when the fusional impulses are withdrawn. Depending upon whether the right or the left axis tends to deviate upwards it is termed right or left hyperphoria, respectively. Even routine testing will show this tendency to be present in 15-30% of normal persons. It is strenuous to keep the vertical deviations in check by fusion. These deviations, therefore, produce symptoms of eye strain even if the deviation is small. This deviation may coexist with a horizontal error and may escape notice. Non-realisation of the presence of vertical deviation along with horizontal deviation may produce disappointing results of the therapy of horizontal deviations.

Double or alternating hyperphoria is not an uncommon entity. In this connection if one eye fixes and the other is occluded, the covered eye deviates upwards.

### Aetiology

Unlike horizontal phorias, accommodational influences do not seem to enter into the production of vertical imbalances. It may be due to certain congenital anatomical peculiarities of intraocular muscles in the form of paresis or spasm. Alternating hyperphorias seem to be due to some innervational anomalies.

### Symptoms

Even relatively small vertical deviation may produce incapacitating symptoms. There may be pain, headache and general fatigue. The patient may develop neurasthenic personality. Objectively, one may see hyperaemia of conjunctiva and lids. Sometimes blepharitis may develop. There may be characteristic head tilt with a drawn expression and with a frowning of the eyebrows. Persistent asthenopia, even after correction of refractive errors and horizontal deviations, should be thoroughly investigated for any vertical muscular imbalance.

### Treatment

After the correction of refractive errors, orthoptic exercises may be tried but these are generally not of much value. For small degree of hyperphoria prescription of prism is very satisfactory. In large degrees of hyperphoria, surgery can give good results.

### Cyclophoria

It is a latent defect characterised by a tendency for the eye to rotate around the anteroposterior axis. It may be in- or excyclophoria.

### Aetiology

Usually it is due to faulty anatomical or innervational anomalies of superior and inferior oblique muscles and has nothing to do with accommodation. Sometimes the presence of cyclophoria may be diagnosed because of the presence of oblique astigmatism (pseudo-cyclophoria).

### Symptoms

It might be symptomless as the amount of cyclophoria that can be corrected varies considerably in different individuals. It may give rise to headache, nausea, and vomiting and rarely may cause upset in balancing the body, there may often be head tilting to neutralise the torsional defect. As a whole the symptoms are far more in cyclophoria than in any other types of phoria. The patient may get a distorted orientation which may result in a profound reflex labyrinthine disturbance. The patient may assume an awkward posture and may become neurasthenic.

### Treatment

Correction of cylindrical error adequately relieves the cyclophoria due to astigmatism. In other cases, surgery on the oblique muscles is quite effective in dealing with this condition.

### Fixation disparity

It may be defined as a sort of esophoria in which there is lack of bifoveal fixation. In addition there is also a small amount of heterophoria. Clinically it is detected by cover test which shows that the eye showing manifest small angle squint deviates more nasally when put under cover.

The condition is characterised by the presence of binocular functions though stereopsis may be defective. It is associated with abnormal retinal correspondence and has invariably different grades of amblyopia in the squinting eye. There may be cases of fixation disparity with hardly any detectable squint on cover test with above functional abnormalities. They are termed as microtropia.

### Treatment

It needs no treatment except for amblyopia.

# CHAPTER 25

# Heterotropia

The eyes try to maintain parallelism of visual axes by an involuntary effort in spite of partial or total abolition of fusional reflexes due to imperfect muscular balance; but not withstanding the effort, deviation of eyes from parallelism may not be overcome. Such a state of imperfect muscular imbalance is termed heterotropia. This may be due to paresis or paralysis of one or more extraocular muscles or this may be due to other causes which do not affect the ocular movements. The former is called paralytic heterotropia and the latter is termed concomitant heterotropia.

Paralytic squint and its treatment is outside the scope of a textbook like this. The only importance of this type of squint is that in some cases it is confused with concomitant squint and such incomitance has to be distinguished from the comitant one. The points of differences are given in Table 25.1.

## Concomitant strabismus

It is defined as a dissociation of the eyes wherein the deviation remains the same in all directions of gaze.

*Aetiology* : In the development of concomitant squint more than one factors may be operative. The obstacles which lead to the causation of squint may be sensory, motor or central.

**Sensory obstacles :** These are essentially optical in nature so that a clear image is not formed on the retina. In early life muscular dissociation leading to squint is almost an inevitable result of the formation of grossly dissimilar images on the retina by the eyes so that they cannot be successfully combined in a single mental impression. These may be due to high refractive errors, incorrect glasses, anisometropia and aniseikonia, etc. This may be due to ptosis, prolonged

**Table 25.1. Differences between paralytic and concomitant squint**

| | | Paralytic | Concomitant |
|---|---|---|---|
| 1. | Angle of deviation (Figs. 23.20 and 23.21) | The angle of primary deviation is smaller than the angle of secondary deviation. This difference tends to disappear in ocular palsy of long-standing. | The angle of primary deviation is equal to the angle of secondary deviation. |
| 2. | Ocular movements | There is limitation of movement in the direction of paralysed muscle. In cases of mild paresis, this may not be easily evident. In long-standing cases it may be difficult to assess. | The ocular movements are normal. |
| 3. | Diplopia | Diplopia is present and it usually gives an indication of the paralysed muscle. In addition, dissociation of the two eyes in Hess screen gives examination more detailed analysis of the paralysis and its sequelae. | Diplopia is usually absent. |
| 4. | False projection and false orientation | False projection and false orientation are positive, i.e., the patient cannot correctly locate the object in space when asked to see in the direction of the paralysed muscle in early stages. | Projection and orientation are accurate. |
| 5. | Head posture | A particular type of head posture is adopted. | No head posture. |
| 6. | Other symptoms | Nausea, vertigo, etc. may occur. | No such symptoms. |

bandaging of the eye, opacities in the cornea or other ocular media (cataract, etc.) and retino-neural obstacles which are the defects and diseases of the retina and the optic nerve.

**Motor obstacles :** The eyeball may be mechanically displaced, e.g., in asymmetry of the orbit, or fracture of the bones of the orbit. The motor obstacles may take the form of muscular defects, developmental or paralytic which actually manifest as paretic squints rather than as concomitant ones. These obstacles may also be due to convergence-accommodation dissociation, e.g., in moderate hypermetropes, accommodation excites excess of convergence leading to convergent squint.

**Central obstacles :** These factors, except for paralytic squint, are rather ambiguous and have not been proved to be a cause of squint. It has been suggested that centrally excited retinal rivalry may result in monocular inhibition leading to squint. During the phase of general hyperexcitability of nervous system the normal muscular imbalance may give way and lead to a concomitant squint. Hysteria may produce severe concomitant squint. A few cases may be due to malingering.

The slow organisation of the central nervous system as in feeble-mindedness or in congenital idiocy, may either not permit the full development of binocular reflexes or may make these reflexes unstable leading to their breakdown and muscular imbalance may be the ultimate outcome.

### Concomitant right or left squint

The concomitant squint may be such that one eye constantly deviates while the other is used for fixation when both eyes are used simultaneously. The squinted eye takes up fixation when the fixing eye is covered (uniocular squint). The deviating eye either converges (convergent squint) or diverges (divergent squint). The ocular movements are unaffected. The squint may be such that when one eye fixes, the other deviates but any eye may take up fixation. At one time the right eye fixes and the left deviates while at other times the left fixes and the right deviates. Thus the fixation and deviation come indiscriminately. Such a squint is alternating squint. The deviation may be convergent of divergent.

### Concomitant convergent squint

This squint is usually accommodational in origin but in about 1/3 of the cases no definite cause can be determined. The most usual cause of this type of deviation is increased convergence innervation, usually accommodative in origin as in hypermetropes, but sometimes it may be seen in myopes. These squints almost always show an inadequacy or absence of fusional reflexes and, therefore, develop early in life. In these cases excessive accommodation is used firstly to correct hypermetropia and secondly to accommodate for varying distances. The squint usually develops in the formative years of life, i.e., when the child is intelligent enough to appreciate the advantages of clear vision and he is small enough for the reflexes to be stable. The squint may at first be periodic and intermittent but later becomes permanent and fixed. The development of squint may be aided by one of the following factors :

• Too early an application to near work.

• Anisometropia or aniseikonia.

• If the binocular vision is rendered difficult

**Classification of squint**

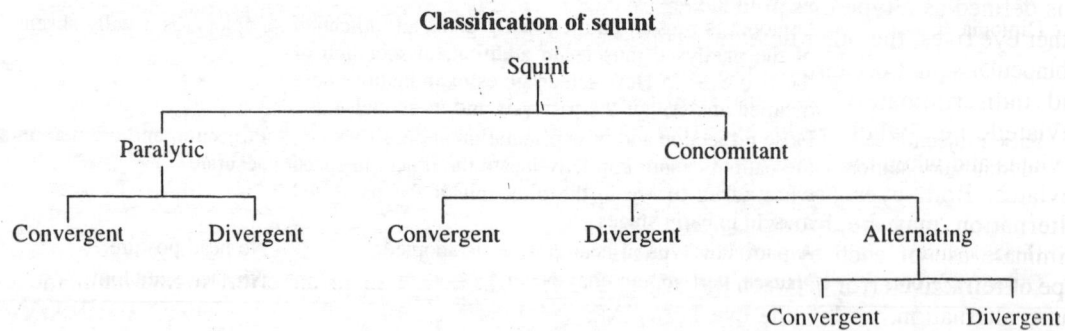

as by high astigmatism or by opacities in the media.

- Lowered general health as in convalescence.

These factors often convert a phoria into a tropia by putting extra burden on an already strained and unstable ocular muscular balance.

### Concomitant divergent squint

Divergent squint is said to be less frequent than convergent squint but in our experience reverse seems to be true. Contrary to convergent squint in hypermetropia, divergent squint is commonly seen in myopes. These are once again due to convergence and accommodation dissociation. There is less accommodation required for the near point as a result of which there is lack of convergence stimulus resulting in divergence. They are more common in females. Due to this development at a later age, the binocular functions have already developed and the patients can bring them into service again once the visual alignment is corrected. The condition is an exaggerated form of exophoria. In exophoria the visual alignment is brought by a desire and capability to fuse the images. If the power of fusion becomes weak divergent squint results. Since the position of rest is divergent, whenever a fusion stimulus is absent the eye tends to take up a position of rest, therefore, divergence occurs in blind eyes. Asymmetry of the orbits, wide interpupillary distance, brachycephaly, enophthalmos and large size of the globe also cause divergence.

Psychopathic squints are uncommon.

### Alternating squint

It is defined as a type of squint where whenever either eye fixes, the other deviates. This is called a binocular squint because both eyes intermittently and indiscriminately take up fixation or get deviated, i.e., when right eye fixes the left deviates and when the left eye fixes the right eye deviates. Both eyes are capable of deviating. Alternation may be brought about by indiscriminate use of each eye. A difference in the type of refractive error between the two eyes may cause alternation, i.e., if one eye is myopic and

the other eye hypermetropic, the myopic is used for near and the hypermetropic for distance with the result that when one eye is being used the other squints. A large number of squints are secondary in type and are essentially due to a paretic factor. As these cases originate early, binocular functions are usually not developed, and in some of them there may be a congenital absence of fusion faculty. These are known as essential alternators which have the following characteristics :

- Both eyes have equal and usually good vision.
- Both eyes show equal angle of deviation.
- Both eyes have central fixation.
- Both eyes generally have no or low and equal refractive error.
- There is no binocular vision.
- The deviation is usually large.
- In convergent squint the right eye fixes in the left field and the left eye fixes in the right field
- There is abnormal retinal correspondence.

Abnormal retinal correspondence is essentially a binocular condition in which both the fovea which usually correspond are unable to do so because of constant deviation. Thus a fovea of one eye corresponds with the extra foveal point of the other eye. The fovea of each eye remains the visual point of par excellence. The extra foveal point, thus, gets the projectional value of fovea and accordingly there is a shift of the projectional values of all the other retinal points. It is for this reason that the objective angle of squint differs from the subjective angle and the angle of anomaly is detectable. The alternating squints are best treated by surgery. It is noteworthy that fovea of each eye is still the point of par excellence of vision.

### Hypertropia

It is not an uncommon condition and is often the manifestation of hyperphoria under conditions of fatigue. It may lead to symptoms of eye strain. Diplopia, headache, and other functional troubles are quite common, more so if hypertropia is intermittent due to an effort to maintain the parallelism of visual axis the stimulus being provided by the desire and capabilities to fuse. If hypertropia becomes permanent, suppression and amblyopia may develop. An anomalous retinal correspondence may be established and consequently relief of symptoms occurs. A compensatory head tilt is evident depending upon the type of hypertropia. Hypertropia is commonly associated with a horizontal component. The squint may either be primary vertical squint with a secondary horizontal component or it may be primary horizontal squint and the vertical component is secondary. In the first type of cases dissociation of binocular functions is secondary to a vertical deviation and due to dissociation of binocular functions a horizontal strabismus occurs. In the second type of cases dissociation of binocular functions is due to horizontal squint and there is an associated secondary vertical element. Common secondary vertical elements are elevation in adduction or abduction due to imbalance of the vertical (superior rectus and inferior rectus) and cyclovertical muscles (superior oblique and inferior oblique). Concomitant vertical deviations are rare and most of the cases are paretic in origin.

## Cyclotropia

These are torsional defects and are extremely rare. These are usually paretic in nature or they are due to congenital defects.

# CHAPTER 26

# Principles of Therapy in Squint

For successful treatment of any type of squint it is essential to understand and diagnose the condition accurately and to plan out the treatment properly considering the age of onset of squint, its duration, association with amblyopia, intelligence of the patient and the cooperation and keenness of the patient.

The normal development of binocular reflexes is hindered due to certain obstacles resulting in squint or it may occur due to certain mechanical or other factors although the binocular reflexes are still present. The treatment of squint, therefore, is based on the detection and removal of these obstacles and correction of deviation. The binocular reflexes are fully developed by the age of five years and get firmly established by six years of age. The squint of short duration occurring after five years of age carries very good prognosis but squint occurring before the age of five years requires very early treatment to avoid certain complications, i.e., amblyopia, abnormal retinal correspondence and secondary musculofascial changes.

It is of paramount importance to decide the plan of treatment keeping in view whether the case can be treated from a functional point of view or only cosmetically.

Thus the ultimate aim of therapy is :
- to restore normal binocular single vision with fair degree of amplitude of fusion and stereopsis; and
- to bring the visual axis to normal state of parallelism.

The management of the case of squint may be discussed under the following headings :

**Refraction :** Every case of squint (except obvious paralytic) must be subjected to refraction under effective cycloplegia (1% atropine three times a day for three days in children). In purely accommodative type of squint of short duration simple full correction of the refractive error is good enough to cure the condition. In other cases refractive error may be partially responsible for the squint and due correction of the refractive error may considerably modify the degree of the squint. It is essential to correct the refractive error before any further step is undertaken and reassessment of the case be done with regard to the improvement of vision (detection and confirmation of the cases of amblyopia) and the degree of squint.

Cases of accommodative squint may be totally cured with proper prescription of glasses only or may considerably improve with regard to their angle of deviation.

As the children grow older they lose some of their hypermetropia and this makes it imperative to reduce the hypermetropic correction accordingly. The prescription of glasses needs certain modifications in special types of cases.
- In esophoria with hypermetropia, full or even over-correction of hypermetropia may be made compatible with good binocular vision.
- In esophoria with myopia, under-correction of myopia should be done compatible with good binocular vision.
- In exophoria with hypermetropia, under-correction should be done compatible with good binocular vision.
- In exophoria with myopia, full or even slightly over-correction may be given compatible with good binocular vision.

In all cases astigmatism should be corrected fully. After refraction and use of proper glasses, if amblyopia is discovered, it should be adequately managed depending upon its nature.

**Amblyopia :** This is a very common feature associated with squint. It may be defined as functional loss of vision without any demonstrable organic pathology in the fundus and not improvable by correction of refractive error. It may be of following varieties :

**Strabismic amblyopia :** Associated with squint and occurring as a result of central inhibition on the affected eye to avoid diplopia.

**Anisometropic amblyopia :** It is due to the presence of marked anisometropia causing difficulty in fusion of the two images and suppression which may subsequently cause squint or be as such associated with it.

**Amblyopia exanopsia :** This is due to the disuse of the eye during its development phase. Prolonged lack of visual stimuli due to any cause results in this type of amblyopia.

**Ametropic amblyopia :** It may occur in one or both eyes in persons who have significant refractive error without adequate correction.

**Congenital amblyopia :**
* May be associated with nystagmus.
* Amblyopia may also be present due to congenital achromatopsia or due to some subclinical damage to the macula.

First of all, it should be ascertained whether the fixation is central or eccentric (it means on uniocular fixation a point other than the fovea fixes a target). The type of fixation can be ascertained by an instrument known as the visuoscope. It is a type of ophthalmoscope provided with a disc which can be brought in front of the lighting beam so that a star can be focused on the retina. The patient is asked to fix the projected star. If the patient fixes the star and the observer finds that the patient has fixed it foveally then the case is of central fixation. If the observer notices the fixation is on extra foveal point then the case is of eccentric fixation which may be of one of the following types as described earlier :
* Erratic
* Parafoveal
* Paramacular
* Paracaecal
* Centrocaecal
* Temporal fixation
* Non-fixation (Fig. 26.1)

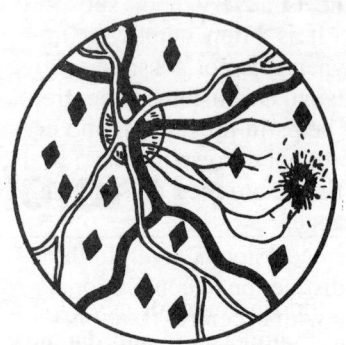

**Fig. 26.1.** Non-fixation.

### Amblyopia with central fixation

**Occlusion :** Total occlusion of the normal eye (conventional occlusion) is the most effective way of eradicating amblyopia, which may be achieved either with an occluder (Fig. 26.2) or with an elastoplast. Sometimes partial occlusion

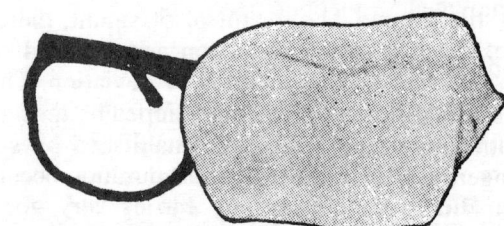

**Fig. 26.2.** Occluder.

(allowing formation of an image but with reduced visual acuity) of normal eye may be utilised towards the end of the treatment when amblyopic eye has almost equal vision with the normal eye and alteration of fixation can be achieved. If occlusion shows no improvement even after 3 months, prognosis should be taken to be poor. Sometimes when occlusion has failed, active pleoptic exercises (described below) can yield beneficial results, or can also speed up recovery. Occlusion is contraindicated in the presence of latent nystagmus.

Sometimes in very young children when it is not possible to assess the visual acuity, a unilateral squint must be suspected to have amblyopia and occlusion therapy should be started till the squint reaches the state of alternation showing that almost equal visual acuity has been achieved in both eyes.

Atropine is a very poor substitute for total occlusion. It is often employed in very young children when it is not possible to give effective total occlusion. Occlusion besides treating amblyopia, also helps in prevention and eradication of abnormal retinal correspondence. It also helps in avoiding the occurrence of secondary musculo-fascial changes.

Inverse occlusion is given to the affected eye, in contra-distinction to conventional occlusion, in amblyopia with eccentric fixation.

### Amblyopia with eccentric fixation

In children below the age of 5 years, conventional occlusion proves quite effective in eliminating amblyopia even with eccentric fixation, although a check on fixation must always be kept to see that eccentric point is not getting further strengthened by occlusion. In older children inverse occlusion should be used prior to the employment of pleoptic treatment.

### Pleoptic treatment

It is a highly specialised and intricate form of treatment of amblyopia and was advocated by Bangerter. He advocated scotomisation of the peripheral retina including the area used for eccentric fixation and subsequent stimulation of normal macula by light. Cüppers' modified Bangerter's pleoptic technique which was complicated and difficult to practice and devised certain small instruments, which were easier to manipulate and were also cheaper. The principle of Cüppers' technique is based on appreciation of negative after-image and has become a popular technique all over the world.

Instruments used by Cüppers in the treatment of eccentric fixation are :

- Euthyscope
- Cüppers' coordinator

### Euthyscope

It is a type of ophthalmoscope with additional special features. Apart from its use as a retinoscope and an ophthalmoscope which emits a strong beam of light to make the examination possible in the presence of hazy media, it is chiefly

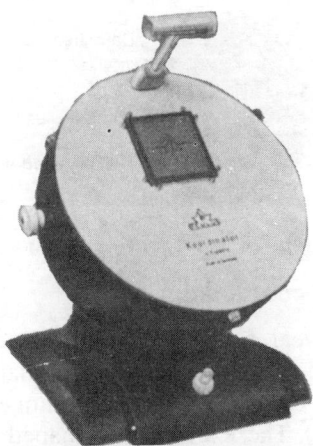

**Fig. 26.3.** Cüppers' coordinator showing the aeroplane slide inserted in front of the aperture.

used in the treatment of eccentric fixation by creating an after-image.

The retina of amblyopic eye is illuminated by using light field of 30° and a correcting spot of 3° or 5° is placed on the normal foveal region. This causes a ring-shaped positive after-image with a dark centre (Fig. 26.4).

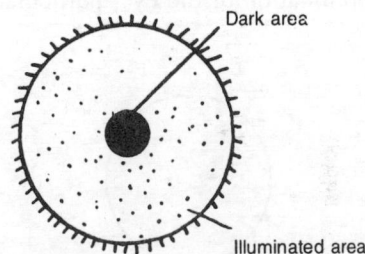

**Fig. 26.4.** Positive after-image.

The next step is to convert the positive after-image into a negative one by asking the patient to look at a white lighted screen. The screen should be intermittently illuminated by a flashing device in order to overcome inhibition. The negative after-image shows a central light field in the middle of the dark grey ring (Fig. 26.5). The light area corresponds to fovea centralis or to the macula. In this way the patient is made conscious of the position of his fovea. For better understanding the patient should be trained to create a negative after-image by doing the test first on non-amblyopic eye (normal eye).

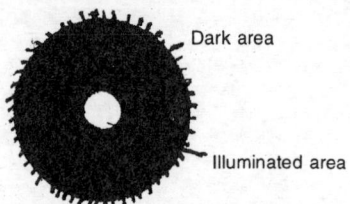

**Fig. 26.5.** Negative after-image.

## Cüppers' coordinator

When foveal fixation has been re-established, other subjective methods of stimulating central vision are employed such as Haidinger's brushes (Fig. 26.6). These are spindle-shaped apparitions of polarized light and their visibility is probably strictly engaged to foveal region. Exercises with Haidinger's brushes aim at stabilization of the recovered foveal fixation. In cases of low eccentric fixation, i.e., 1° to 5° para-foveal, change of fixation and localisation can be brought about by the coordinator. This does not help to cure suppression which can be achieved only by euthyscope. The chief use of the coordinator after establishing central fixation is to re-establish the motor coordination of the eye, particularly with the hand.

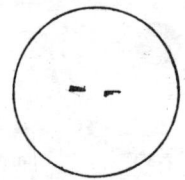

**Fig. 26.6.** Haidinger's brushes.

## Projectoscope (Fig. 26.7)

It is an instrument which can utilise both Cüppers' and Bangerter's principle of therapy. It is used in the same way as the euthyscope so that the star is placed on the fovea objectively. On pressing a trigger switch the star is replaced by a shielding disc and also an increase in the illumination takes place which results in the formation of after-images. A flashing unit is also attached along with, which helps in scotomisation of the entire extramacular field including eccentrically fixing area.

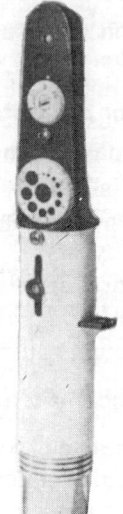

**Fig. 26.7.** Projectoscope (Keeler).

## Red filter treatment

By this means the only light to which cones are sensitive reaches the retina so that peripheral fixation involving rods is prevented. The requisite filter is Kodak No. 92 which is fixed to the glasses in front of the eccentrically fixing eye with total occlusion of the normal eye. Reports in the literature suggest that the results are equivocal.

## Use of prisms

In amblyopia with eccentric fixation in recalcitrant cases prisms associated with conventional occlusion can be given. Pleoptic therapy in the form of after-images etc. may be superadded. The prisms help in changing the muscle balance, thus change in motor innervation is able to bring about a sensory change in the form of a change of fixation.

## Orthoptics

After the successful treatment of amblyopia, orthoptic exercises are instituted to overcome suppression, abnormal retinal correspondence (ARC), and to develop range of fusion and stereopsis. These exercises do not aim at correction of any ocular deviation. Any change in the degree of squint which may follow the acquirement of correction of visual habits is merely coincidental.

### Cases suitable for orthoptic exercises

- Good general and mental health.
- Good vision in both eyes achieved by refractive correction, occlusion or pleoptic treatment.
- Age below 8 years.
- Some evidence of fusion carries good prognosis.
- Squints with late age of onset.
- Divergent squints are usually more amenable to orthoptic exercises because of the late age of onset.
- Convergence insufficiency.
- Exophoria.
- Esophoria.

### Cases unsuitable for orthoptic exercises

- Conditions where there is no likelihood of development of binocular vision.
- Patients over the age of 8 years with no evidence of fusion.
- Presence of insuperable dense amblyopia with or without eccentric fixation.
- Essential alternating squint.
- Squint associated with paretic element.
- Mentally deficient and uncooperative patients.
- Children below 5 years of age.

In certain types of cases orthoptics alone can achieve cure, viz.,

- Convergence insufficiency.
- Small degree of eso- and exophoria.
- Sometimes very small degree of hyperphoria.

Orthoptics may be needed in addition both as pre- and post-operative measure with the object of maintaining binocular faculties and to increase the range of fusion. Usually a two week course of orthoptic therapy is sufficient to secure these aims.

Orthoptic treatment is not aimed to achieve correction of deviation itself but is aimed to control the deviation by efficient binocular functions if present or to develop these functions normally in cases where anomalies like suppression and abnormal retinal correspondence are present.

Orthoptic exercises can be given either in the clinic or home. Exercises may be supplemented for the correction of suppression and improvement of the range of fusion.

### Treatment of abnormal retinal correspondence

*Occlusion* of the dominant eye or of alternate eye helps to weaken abnormal retinal correspondence and it may be given for four weeks or longer.

*Orthoptic* exercises for the treatment of abnormal retinal correspondence consists in

- Giving kinetic stimulations of corresponding biretinal points on the synoptophore. Some patients may superimpose and fuse them when the tubes are stationary.
- In difficult cases after-images on the synoptophore are utilised to bring about normal retinal correspondence. Once normalcy has been achieved with after-images, then the real objects in the form of slides may, in addition to after-images, be presented to the patients.

*Prisms* may be utilised to bring about changes in retinal correspondence. A little over-correction of prism for the neutralisation of the angle of squint is prescribed for many months which may result in normalisation of retinal correspondence.

*Surgery :* In many cases where preoperative orthoptic exercises fail to achieve normal retinal correspondence, surgery for the correction of deviation is able to achieve normal retinal correspondence. The case may need a few postoperative orthoptic exercises.

### Treatment of suppression

Anti-suppression exercises with the help of simultaneous perception slides or fusion slides are given or it may be treated with the help of cheiroscope. On synoptophore, chasing exercises are given or alternate flashing may prove useful.

Once the suppression has been treated, fusion exercises may be started on the synoptophore which needs an increase in its range by the following exercises :

- Adduction
- Abduction
- Supraduction

### Adduction exercises

These exercises are usually given with fusion slides, i.e., pictures with central control. Adduction requires great concentration. The more compact are the pictures the easier it is to maintain fusion. If the patient feels difficulty in adduction due to suppression and loses binocular fixation, it is advisable to treat him by kinetic stimulation of corresponding bi-retinal points. In other patients, where adduction is found to be difficult, one can make the patient exert his accommodation and thereby convergence by inserting a concave lens of 3 to 4 dioptres in the lens holder, provided the patient is not a presbyope. Exercises with added concave lens should not be performed for more than five minutes to avoid spasm of accommodation.

A healthy adult will not find it difficult to raise his adduction to 35° to 40° but children and elderly people may not be able to attain this standard. The patient should be asked to keep the picture clear as far as possible while he is converging so that he does not exert excessive accommodation. Later, adduction exercises should be given by simultaneous perception pictures. By this the patient learns voluntary adduction. This, when developed, ensures cure although some patients may not be able to develop it and still become asymptomatic. It is also important that the patient should be taught to relax from the position of maximum convergence to come gradually to zero.

### Abduction exercises

The normal abduction is from 3° to 7°. In teaching abduction the patient should be encouraged to relax and to feel that he is gazing beyond the pictures in the synoptophore. These exercises are performed with larger and less detailed fusion slides. For good results one would do well to start with adduction exercises. The patient will find maintenance of binocular fixation easier with stereoscopic pictures than with ordinary fusion pictures.

### Supraduction exercises

The degree of supraduction varies considerably and exercises are given with fusion slides. To prevent suppression and to improve lateroversion these exercises should be accompanied by side movements.

### Home exercises

These exercises are an important adjunct to clinic exercises on synoptophore in cutting short the duration of the therapy. The patient should be explained that the success and speed of the treatment depends largely on his own effort and perseverance. Such exercises, if at all, require very simple apparatus which the patient can use correctly and easily. A few simple exercises performed for about 5 to 10 minutes two to three times a day are quite sufficient. The following is usually advised to be carried out at home.

### Physiological diplopia

This is to aid in teaching the patient to know the relative position of his eyes and to control them. This also helps in eliminating suppression, if present.

**Physiological diplopia for distant objects :** The patient is asked to fix on a distant small spot, light or a bright object or at the moon. He then interposes a finger or a pencil at a distance of one foot and fixes at the top end of this. The distant object will then appear as two; one on either side of the pencil forming uncrossed diplopia (Fig. 26.8A). Next the observer moves the pencil closer to him and will note that the images move apart. Once he has learnt this and performs it easily, he is asked to maintain diplopia when the pencil is removed. Eventually he should be able to see double at will without interposing a pencil.

**Physiological diplopia for near objects :** The patient fixes at a distant object and interposes a pencil in front as before, but keeps his gaze fixed at the distant object so as to see the pencil as double, one on either side of the light (Fig. 26.8B). Then he moves the pencil to and from the eyes maintaining diplopia, which is of the crossed type. Certain patients find difficulty in appreciating physiological diplopia particularly for near. Ask the patient to hold the pencil in front of the light and to see it first with one eye and then with

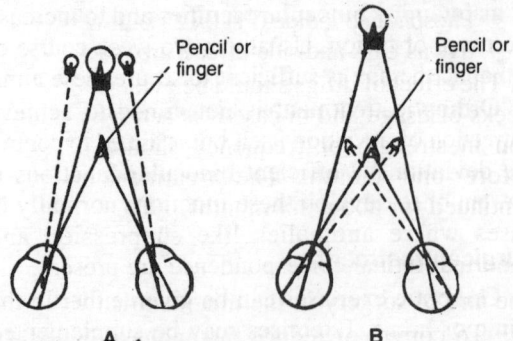

**Fig. 26.8.** Physiological diplopia for distance and near. A, uncrossed; B, crossed.

the other. The change of positions and crossing-over of the image would facilitate him to see double with both the eyes. He should try to maintain diplopia for near object by gazing into the distance without fixing at any distant object.

## Convergence to a near point

A sharp pencil is held at a distance of one to one and half feet from the eyes, its tip is viewed and is steadily moved nearer until it is seen as double or gets blurred. This exercise is better done after the patient is able to appreciate physiological diplopia.

## Physiological diplopia with a stereogram

This exercise has an additional advantage of involving the voluntary use of accommodation.

Various other instruments like diploscope, cheiroscope and stereoscope are used for giving home exercises.

## Miotic therapy

This therapy is indicated in accommodational squint or where there is abnormal AC/A ratio. Sometimes it is used in postoperative period for residual esotropia. These drugs cause ciliary body spasms and thus fix up accommodation. It obviates the use of frontal accommodation thereby removing concomitant stimulus. The commonly used drugs are :

- Pilocarpine 2-4% three times a day. It is not found to be effective and can be useful in slight post-operative residual angles.
- Di-isopropyl-fluorophosphate (DFP) 0.025%. The strength of the drug may be reduced from time to time. The side-effects of this drug are headache, conjunctival congestion and iris cysts.
- Phospholine iodide (PI) 0.125%. It is as effective as DFP and side-effects are much milder.

The effect of drugs should be evident after two weeks of usage and in case it is acting no reduction in strength or frequency should be made before one month. The treatment may be continued for about six months.

## Surgical treatment

The aim of surgery in the treatment is two-fold :
1. To correct or reduce the angle of deviation and thereby help other methods like orthoptics to develop binocular vision. In young patients, where other measures cannot be employed, surgery alone brings the visual axes in normal parallelism thus helping the natural development of binocular reflexes.
2. To correct the squint cosmetically when development of binocular single vision is not feasible either due to its non-development since birth, or due to an incurable amblyopia.

In congenital squint, early surgical correction helps development of binocular reflexes, does not allow abnormal retinal correspondence to develop, and is a single procedure with lesser complications than when performed at a later stage. In children undergoing orthoptic treatment, if there is inability to develop binocular reflexes because of greater angle of deviation, surgical correction of squint helps in the development of reflexes by post-operative exercises.

In convergent squint with considerable loss of vision in one eye there is a tendency of the eye to diverge and, therefore, if for psychological reasons operation is contemplated, an under-correction is advisable.

In alternating type of squints, operation should be preferably symmetrical particularly in adults. In alternating divergent squint bilateral recession of lateral recti is performed. Another point to be considered at the time of planning surgery is the position of the eyeball. In slight enophthalmos lengthening or weakening operation is recommended and in exophthalmos a shortening or strengthening operation is recommended.

## Concomitant convergent strabismus

Irrespective of age of the patient, history and the duration of squint, there is always something that can be done for these patients. The aim of the treatment is to restore binocular single vision, wherever possible, failing which at least to give a cosmetic correction. The outline of treatment for convergent concomitant squint is given in Table 26.1.

## Concomitant divergent squint

### Intermittent divergent squint

*Correction of refractive error :* Usually there is no significant refractive error, but if a refractive error is present hypermetropia is undercorrected and myopia is fully corrected, so as to exercise accommodation and convergence.

**Table 26.1. Management of concomitant convergent squint**

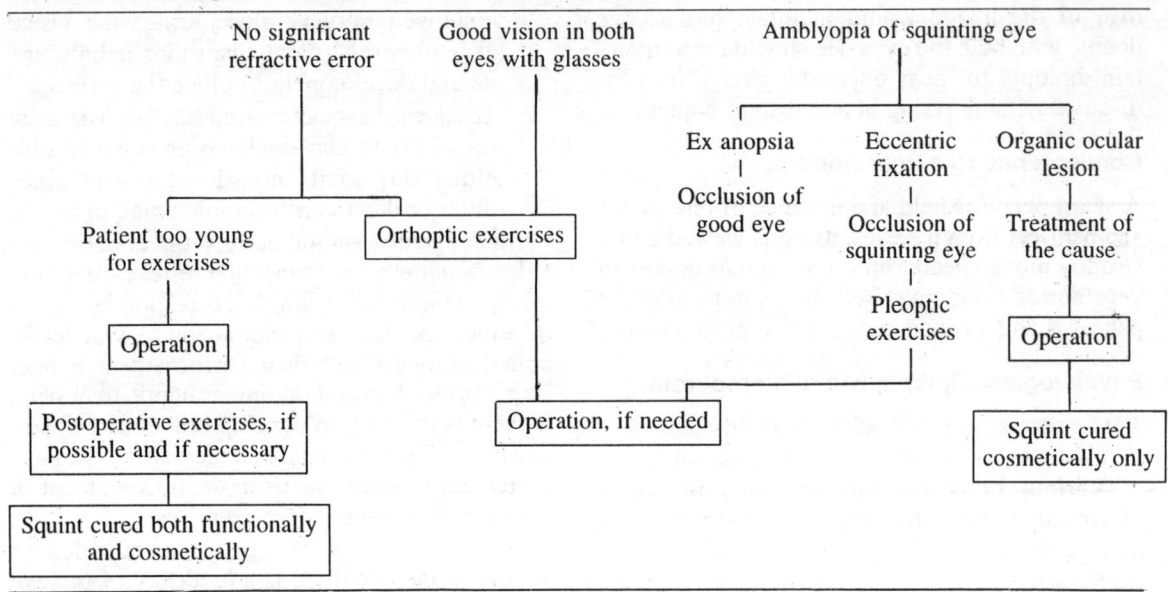

**Table 26.2. Management of concomitant divergent squint**

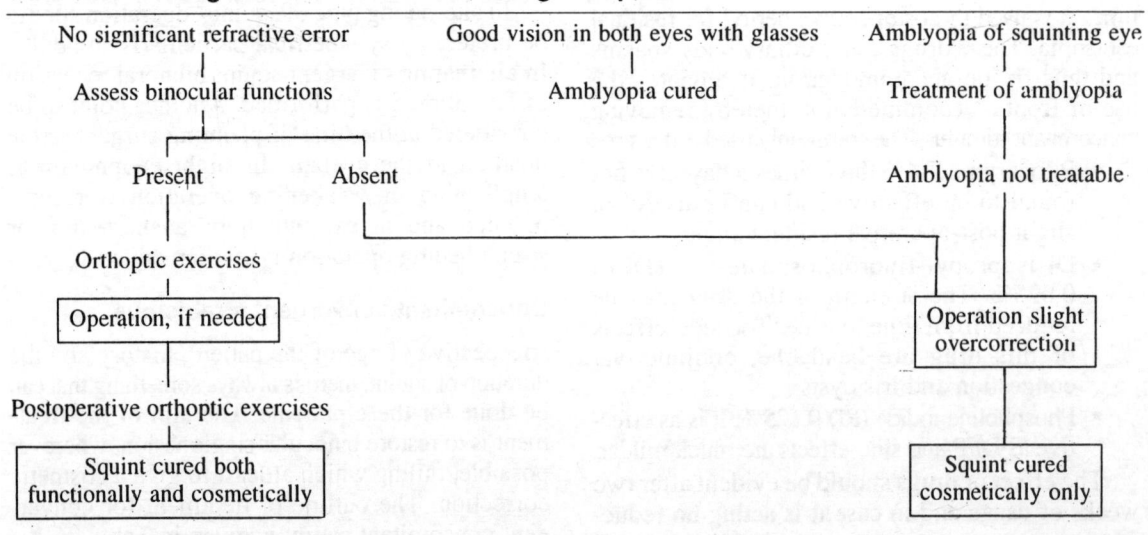

*Orthoptic treatment :* To improve convergence, it is usually effective as a pre-operative measure and also effective if given post-operatively.

*Surgery :* Operation on horizontal recti should be contemplated depending upon the degree and type of squint.

### Constant divergent squint

The line of treatment depends upon the state of the diverging eye and the visual acuity with glasses. These cases may be divided into three groups for purposes of further management (Table 26.2).

SECTION VII

# Contact Lenses and
# Low Vision Aids

# CHAPTER 27

# Contact Lenses

Contact lenses as refractive aids are becoming more and more popular.

## History

Leonardo da Vinci (1508) conceived the idea of neutralising the front surface of the cornea by immersing his face in a bowl of water. Descartes (1637) also suggested the possibility of neutralising corneal surface by applying a tube of water, at the end of which was attached a watch glass with curvature like that of cornea, to the eye. Thomas Young (1801) attempted to neutralise his own irregular corneal surface by a similar device but at the end of the water tube instead of glass he fitted a microscope lens. Herschel (1827) suggested the application to the eye of a glass capsule containing animal jelly in front of the cornea to eliminate astigmatism. Nothing further happened till F.E. Müller (1889) made a glass shell for a one-eyed patient as there was an apprehension of loss of sight in the remaining eye due to exposure since the lids had been removed. It proved to be an outstanding optical protective device.

Fick (1888) introduced the term of contact lenses and used the device of moulded lens for optical treatment of conical cornea. This led to problem of intolerance yet the idea caught on. Several others (Gatt, Saltear) simultaneously tried to experiment but with indifferent result due to excessive thickness and weight of the lenses. Müller (1889), Kalt (1889), Sulzer (1892), Keil (1929), Dallos (1933) are the pioneer workers who devised various types of contact lenses in order to improve vision and increase tolerance. Mostly glass was used as the material of choice.

Till 1932, all ophthalmic literature refers to the use of two types of contact lenses, namely

• Ground contact lens (Figs. 27.1 and 27.2)

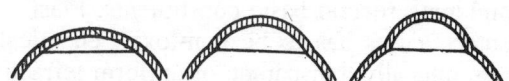

**Fig. 27.1.** Ground contact lens of different corneal and scleral curvatures.

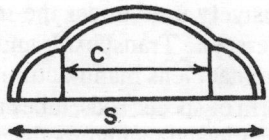

**Fig. 27.2.** Parts of the ground contact lenses. C, corneal curve; S, scleral curve.

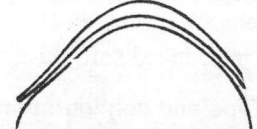

**Fig. 27.3.** Moulded contact lenses.

• Blown or moulded contact lens (Fig. 27.3)

Both the types were made of transparent glass, having spherical corneal and scleral curves. With these lenses it was not possible to get optical perfection or to add desired refractive power. Moreover, they were difficult to fit and could not be worn for a long time. This led to the development of moulded contact lenses (Fig. 27.3) which conform to the shape and size of the eye. Dallos (1933) was the one to realise the importance of making a cast of the living eye in order to improve the effectivity and tolerance of contact lenses.

Glass contact lenses being heavy and breakable, search for a better material started. Plastics, which are capable of being moulded by application of heat pressure and action of catalysts were tested to a large extent. Plastics are natural and synthetic organic materials produced by chemical condensation or polymerisation of cellulose, resin, protein and other organic substances. Chemically, they are distinguishable as celluloses, acrylics, phenolics, butyrates, formaldehydes, styrenes, vinylates and melamines, depending upon the basic material of which they are made. Plastics exhibiting different qualities can be prepared by subjecting them to different treatments or by combining several basic constituents. Plastic of contact lenses has to be non-toxic, chemically inert, optically transparent, of uniform refractive index and scratch resistant. Some more properties which need to be considered are stability, surface hardness, moulding ability and resistance to chemical and heat. Pure methyl methacrylate is almost exclusively used under the trade name of Plexiglas, Perspex, Transpex I and Lencite by most of the contact lens manufacturers. It is available in the form of sheets, rods, tubes and moulding powder. Prefabricated methyl methacrylate contact lenses with known curvature and power are also available. Slight modification, if needed, can be easily made on the anterior and or posterior surfaces of the lens.

Wichterla introduced soft plastic lenses made of a hydrogel, chemically known as polydiaxthlene methacrylate. It moulds to the shape of the eye and can be squeezed like a sponge.

Table 27.1 gives the present day picture of type and configuration of lenses. Evolution has not ended and surgery on the cornea may overtake the use of contact lenses.

## OPTICAL CONSIDERATION OF CONTACT LENSES

### Optics of contact lenses

The aim of contact lens is to eliminate the anterior surface of cornea as an optical system. In fact, with the lens in place, anterior corneal surface becomes almost optically non-existent because it forms the posterior surface of liquid lens, formed by a thin tear film between the cornea and the contact lens. It has the same refractive index as the cornea. The fluid lens may thus be considered as a forward extension of the cornea.

If the curvatures of the two surfaces of the contact lens are equal it is known as afocal contact lens (Fig. 27.4). If the curvature is the same as that of cornea these lenses become optically inert. Otherwise the effective power of the combination becomes reduced to that of the fluid lens. Such

**Table 27.1. Type and configuration of contact lenses**

| Category (scleral or corneal) | Type | Configuration and type of wear |
|---|---|---|
| *Scleral* | | |
| Scleral lenses | Ground | Spherical |
| | Moulded | Toric back surface |
| | Cosmetic | With clear pupil |
| | | With black pupil |
| *Corneal* | | |
| Corneal lenses fabricated in PMMA or oxygen permeable material | In clear or tinted material | Toric periphery |
| | Toric | Bitoric |
| | Bifocals | |
| Corneal cosmetic lenses fabricated in PMMA material only | Clear pupil with painted iris | |
| | Black pupil with clear periphery (occluder lens) | |
| | Black pupil with painted iris | |
| Soft lenses | In clear material with varying water content | Daily wear |
| | | Extended wear |
| | Tinted lenses with clear pupil and clear periphery | Permanent |
| | | Painted iris with clear pupil and clear periphery |
| | Toric lenses | Black pupil with painted iris and clear periphery |
| | Bifocal lenses | |
| | Iris lenses | |

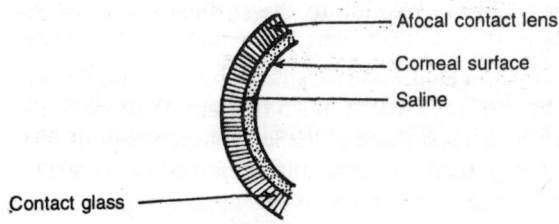

**Fig. 27.4.** Afocal contact lens.

afocal contact lenses are indicated in eyes with corneal irregularities but axially emmetropic.

The contact lens system may either be liquid lens (fluid lens) system or glass lens system depending upon which one of the two imparts power.

**Liquid lens :** The anterior surface of the liquid lens is formed by the posterior surface of the contact lens while the posterior surface is formed by the anterior surface of the cornea. The power is given to the posterior surface of the contact lens (Fig. 27.5).

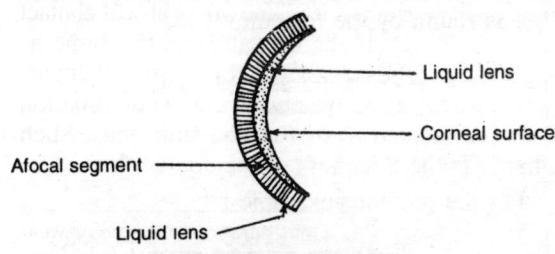

**Fig. 27.5.** Liquid lens.

**Glass lens :** When the spherical correction is made by modifying the curvature of the anterior surface of the contact lens, it is termed a glass lens (Fig. 27.6).

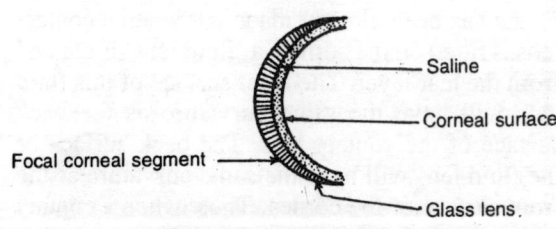

**Fig. 27.6.** Glass lens.

**Combined liquid and solid contact lens :** The power of such a lens is resultant of the power of both of them (Fig. 27.7).

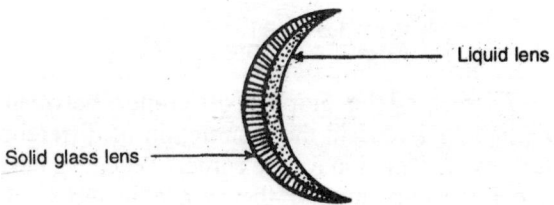

**Fig. 27.7.** Combined liquid and solid contact lens.

The ametropic eye is corrected by a combination of the power provided by the curvatures of the glass lens and the liquid lens. The effective power of the afocal lenses can be changed by altering its curvature from that of the cornea. The effective power of this system depends upon the power of the liquid lens. If the afocal lens gives the remaining effective power which is ground on the anterior surface of the lens, the residual astigmatism, when present, can be ground on the posterior surface of the lens, thus converting it into a combined lens.

In order to design an optical contact lens an accurate estimation of corneal curvature is of utmost importance. This is done with the help of keratometer. Modern keratometers are designed to measure the corneal curvature in different zones. This is one of the biggest breakthroughs in the designing and fitting of contact lenses.

### Optics

Now let us consider the optics of finding out the power of cornea, knowing its radius of curvature and refractive index. The power of any surface in air is found from the formula

$$P = \frac{n-1}{r}$$

where $n$ is the index of refraction of the surface in question and $r$ is the radius in metres. Most types of keratometers are calibrated for an index ($n$) of 1.3375, which is the assumed index of the cornea. When measuring the corneal curvatures with the keratometer, the formula is written as

$$P_K = \frac{1.3375 - 1}{r}$$

Most of modern keratometers are designed to give the surface powers directly in dioptres.

Taking the index of the cornea ($n$) as 1.376, the power formula for the cornea becomes

$$P_C = \frac{1.376 - 1}{r}$$

Therefore, the dioptric difference between $P_K$ and $P_C$ is due to the assumption of different indices of refraction for the cornea. When we talk about the curvature of the cornea in terms of dioptres of $K$ reading (DK) we are not talking about the 'true' dioptral corneal curvature surface power, e.g., a particular cornea measures 44.0 DK on the keratometer.

Rewriting the $P_K$ formula as

$$r = \frac{1.3375 - 1}{P_K}$$

the radius of the cornea is found to be 7.67 mm. Since the corneal radius is constant, the power of the cornea from the $P_C$ formula for $r = 7.67$ is 49.02 D.

When a practitioner specifies the base curve of a lens in terms of dioptres of 'K', both he and the laboratory must understand that this dioptric value refers to the corneal radius as derived from the $P_K$ formula. Although the base curve may be specified in millimetres of radius, the dioptric power ($P_1$) of this surface will be different from both $P_K$ and $P_C$. For an index ($n_1$) for plastic of 1.49, the surface power of a contact lens with a radius of 7.67 mm would be

$$P_1 = \frac{1.49 - 1}{0.00767} = 63.89 \text{ D}$$

When measured on the keratometer the same lens will give a power reading of 44.0 DK. This occurs because the karatometer is designed to measure the curvature of a reflecting surface and is calibrated for a set index of refraction as has already been mentioned. The dioptric reading will be slightly in error because the kerotometer is designed to measure convex, and not concave surfaces. For most clinical purposes this error is insignificant. Conversion charts of the true radii are available when accuracy is required.

Before trying to understand the power relationships between the contact lens and the cornea, the reader should be familiar with the purely optical aspects of contact lens. Although physically thin, a contact lens cannot be considered as a thin lens in power calculations. By optical definition a lens is considered thin when it is thin in relation to the surface power of the lens.

This can best be illustrated by an example. Say that we have a lens of –5.0 D and 0.2 mm thick. If the back surface of the lens has a power of 65.0 D ($P_2$), then the front surface power ($P_1$) must be +60.0 D. According to the approximate or thin lens formula, $P = P_1 + P_2$. However, if we use thick lens or effectivity formula ($P_e$) where

$$P_e = P_1 + P_2 - \frac{t}{n} P_1 P_2,$$

it is evident that thickness of a contact lens ($t$) is a significant factor and must be taken into account. In this example,

$$P_e = 60 + (-65) - \frac{0.0002}{1.49} \, 60 \times (-65)$$
$$= -5.0 \text{ D} + 0.52 \text{ D}$$
$$= -4.48 \text{ D}$$

In the contact lens fitting we are mainly concerned with the back vertex power of the lens at the corneal plane. The back vertex power $P_{BVP}$ is found by the formula :

$$P_{BVP} = \frac{P_1}{1 - \frac{t}{n}(P_1)} + P_2$$

where $t$ is the thickness of the contact lens.

For the previous example :

$$P_{BVP} = \frac{+60}{\dfrac{1 - 0.0002}{1.49}(+60)} + (-65)$$
$$= \frac{+60}{1 - 0.008} + (-65)$$
$$= 60.48 - 65$$
$$= -4.52 \text{ D}$$

As has been already made out when a contact lens is fitted on the cornea, a 'fluid lens' is created from the tear layer. The front surface of this fluid lens will have the same curvature as the back surface of the contact lens. The back surface of the fluid lens will have the same curvature as the front surface of the cornea. Thus, when a contact lens is placed on the eye, a two-lens system is formed consisting of the contact lens and the fluid lens. It is the back vertex power of the two lens systems at the corneal plane which corrects the refractive error of the eye.

It would be a very time-consuming task to calculate the exact power of such a lens system for each patient. For clinical purposes, in determining the power of the contact lens to be prescribed, we can make use of certain principles and assumptions. One important principle is that two lenses each having the surface of the same radius of curvature but of different sign will have the same total power, whether they are placed together or separated by a layer of air; that is,

$$P_{Total} = P_{L1} + P_{L2}$$

For example, the refractive power at the corneal plane of a contact lens whose base curve is equal to the corneal curvature will correct the refractive error of the eye whether it is placed on the cornea or separated from it by a thin air space.

In reality there will be a tear layer between the lens and the cornea. As with the contact lens this tear layer or fluid lens cannot be considered thin in relation to its surface power. If the lens is fit on K, then the tear layer thickness is negligible. If the lens is not fit on K, then the fluid lens thickness becomes significant. However, for clinical purposes this difference can be considered negligible.

Using the principle previously mentioned, the parts of the lens-corneal system can be separated in air; that is, the contact lens, the fluid lens, and the cornea can be considered as separated by a thin layer of air. The total power of the lens-corneal system will be equal to the power of the contact lens ($P_{CL}$) at the corneal plane in the air, and the power of the cornea ($P_e$) (refractive power of the eye at the corneal plane) in air. Since the system is designed to negate the refractive error of the eye, the desired total power of the system is 0, and the formula is $P_{CL} + P_{FL} = P_e$.

This is known as the exact or lens method of power calculation. For refractive errors greater than +4.0 D effectivity is significant, and the true back vertex power must be calculated. The power of the fluid lens (ignoring thickness factors) is simply the dioptric differences between the curvature of the base curve ($K_L$) and the curvature of the cornea ($K_C$) for each of the principle meridians; i.e., $P_{FL} = K_L - K_C$. Once the refractive power of the eye and the base curve are known, $P_{CL}$ can be calculated from the above formula.

**Example 1 :**
    $R_x$    –2.0 D at 11 mm vertex distance
    $K_C$    44.0 DK sphere
    $B_C$    44.0 DK
    $P_e$    –2.0 D
    $P_{FL}$    0
    $P_{CL}$    –2.0 D

**Example 2 :**
    $R_x$    $- 2.0 - 1.0 \times 180$
    $K_C$    44.0/180, 45.0/90
    $B_C$    44.0 DK
    $P_e$    $- 2.0 - 1.0 \times 180$
  (–) $P_{FL}$    $0 - 1.0 \times 180$
    $P_{CL}$    –2.0 D

**Example 3 :**
    $R_x$    $+ 2.0 - 1.0 \times 180$
    $K_C$    44.0/180, 45.0/90
    $B_C$    44.5 DK
    $P_e$    $- 2.0 - 1.0 \times 180$
  (–) $P_{FL}$    $+ 0.5 - 1.0 \times 180$
    $P_{CL}$    –2.5 D

**Example 4 :**
    $R_x$    $+ 4.0 - 1.0 \times 180$ at 13 mm V.D.
    $K_C$    44.0/180, 45.0/90
    $B_C$    44.5 DK
    $P_e$    $- 3.8 - 0.89 \times 180$

For clinical purposes each principle meridian can be taken to the nearest 0.12 D.
    $P_e$    $- 3.75 - 0.87 \times 180$
    $P_{FL}$    $+ 0.5 - 1.0 \times 180$
    $P_{CL}$    $- 4.25 + 0.12 \times 180$

**Example 5 :**
    $R_x$    $- 4.0 - 1.0 \times 180$ at 13 cm V.D.
    $K_C$    45.5/180, 45.0/90
    $B_C$    45.25 D
    $P_e$    $- 3.75 - 0.87 \times 180$
  (–) $P_{FL}$    $\dfrac{+ 0.25 - 0.5 \times 90}{0}$

When the axes are 90° apart, convert the spectacle correction to plus cylinder form.
    $P_e$    $- 4.62 + 0.87 \times 90$
    $P_{FL}$    $+ 0.25 - 0.50 \times 90$
    $P_{CL}$    $- 4.87 + 1.37 \times 90$

**Example 6 :**
    $R_x$    $+ 12.0 - 1.0 \times 165$ at 11 mm V.D

$K_C$   42.0/165, 46.5/75
$B_C$   43.5 DK
$P_e$   $+ 13.87 - 1.37 \times 165$
$(-) P_{FL}$   $+ 1.5 - 4.5 \times 165$
$P_{CL}$   $+ 12.37 + 3.12 \times 165$

In the first three examples the calculated lens power is what would generally be prescribed. In example 4 to 6, astigmatism is a complicating factor in determining the power of the lens. Since most contact lenses are fit with a spherical base curve, there will frequently be a residual astigmatism. In examples 4 to 6 the astigmatic component of $P_{Cl}$ is known as the predicted residual astigmatism. It is the difference between the total astigmatism of the eye (i.e., the astigmatic component of the spectacle correction), and the corneal astigmatism (i.e., the corneal tonicity as measured on the keratometer). This is true for all cases regardless of the spherical component.

The contact lens power that is to be specified is determined from $P_{CL}$ by making use of the principle of equivalent sphere which is found by taking one-half of the cylinder power and adding this to the sphere with the same sign. In example 5 the predicted residual astigmatism, would be $+1.37 \times 90$ and the equivalent sphere would be $-0.75 + 1.37 \times 90$. The equivalent sphere will provide the best spherical correction.

## Types of contact lenses

**Scleral or haptic**, better called corneo-scleral contact lenses. These are being widely used for therapeutic, and less often for optical, cosmetic and diagnostic purposes.

**Corneal :** Contact lenses on the other hand are mainly used for visual improvement. Tuohy (1943) introduced a corneal contact lens equal to the diameter of the cornea (11.5 mm) and a back curve which was 1.5 dioptres flatter than the cornea. Such a lens was available in a prefabricated state, was easy to fit and handle by the patient. The main disadvantage it suffered was that it could not be worn for a long time due to development of corneal oedema. Fenestration, faceting, grooving or channelisation of the back surface of the lens were employed to increase the tolerability of such a lens.

Micro-corneal contact lens of the diameter of

9.5 mm and a single back curve 2.5 mm flatter than cornea was simultaneously developed by Dickinson, and Sohnges (1954). The diameter of present day contact lenses varies from 7.5 mm to 9.5 mm.

According to the back curve, contact lenses can be categorised into monocurve, bicurve, tricurve and multicurve lenses. The monocurve lens which is very rarely used today, consists of a single curve on both the surfaces of the lens. The bicurve lens (Fig. 27.8) consists of a central base curve and a flatter peripheral curve. The tricurve lens is similar to the bicurve except that

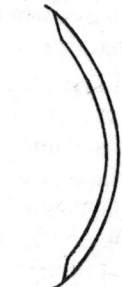

**Fig. 27.8.** Bicurve lens.

it has an intermediate curve in between the base curve and peripheral curve. A multicurve lens has more than one intermediate curves. Special lens types have been developed to achieve a good lens fit in special fitting problems. A highly toric cornea needs to be fitted with a contact lens that has a toric back surface. Since it is often impossible to eliminate significant residual astigmatism in these cases, it is frequently necessary to incorporate a cylinder in the front surface of the lens, creating a 'bitoric' contact lens. For an eye with a high degree of astigmatism and low corneal toricity, the cylinder is incorporated on the anterior surface of the lens. The rotation of the lens in these cases is prevented either by using a prism ballast lens which is heavier at the bottom or by truncated lens which is supported by the lower lid.

The various optional lens shapes used to discourage rotation are used in high corneal astigmatic errors and usually help to improve vision (Fig. 27.9).

The lenticular contact lens (Fig. 27.10) is best

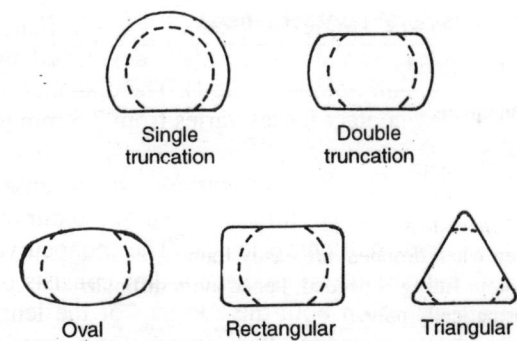

Single          Double
truncation      truncation

Oval        Rectangular       Triangular

**Fig. 27.9.** Various optional lens shapes used to discourage rotation.

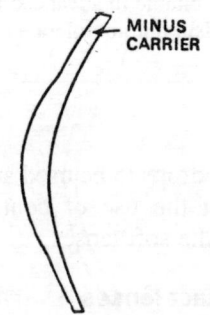

MINUS
CARRIER

**Fig. 27.10.** Lenticular contact lens.

known for its use in aphakia. Such a lens design greatly reduces its weight and gives an optimum edge thickness to a high plus lens. The lenticular lens can also be used in very high myopes. In these cases a plus carrier can be used on the lenticular lens to keep the edge thickness at a minimum.

Several types of bifocal contact lenses (Fig. 27.11) have been designed; none has proven to be generally applicable to the majority of presbyopes. The patients may experience blurred vision, jumps and doubling. The prism ballast bifocal may bump against the lower lid.

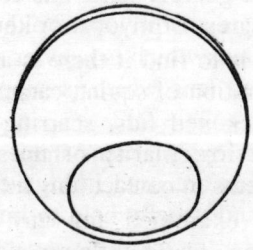

**Fig. 27.11.** Bifocal contact lens.

Lenses are prone to warpage and segment separation. A bifocal trial set is necessary for fitting the patients and it is an expensive proposition.

## Advantages of contact lenses over spectacles

The contact lenses have the following advantages over the spectacles :

- The disadvantages of spectacles having meridional distortion in oblique cylinders is avoided with the use of contact lenses. The irregular astigmatism, which is not possible to correct with glasses, can be easily corrected.

- Provides the normal field.

- Aberrations associated with spectacles are eliminated, e.g., peripheral aberration, chromatic aberration and prismatic distortion.

- The size of image is reduced with plus correction while it is enlarged with minus correction. It is an advantage to myopes. It is also used to diminish aniseikonia in anisometropia and unilateral aphakia which renders the binocular vision easier.

- The amount of accommodative and convergence effort used is proportional to the achievement of results. It is an advantage to hypermetropes.

- Rain and fog do not condense upon contact lenses as they do on spectacles for they are kept at body temperature.

- Cosmetically more pleasant.

There are specific indications and contra-indications for either the use of corneo-scleral or micro-corneal contact lenses; the advantages and disadvantage of either type when used in a particular case are given in Table 27.2.

In order to fit contact lenses the following steps are rewarding :

### Selecting the patient

Careful screening will enable one to choose patients who have a good chance of achieving success. One should discuss potential problems honestly and openly with them.

**Table 27.2. Differences between microcorneal and corneoscleral contact lenses**

| Microcorneal | Corneoscleral |
|---|---|
| 1. Flushing and replenishing of tear film is easy due to constant movement of the lens. | Inadequate. |
| 2. They pose problem of mechanical abrasion of cornea due to direct contact of the edges. | Less frequent. |
| 3. Tolerance is better. | Tolerance less. |
| 4. Lost easily under the lid or out of the eye. | Even when dropped, are easily found. |
| 5. Easy to manufacture, fit and use. | Custom fitting is needed; hence more difficult. |
| 6. Cosmetically excellent. | Cosmetically poor. |
| 7. No artificial fluid is needed. | In most instances artificial fluid is needed. |
| 8. Not good for old, virtually blind, handicapped, athletes, swimmers, boxers, etc. | Give better service in old, virtually blind, handicapped, athletes, swimmers, etc. |
| 9. Not suitable for irregular corneas, advanced keratoconus, high astigmatism and therapeutic purposes. | The lens is more suitable in advanced keratoconus, irregular astigmatism but not tolerated well. |

An ideal choice of a patient is :

• One who is motivated, which implies that he wishes to see properly and effectively. He also desires to be seen without glasses. Girls are the subjects who eminently answer this description.

• The patient preferably should be young or one who has been using contact lenses. At presbyopic age even with good fitting reading problems will remain. Bifocals may be the answer but in many instances it is inadequate. At this age group there are problems of dry eyes and general health problems. They must also know that contact lenses do not prevent myopia from progressing.

• The work of the patient, particularly hazardous occupations like construction workers, mechanics, chemical workers and whole time cooks limit the success of contact lenses.

• Sports persons may be ideal for these lenses except swimming. Soft lenses may be preferable.

• Toric contact lenses, even amongst soft lenses, permit patients with astigmatism to use them.

• How painstaking can a patient be with the hygiene of the lens.

• Past history of eye disease or general health like diabetes may limit the choice.

• Local eyedrops to be used at frequent intervals limit the use of contact lenses particularly the soft lenses.

**Fitting of contact lenses**

It follows that it is essential to have a pre-fitting consultation with the client. It serves a dual purpose : the fitter can know about the degree of motivation of the patient and the patient receives correct information regarding contact lenses. The percentage of successful contact lens wearers depends as much on the motivation of the patient as on the fitting. Roughly the success rate is 90 percent. The advantages and disadvantages of contact lenses wear should be clearly told to the patient. The usual adaptation period is about two months. However, the sensation of wearing persists, even after the adaptation period, in majority of cases. Contact lenses improve the visual acuity as much or better than spectacles but contrary to the general belief it is doubtful if they arrest the progress of myopia or keratoconus.

Next step is to find if there is any history of injury or operation of squint, cataract or corneal grafting. Thickened lids, scarring of the conjunctiva and irregularity of the cornea pose special problems in contact lens fitting.

Lids are examined for any meibomitis, dandruff, ulcers, warts, inflammation and use of cosmetics. An estimate of lid tension is made by grasping the lid between the thumb and finger, thus noting the resiliency as the lid springs back into space.

Blink rate is also noted; normally it is 12 to 20 per minute. Any abnormality regarding tear film is also looked for.

In conjunctival lesions such as kerato-conjunctivitis sicca scleral contact lenses are prescribed. Lesions near the limbus like filtering bleb of glaucoma operation, pinguecula, operated or unoperated pterygium or limbal growth are noted.

*Corneal diameter* is measured. It is· the horizontal diameter that is more important.

*Radius of curvature* of the cornéa is measured in different meridians with keratometer.

*Visual acuity* without and with glasses is recorded. Prescription of refractive error is noted with cylinder of minus power.

Near point of accommodation and convergence is also recorded.

Pupil diameter is measured in low illumination with a ruler on an infrared photograph or on Goldmann's perimeter.

### Fitting of corneal contact lenses

The lenses are of three types :
1. Rigid lenses
2. Gas permeable lenses
3. Soft lenses or hydrogel lenses

#### Rigid lenses

The rigid lenses may be corneal or scleral.

#### Corneal rigid lenses

The posterior surface of a rigid contact lens consists of :

Base curve or central posterior curve on which the power is ground and is called the optical zone (Fig. 27.12).

Intermediate curve or blend : This curve blends the junction between adjacent curves on the posterior surface of the lens (Fig. 27.13).

Secondary curve or peripheral curve : It is a flatter curve (the curve has a longer radius) adjacent to base curve which is designed to simulate the corneal contour as cornea gradually

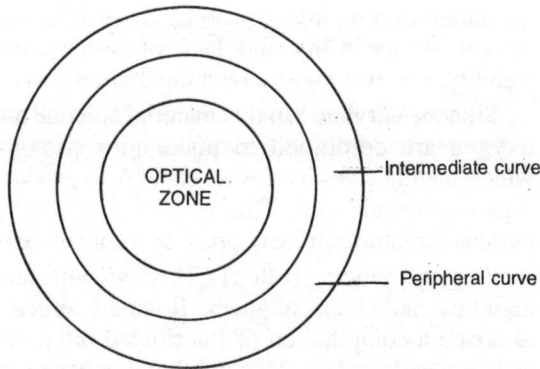

**Fig. 27.12.** Base curve of rigid contact lens

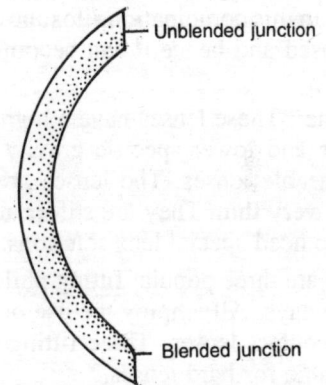

**Fig. 27.13.** Intermediate curve.

flattens off towards the periphery. It may vary from 0.50 mm to 5 mm.

This curve provides a better contact lens/cornea relationship and assists in chanelling fresh oxygenated tears to the cornea.

### Materials for rigid contact lenses

The materials used are :

PMMA : It is a stable material that resists warpage, wets well and cleans easily. Its major drawback is its lack of permeability to oxygen. The oxygen to cornea in these lenses is provided by tear exchange phenomenon.

#### Gas permeable lenses

These are essentially rigid lenses. The materials used for gas permeable lenses are :

Cellulose acetate butyrate : In this cellulose is combined with acetic and butyric acids. The material has fallen into relative disuse because of its low oxygen permeability and lack of dimensional stability, i.e., warpage, scratching and coating.

Silicone/acrylate : In this material silicone and oxygen are combined to make into siloxane which then is combined with PMMA to produce a gas permeable lens. This is used in preparing buttons for lathe cutting to produce a contact lens.

Fluoropolymers (Teflon) : This can withstand high heat and chemical attack. It would be better to create a combination of fluorinated monomer and silicone/acrylate. This will have better resistance to deposits and better in-eye wettability. Due to this it may also reduce the incidence of red eyes. In this combination siloxane content can be increased and hence it can become more gas permeable.

Styrene : These lenses have a higher index of refraction and lower specific gravity than other gas permeable lenses. The lenses are thus very light and very thin. They are stiffer and wet better. These need special lens solutions.

There are three popular fitting philosophies in use these days. All employ the use of bicurve or tricurve contact lenses. Three fitting techniques are the same for hard lenses.

Modified contour fitting philosophy : The lenses have an optical zone with base curve close to the flattest corneal radius of curvature. This zone is relatively small as compared to the wide peripheral zone which is slightly flatter than the base curve. The lens is primarily supported in the optical zone range of 7.0 to 7.8 mm.

Sphericon philosophy : It is similar to modified contour one. The lens here has a relatively large optical zone diameter with a narrow, and flat peripheral curve. The lens is supported mostly in the optical zone region. The peripheral curve is 0.4 mm wide with a standard radius of curvature of 12.25 mm. The total diameter of the lens is usually 9.2 mm.

Palpebral aperture or small thin lens philosophy : In this the lens rides within the palpebral aperture. The diameter ranges from 7.5 to 8.8 mm with an optical zone diameter of about 6.7 to 8.4 mm. The base curve is slightly steeper than the flattest corneal radius of curvature. The peripheral curve is moderately wide and flatter

than the base curve. Here again the lens is supported in optical zone and secondary curve, if present.

Whatever fitting philosophy is used there are two basic fitting procedures to determine the dimension of the lens to be prescribed.

**Keratometric method**

Reading of radius of curvature of cornea in two principal meridians and the spectacle correction are used to determine the dimensions of the lens, depending upon the fitting philosophy. The total diameter is primarily determined by the vertical width of the palpebral aperture and the horizontal diameter of the cornea. The effect of the lid position and lid tension on the lens-cornea bearing relationship should also be taken into account. The diameter of the optical zone is determined from the diameter of the pupil. It should be at least the size of the pupil in low illumination and generally slightly larger as the lens moves on the cornea. The base curve of the lens is determined from the keratometric reading (K). It is flatter or steeper than K, depending upon the fitting philosophy. The width and radius of curvature of peripheral curves are determined by the fitting philosophy and the lens type used. Determination of lens power is discussed under optics of contact lenses.

**Trial lens method**

It consists of trying various types until appropriate base curve and a good lens cornea bearing relationship is achieved. The total diameter, optical zone diameter, base curve, and peripheral curve radius and width are determined from the trial lens specifications. In most cases the power can be determined by the amount of additional power that must be added to the power of the trial lens, plus any differences that must be compensated for, due to a difference in the base curve of the trial lens and that of the lens to be ordered.

Both the methods have inherent faults. The keratometer method suffers as cornea is not a spherical surface, it tends to flatten towards the periphery.

The trial lens method has a disadvantage of being cumbersome and not very accurate. Moreover it needs a very large trial set.

PLATE III

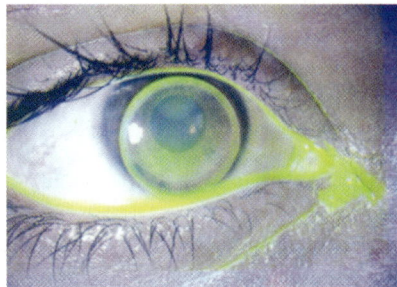

**A.** Alignment fit with adequate clearance at periphery

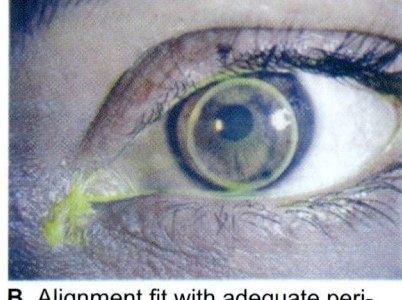

**B.** Alignment fit with adequate peripheral clearance.

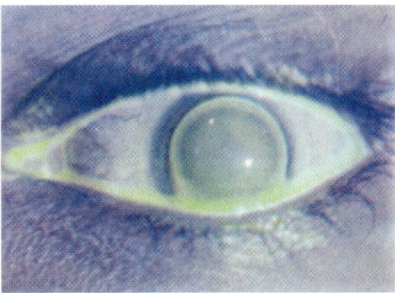

**C.** Optimum fit—evenly distributed fluorescein all over in central zone and adequate edge fit.

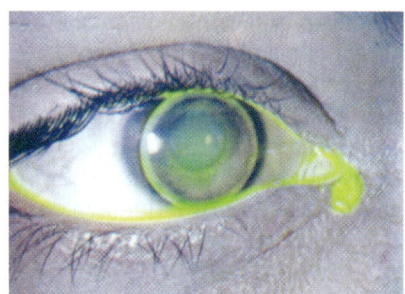

**D.** Optimum fit.

**Fig. 27.15.** Optimum fit and alignment.

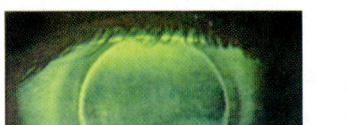

**A.** Fit in highly toric cornea. Parallel to "K" fitting pattern shows equal distribution in horizontal meridian.

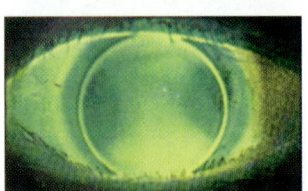 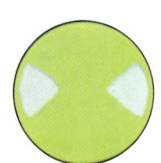

**B.** Fit in highly toric cornea. BCOD steeper than K (astigmatism with the rule)

**Fig. 27.16.** Steeper fit.

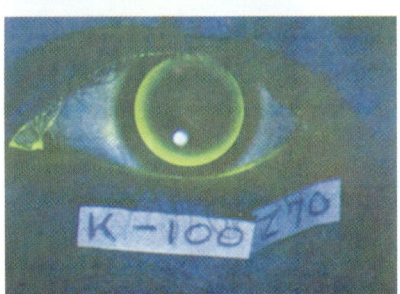

**Fig. 27.17.** Flat fit. Central grey zone manifesting lens contact with corneal surface.

A combination of the two methods is generally employed.

The lenses are examined under fluorescein with a slit biomicroscope or an ultraviolet lamp after initial lacrimation has subsided. If the lens is found too flat or too steep it must be exchanged with another one from the trial set with a steeper or flatter radius as the case may be.

A small drop of 1% solution of fluorescein is applied to the upper limbus. Strips of fluorescein are now available which have made application of fluorescein quite simple. The lamps or filter used in the slit-lamp which permit shorter wavelengths of light at the blue end of visual spectrum cause fluorescence of fluorescein. The lacrimal fluid behind the lens and in front of the cornea is observed. This essentially is the examination of the tear film under magnification (Fig. 27.14). The fit can be judged by the fluorescein pattern (Figs. 27.15, 27.16 and 27.17). Fig. 27.15 shows the optimum fit, Fig. 27.16 shows the flat fit, and Fig. 27.17 shows the steep fit.

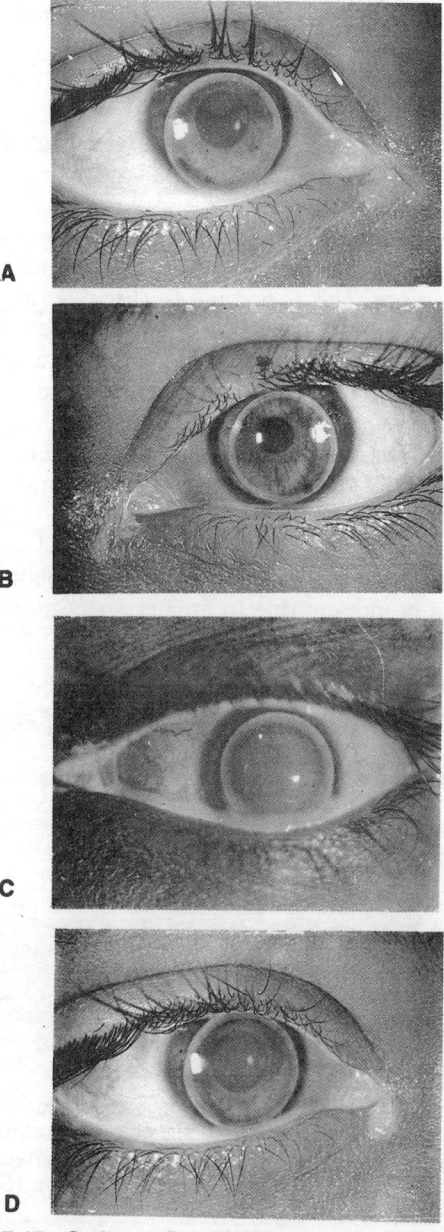

A

B

C

D

**Fig. 27.15.** Optimum fit and alignment. **A.** Alignment fit with adequate clearance at periphery. **B.** Alignment fit with adequate peripheral clearance. **C.** Optimum fit—evenly distributed fluorescein all over in central zone and adequate edge fit. **D.** Optimum fit. (*See also* Plate 3)

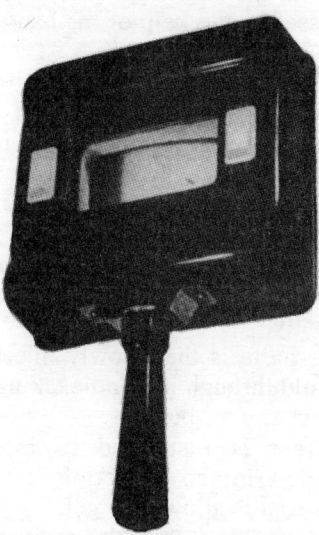

**Fig. 27.14.** Ultraviolet lamp.

Slit-lamp or biomicroscope should be used for examining the contact lens and its fit. The apparatus can be used for examination under white light and for fluorescein pattern under UV light by manipulating the required filter in the pathway of light.

In all fittings some degree of the mobility of a corneal lens should be expected. With temporal movement of the eye the lens moves towards the nasal limbus; with upward movement the lens moves downwards; and with downward movement of the eye the lens moves upwards. In all cases, however, the movement should be a glide without disturbance of centration otherwise visual confusion will result.

The fitting is described as tight when the lens moves little on blinking. The lens fitting is loose when the movements of the lens are excessive. The lens may even fall down. The relationship generally favoured is that of minimal apical clearance. This is optimal fit (Fig. 27.15). In this case a uniform tear film intervenes between the cornea and the lens at their optical zones. The film becomes darker in the intermediate zone because it is in this zone that more support is given to the lens by the cornea and at the periphery green colour again becomes more intense. In steep fitting (Fig. 27.16) a thick pool of fluorescein can be seen in the central area confined to about 2-4 mm. A small air bubble may also be present due to greater space in between the lens and the cornea.

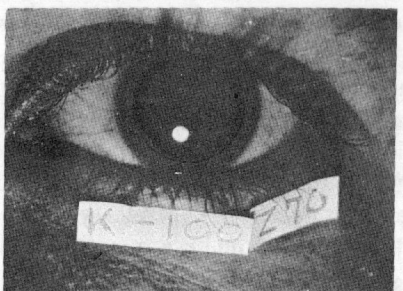

**Fig. 27.17.** Flat fit. Central grey zone manifesting lens contact with corneal surface. (*See also* Plate 3)

- The patient lies in a supine position.
- The conjunctival sac is anaesthetised by topical use of anaesthetic with adrenaline.
- The patient is instructed to fix his gaze so that the concerned eye is in neutral (lower limbus in line with the lower lid margin) or desired position of gaze. It is better to block the eye to be moulded and its position adjusted by fixing the gaze with uncovered eye. In case the uncovered eye has a poor vision, the same is aided by patient's own glasses or the help of his hand or a strong source of light.
- Moldite powder is made into a uniform paste with requisite amount of distilled water, by spatulation for two minutes in a plaster bowl.
- The paste is poured into a 10 ml syringe with a spatula.
- The moulding shell is placed on the eyeball under the lids, with the horizontal line nasally.
- The paste is then slowly injected into the mould through its handle taking care not to inject any air bubbles.
- Patient is instructed to look into the predetermined direction of gaze. The material is allowed to gel.
- The moulding shell along with the mould is gently removed.
- The negative mould thus prepared is then allowed to harden.
- Positive mould is made by filling the hollow of the negative mould with paste made out of the hard dental stone powder.
- It is the positive mould from which methyl methacrylate sheet takes shape of contact lens.

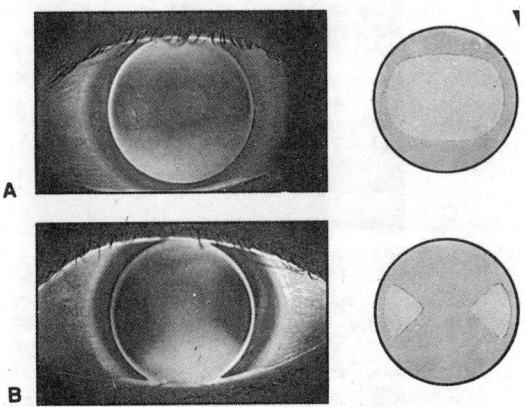

**Fig. 27.16.** Steeper fit. **A.** Fit in highly toric cornea. Parallel to 'K' fitting pattern shows equal distribution in horizontal meridian. **B.** Fit in highly toric cornea. BCOD steeper than K (astigmatism with the rule). (*See also* Plate 3)

In flat fitting lens (Fig. 27.17) a greyish reflex is seen in the centre indicating central touch while fluorescein extends over a wide area at the periphery.

### Fitting of scleral contact lenses

Moulds are made for the individual eye. The technique of making negative and positive moulds is as follows :

The scleral contact lenses could be flush fitting or afocal (without any power). When power is to be given, same principles as for corneal lenses, are applicable.

### Post-wear check-up

Visual acuity, orthoptic check-up and slit-lamp examination with and without contact lens should always be done. Frequency and quality of blink is noticed best under the slit-lamp. Deposits of extraneous matter, mucus or meibomian secretions over the lens, if any, are noted. Drying of the anterior surface of the lens indicates a bad quality or inadequate blinking.

Position of the lens, whether it is central, eccentric or dislodged is noted. Normally lens rests over the apex of the cornea and rides the steeper meridian. Also note how much of the lens is covered by the lids. Movement of the lens is very important for tear circulation beneath the lens. A lens may move too much or too little or may remain stationary. Normally with a blink, it should move up and then gradually slide down over the cornea. Any abnormality in the edge and anterior surface, for example chipping of the edge or scratches over the anterior surface, are noted.

Slit-lamp examination with fluorescein is done to study the lens-cornea relationship and any staining areas over the cornea or limbus. Fluorescein is then observed with ultraviolet light; areas of touch or pooling are indicated by blue and green areas respectively. Staining of the uncovered areas, if any, is also brought out.

Slit-lamp examination after removal of the lens is done to find out any areas of oedema, stippling or abrasion over the cornea.

Check-up of the lens is done with regard to the following points :

- Base curve is noted by radiuscope Figs. 27.18 and 27.19 and keratometer. The latter method is less accurate and measures only the central portion.

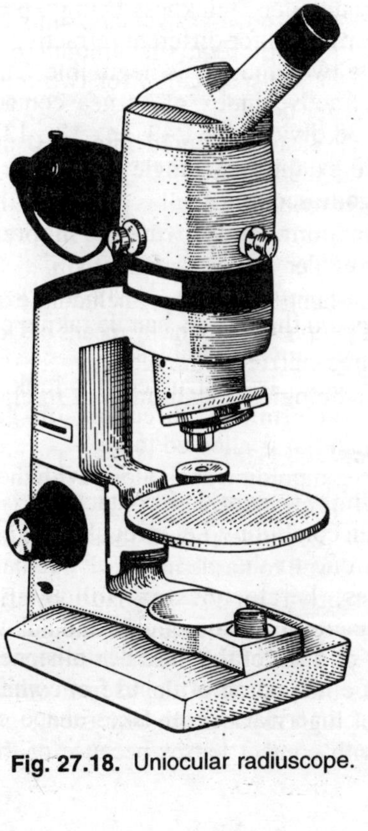

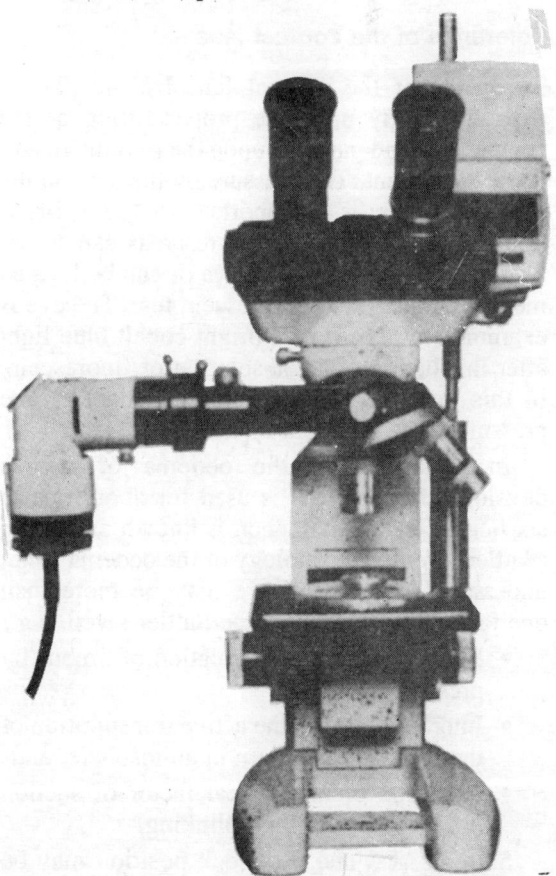

**Fig. 27.18.** Uniocular radiuscope.

**Fig. 27.19.** Binocular radiuscope for measuring back and front curvature of the contact lens.

- Power is seen by focimeter or lensometer. It is back vertex power which is measured. This is done by examining the lens with convexity facing the telescope.
- Diameter is measured by vernier calliper, V-slot gauge or slipscale, a measuring lens magnifier or shadowgraph.
- Thickness is recorded in one-tenth of a millimetre by dial thickness gauge.
- Quality of the anterior surface is seen by radiuscope. The curve of the anterior surface should be uniform in the centre as well as periphery.
- Quality of the edges is noted by uniocular magnifying loupe.
- The radius of curvature of secondary and peripheral curves is measured by radiuscope.

## Tolerance of the contact lens

Tolerance of the contact lens by the patient depends mostly upon the proper fitting of the contact lens and partially upon the psychic make-up of the patient. The pressure by the lens on the cornea or sclera is an important source of irritation to the eye. These pressure areas can sometimes be seen by the naked eye or can be located more accurately with fluorescein test. The eye is examined by means of a bright cobalt blue light after instillation of a 2% solution of fluorescein. In this light the eye fluoresces brilliantly. The pressure areas stand out blanched.

In certain cases the oedema of cornea develops after the lens is used for about one to six hours. The phenomenon is known as veiling (Sattler's veil). The etiology of the oedema is not understood properly. There may be more than one factor responsible for the Sattler's veil, e.g.,

- Embarrassment of circulation of limbus by pressure;
- Interference with the active transpiration of the corneal epithelium in atmosphere; and
- Abolition of mechanical factor of suction produced by constant blinking.

Staining at 3 and 9 o'clock position may be traumatic in origin or it may be related to drying of cornea when the lens prevents contact between the lids and the globe. This is a serious complication and results from :

- Oedema
- Anomalous conditions
- Greasy and dirty lenses
- Low riding corneal lenses

## Uses and indications of contact lenses

These are ever increasing. For convenience they can be classified into :

### 1. Diagnostic

- To ascertain maximum visual acuity.
- To eliminate aniseikonia for orthoptic check-up.
- To find out whether an eye with an irregular astigmatism is amblyopic.
- Corneal biomicroscopy—Contact lens acts like a cover slip for more effective examination of edges and base of corneal ulcer and allied conditions.
- To determine corneal thickness the usual ratio being Cornea : Contact lens = 4.3 (the contact lens thickness being 0.6 mm). The correction for different refractive indices of the two amounts is negligible. The ratio of refractive index of cornea contact lens is 1.38 divided by 1.49, i.e., 12 : 13.
- To examine the angle of anterior chamber (gonioscopy).
- Examination of fundus in presence of irregular corneal astigmatism.
- Slit-lamp funduscopy including examination of periphery of retina by means of Goldmann's three-mirror contact lens.
- Radiological localisation of foreign bodies.

### 2. Optical

Visual improvement with contact lens is dramatic in certain conditions, i.e., irregular and high astigmatism due to the presence of nebular corneal opacities; keratoconus or following corneal transplantation; anisometropia and aniseikonia as a result of unilateral aphakia or otherwise is also a specific indication of the use of contact lenses. Cases of high myopia are benefited significantly more with contact lenses because of the optical advantage it possesses over spectacle glasses especially of a high number due to the approximation of the size of the image to near normal.

Microcorneal contact lenses are the choice in the above mentioned conditions except in cases of irregular corneal surface and advanced keratoconus. In these conditions only lenses with scleral haptic will fit to give some visual improvement.

Cases of keratoconus with extreme thinning at the apex and those in which acute hydrops has occurred with or without resulting corneal opacity are unsuitable cases for any type of contact lens.

Contact lenses following keratoplasty should be prescribed six to twelve months after the operation. Corneal lenses are preferred. In case there is raising of suture line due to excessive scarring, a contact lens smaller than the graft is fitted to avoid stagnation of tear circulation and collection of air bubble underneath the lens. Scleral lenses are indicated when there is irregular or high degree of astigmatism.

### 3. Protective

Next to optical reasons, contact lenses are used for protective purposes in a wide variety of conjunctival and corneal conditions. The most important being :

- Chemical, especially, alkali burns.
- Non-healing corneal ulcers especially with diminished corneal sensitivity, for instance, recurrent herpetic keratitis, disciform keratitis, neuroparalytic keratitis. mustard gas keratitis, acne rosacea, ulcer with deep corneal crater, recurrent erosion, exposure keratitis and corneal grafts.
- To splint operated symblepharon.
- Cases of ocular pemphigus, xerophthalmia.
- Cases of aniridia, coloboma and albinism to avoid glare.
- For protection from steam, spray and mist in professional people.

### 4. Therapeutic

Use of contact lenses to provide a dose of radiation in cases of melanosis of conjunctiva or following enucleation.

### 5. Cosmetic

The chief function of cosmetic contact lenses is to hide a manifest anterior ocular deformity or the corneal blemishes. Sometimes these are also used to present a different colour of the iris at different occasions. Sometimes along with a good cosmetic effect these lenses also improve the visual function. In view of these varying demands from cosmetic contact lenses, it is obvious that the lens has to be custom made to suit a particular requirement.

The cosmetic lenses can be scleral commonly known as haptic (cosmetic lens or contact shell) or hard corneal contact lenses (which can be tinted, clear pupil, black pupil) or soft contact lenses (tinted iris lens, black pupil iris lens).

In scleral cosmetic contact lenses iris pattern is painted on the corneal zone leaving the pupillary zone clear on which even optical correction can be ground. In what is known as cosmetic shell there is no need to leave a clear pupillary zone which is done for a scleral cosmetic contact lens.

The corneal cosmetic contact lenses also are essentially modifications of optical corneal contact lenses. The tinted lenses are made of tinted PMMA (polymethyl methylacrylate) and can be used to mask various occasions. When they are used for other cosmetic reasons it should be remembered that such material is available in a variety of colours to produce the effect of a different colour iris. In such cases a clear optical zone with necessary dioptric power provided on it like the hard corneal tinted lenses, soft or flexible tinted lenses are also available with clear optical zone.

When the lenses are used purely as prosthesis and where the pupillary zone is blemish free, it may be advisable to leave the pupillary zone optically clear with the dioptric correction if some visual improvement can be obtained. In uniocular cases the iris zone is coloured and painted to match the iris colour and pattern of the fellow eye or else contact lenses can be provided for both eyes to change the colour of the iris in both eyes which serves as excellent prosthesis.

When the pupillary zone itself is sharing blemish and visual improvement is not possible, the pupillary zone need not be optically clear but may be painted black. This can be used also for occlusion in cases of squints. This treatment can be provided to both the soft and hard contact lenses depending upon the initial choice of the material made on tolerance factor.

It is needless to say that the utility and scope of contact lenses is increasing day by day. Many more clients are being helped and many modifications are being made to fulfil the requirements in an individual case.

### Soft contact lenses

In 1950, Wichterle of Czechoslovakia invented gel contact lenses. The lens could be folded from edge to edge without any damage to its physical properties.

Chemically it is hydroxyethylmethacrylate which is cross-linked with ethyldimethylacrylate (EDMA) or with polyvinylpyrrolidone (PVP).

The former is the usual one marketed with water content of about 38% and is termed the daily wear lens. HEMA PVP lenses sold as softcon has a water content of 55%. PVP/MA lenses (polyvinylpyrrolidone-co-methylmethacry-late- c-allyemethacrylate-c-ethylene demethacry-late) are available as Permalens 68% water, Sauflon-70 with 70% water, Sauflon-80 with 80% water, and Sauflon-85 with 85% water. The materials are summarised in Table 27.3.

**Table 27.3. Some soft lens materials and their water content**

| Material | Water content | Purpose |
|----------|---------------|---------|
| 1. HEMA or EDMA | 38% | Daily wear |
| 2. HEMA/PVP (Softcon) | 55% | Prolonged wear |
| 3. PVP/MA | 68% | Permalens |
| (a) Sauflon-70 | 70% | Extended wear or daily wear |
| (b) Sauflon-80 | 80% | Extended wear |
| (c) Sauflon-85 | 85% | Extended wear |

The lenses are prepared in three basic ways :

1. **Spin casting** : Spin cast lenses are formed in a revolving mould that spins liquid plastics at a very high speed. The curvature of the outer, anterior surface of the lens is predetermined by the shape of the mould. The inner posterior surface is dependent upon :

- Shape of the mould;
- Amount of liquid plastic that is injected into the spinning mould;
- Physical properties of the liquid; and
- Rate of spin. The curvature of the lenses will steepen as minus power increases or plus power decreases.

The fitting of these lenses is unpredictable and is not dependent upon the K reading of the patient.

2. **Lathe cutting** : In lathe cut soft lenses, the lens is in a dehydrated state and is like hard contact lens. It is cut on a lathe to exact specifications similar to those of rigid contact lens. It implies that buttons of hydrophilic plastic are machined while in the hard state, using precision lathes. Initially, the posterior surface is ground with a diamond tool then the anterior surface is polished and edged. The power is ground on the anterior surface. The base curve is a true sphere. In this method peripheral curves, blends and intermediate curves can be cut for better lens design. The lens fit does not vary with power changes as against spin cast lenses. At the end of water-free grinding, cutting and polishing the lens is placed in a water bath for several hours where it undergoes swelling and expands to its final state.

Fitting differences are due to differences in edge thickness that occur as the power increases or decreases, and not to the differences in base curve.

The advantages of lathe cut lenses are :

- Wider choice of parameters for better fit.
- Stable visual acuity that does not fluctuate.
- Can mask astigmatism by bordering of lens of special type.
- Toric lenses as per requirement of the patient can be made for correcting astigmatism.
- Better corneal centering possible with proper selection of lenses.

3. **Cast moulding** : In this process casts of anterior, i.e., optical and base curves, i.e., posterior are assembled. Liquid plastic is dropped in the mould and after a cutting process, the mould is opened. The cross linkable lens monomers are directly converted into a finished

surface from the mould. The edges are polished and the lens is hydrated as in lathe cut process.

**Fitting of lens :** The following factors need to be taken into account while fitting soft lenses.

*Base curve :* It is the central posterior curve of a contact lens. In case of spin cast lenses it is called the posterior apical radius.

If contact lenses are conceptualized as a part of a sphere, the base curve is its radius (i.e., from the centre of the sphere to its periphery—Fig. 27.20). The longer the radius, the flatter the lens; the shorter the radius, the steeper the lens.

*Diameter :* It is the distance expressed as chord diameter. This indicates that though the base curve of lenses aa', bb' and cc' are the same yet their diameters differ (Fig. 27.20).

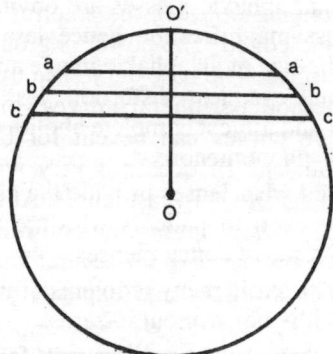

**Fig. 27.20.**

## Determine the lens power

The spectacle correction is written in minus cylinder form. Half the cylindrical power is added algebraically to the spherical power. This power is then chosen.

**Examples :**

   (a) –4.00 D sph./–1.00 D cyl. at 75° axis, the power of soft lens would be

         –4.00 D sph.
 +    –0.50 D sph.

         –4.50 D sph. power of soft lens

   (b) +4.00 D sph./–1.00 D cyl. 45°

         +4.00
 +    –0.50

         +3.50 power of soft lens

## Good fitting

A well-fitted lens should provide at least limbus to limbus coverage in the patient's eye better it is to have a lens extending about 1 mm beyond the limbus in all directions.

The lens may be too tight, i.e., the base curve is less than desirable and needs to be increased (steep lens is made more flat fitting) or the lens may be too loose, i.e., the base curve is more than desirable and needs to be lessened (flat lens is made more steeper). The lens should neither be too tight or steep nor should it be loose or flat.

## Movement

The lenses must move on the eye to oxygenate the cornea and flush the debris out from under the lens. An acceptable movement is not more than 1 mm and not less than 0.5 mm from the limbus in all directions.

The lens may be tight or loose.

*A correct base curve will show*

- Comfort,
- Movement of about 1 mm,
- Stable vision,
- Normal crisp retinoscopic reflex on over-refraction, and
- Undistorted mires on keratometry.

*A tight lens (steep lens) will exhibit*

- Movement of less than 0.5 mm or even if apparent movement is correct a slit-lamp examination will show drag of the limbus conjunctiva.
- Fluctuating vision that momentarily clears on blinking.
- Initially comfortable but becomes progressively uncomfortable with longer time of wear.
- Circumcorneal injection.
- Edge indentation of limbus or sclera.
- Keratometric mires clear on blinking.
- Retinoscopic reflex is fuzzy.

To rectify this defect increase the base curve by 0.2 to 0.3 mm or decrease the diameter by about 0.5 mm.

*A loose lens (flat lens) shows*

- Poor centering
- Movements of more than 1 mm generally

but movements of more than 1.5 mm are surely indicative

- Variable vision which blurs on blinking
- Patient is more and more conscious of lens and experiences discomfort
- Edge stands off
- Ejection of lens
- Air bubble inside the lens
- Blurring of keratometric mires particularly after blinking
- Blinking produces blurring of retinoscopic reflex

Replace loose lens by increasing the diameter by about 0.5 mm to 1 mm or decreasing the base curve by 0.2 to 0.3 mm or prescribing extra thin lenses particularly in those with high refractive errors.

### Advantages of soft lenses

The hydrogel lens has the advantage of
- Comfortable wear,
- Lack of ejection or displacement,
- Foreign bodies not being able to go under the lens,
- Easy adaptation,
- Minimum blur,
- Less glare and photophobia, and
- Regularity in wear is not essential.

### Disadvantages of soft lenses

The soft lenses have the following disadvantages :
- Visual acuity is not stable
- Lens is prone to damage by deposits, absorptions, splitting and tearing
- Presents problems of cleaning and sterilization. It is a cumbersome process and is likely to be skipped by the wearer
- It is difficult to verify the dioptric value of the lens
- Lens fit is difficult to verify and
- May not solve problems of high astigmatism.

### Extended wear contact lenses

Daily or even twice a day wearing and taking out of contact lenses is quite irritating to the patients particularly those of old age group. Even young individuals find it quite cumbersome. An attempt has, therefore, been made to search for materials and designs which can permit a much longer wear and even permit permanent wear. The chief considerations are the water content and oxygen permeability. Three materials are now commercially exploited. Hydro-curve (water content 79%, oxygen permeability 14%), Sauflon (water content 80%, oxygen permeability 47%), and Permalens (water content 71%, oxygen permeability 33%). One can choose according to the tolerance and requirement of the patient.

The most urgent need of these lenses has been felt in aphakics though they are also being used by a fairly large number of myopes.

In aphakics the lens provides a competitive alternative to much practised intraocular lens implantation which provides an ideal correction of the aphakic eye.

The optical advantages of contact lenses over conventional aphakic glasses are obvious which include less magnification hence less disparity between the size of an aphakic image and the size of a normal eye, less distortion, less marginal aberration and almost complete abolition of 'jack in the box' phenomenon.

Extended wear lenses provide the use of contact lenses even in patients who are unable to insert and remove contact lenses.

It tends to avoid many problems of intraocular lenses but it is not without hazards.

All aphakics are not good patients for extended wear lenses. The lenses are more suitable for cases with arthritis, Parkinson's disease, elderly monocular aphakics who have been considered as potential subjects for secondary lens implantation, a child with monocular aphakia as an alternative to secondary intraocular lens implantation. It is perhaps worth a trial in cases where bilateral cataract extraction has been done and only in one eye an intraocular lens has been implanted.

The lenses are contraindicated in aphakics with anterior segment infection, blepharitis, dry eyes, patient with increased risk of corneal infection, patient with poor personal hygiene, uncooperative patients who are unable or unwilling to subject themselves to regular follow-ups.

Extended wear contact lenses are being increasingly prescribed for myopic patients and for children with squints needing optical correction. The advantages are many though precautions are needed. For the time being they may be considered only for such patients who are successful daily wear patients.

The literature on these lenses is being added everyday and those interested in prescribing these types of lenses are referred to a more comprehensive treatise on the subject.

### Day to day management by the wearer

The soft lenses are subject to coating, deposit build up, discoloration and infection. The soft lenses being porous and hydrophilic, they provide excellent medium for growth of bacteria, fungus and viruses.

The soft lenses should be cleaned daily by solutions containing non-ionic surfactant chemicals, oxidants or fat solvents. Household detergents are not recommended because they often leave a film on the lens. They should also be disinfected regularly either by chemical enzymic tablets or by boiling.

Most contact lens solutions contain preservatives to avoid contamination during storage.

Thimerosal, a mercury compound, was at one time used as the preservative. It was found to be responsible for many cases of red eyes and contact lens intolerance. It is being phased out.

Other preservatives used are :

*Benzalkonium chloride :* Only low concentrations should be used as otherwise irreparable corneal damage may occur. It should be in the neighbourhood of 0.004% but never more than 0.1%. It can be used along with other preservatives for its additive sterilizing capacity.

*Chlorbutanol :* It is usually used in 0.5% but it is better avoided as it causes damage to corneal epithelium. It also binds with silicone and causes damage to silicone lenses.

*Chlorhexidine gluconate :* It is a safer preservative with soft lens solutions. It does not cause ocular irritation in clinical dosage. Prolonged use may however cause toxic reactions.

*Phenyl mercuric nitrate :* It is used in 0.002% strength but is useless since it does not have good antimicrobial action.

*Sorbates :* As sorbic acid or potassium sorbate and are less toxic. Their use, however, does not give adequate protection because they are only bacteriostatic. They are used in 0.25% strength.

*Quaternary ammonium compounds (Polyquad) :* It is 99% reaction free. If mixed with sorbic acid, filming of the lens surface may occur.

*Dymed (polyaminopropyl biguamamide) :* It is not absorbed into matrix of soft lens. It has high antimicrobial action at low levels of concentration. It is compatible with all types of soft lenses and does not cause discoloration of lenses.

There are other preservatives that are being developed like trimethoprim a synthetic antibiotic.

#### The ideal preservative

- Should not cause irritation or sensitivity.
- Be non-toxic to human tissue.
- Have a broad spectrum of antibiotic activity.
- Not penetrate into the matrix of the lens.
- Be compatible with thermal as well as cold disinfection.

#### Complications and management

Contact lenses, particularly the soft lenses, may cause

*Microbial keratitis :* Particularly so if it is left unprotected overnight; commonest is Acanthamoeba keratitis (Fig. 27.21). Marginal pathology (Fig. 27.22) and staphylococcal infection (Fig. 27.23) may also be seen.

*Allergic or toxic reactions* may also be seen as thiomersal keratitis (Figs. 27.24 and 27.25) and giant papillary conjunctivitis (Figs. 27.26 and 27.27)

*Microbial keratitis :* This is particularly seen in

- extended lens wear
- permalenses
- neglectful wearing overnight by daily soft lens wearers
- unclean lenses
- unclean habits of lens wearers

The commonest forms are due to *Staphylococcus* and *Acanthomoeba.*

Acanthomoeba keratitis is fortunately uncommon but can be a devastating infection if

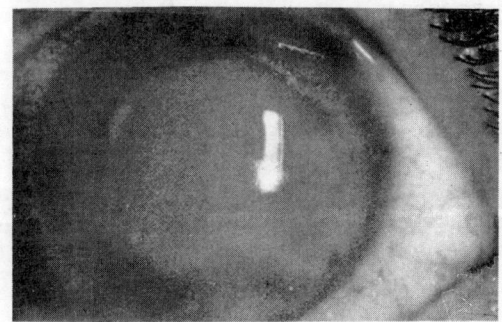

**Fig. 27.21.** Acanthamoeba keratitis. (*See also* Plate 2)

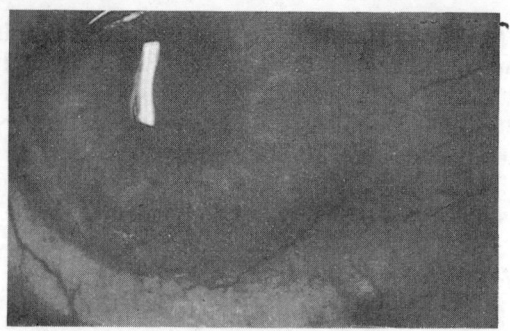

**Fig. 27.22.** Marginal corneal involvement. (*See also* Plate 2)

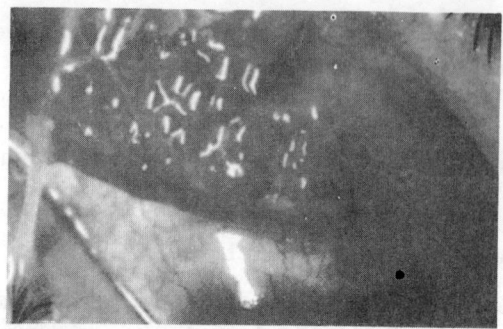

**Fig. 27.25.** An advanced case of giant papillary conjunctivitis. (*See also* Plate 2)

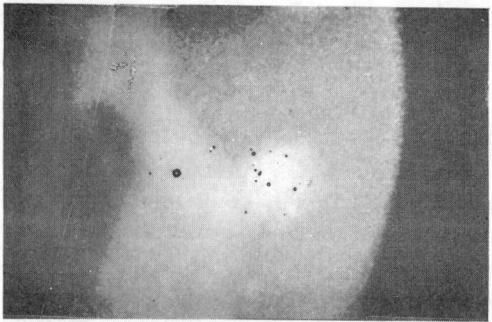

**Fig. 27.23.** Staphylococcal corneal infiltration in a soft lens wearer. (*See also* Plate 2)

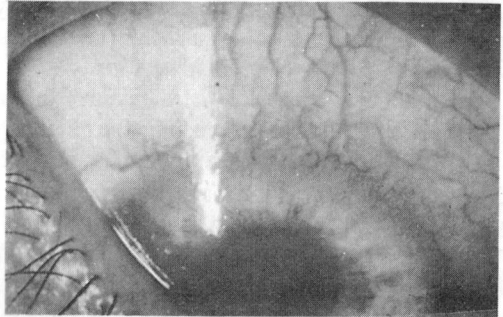

**Fig. 27.26.** Early thiomersal toxicity. (*See also* Plate 2)

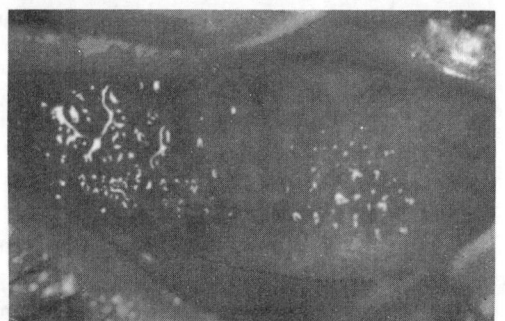

**Fig. 27.24.** Early giant papillary conjunctivitis. (*See also* Plate 2)

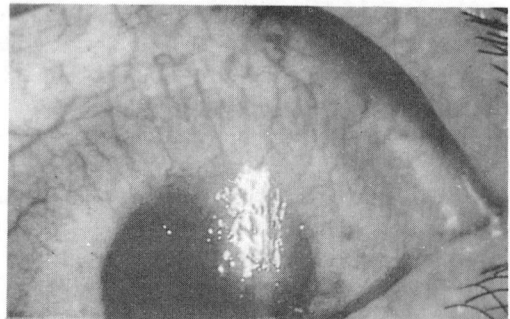

**Fig. 27.27.** Established thiomersal keratopathy. (*See also* Plate 2)

there is no awareness of its possibility in such wearers and early diagnosis is not made.

It is usually unilateral with the formation of a ring infiltrate; it is indolent and the epithelium is intact initially but has a mottled, dendritiform appearance which later breaks down. Ocular pain is severe and is disproportionate to the epithelial lesion. The pain is severe, perhaps due to deep linear stromal infiltrates localized along the corneal nerves. The treatment of choice is propamidine isothionate (Borolene).

The other common lesion is marginal corneal pathology (Fig. 27.2) and staphylococcal infection (Fig. 27.3).

**PLATE IV**

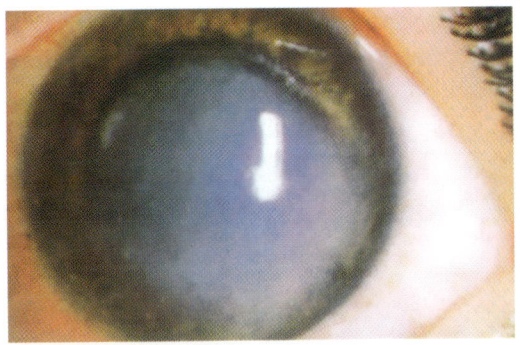

**Fig. 27.21.** Acanthamoeba keratitis.

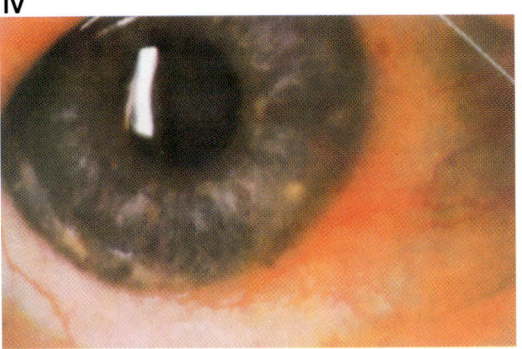

**Fig. 27.22.** Marginal corneal involvement.

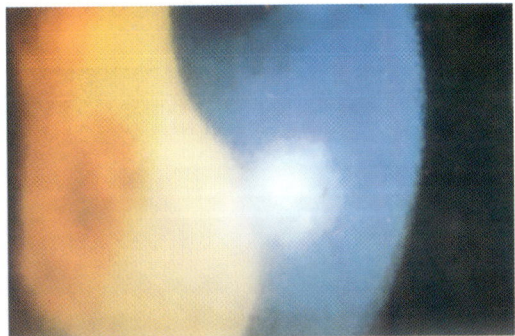

**Fig. 27.23.** Staphylococcal corneal infiltration in a soft lens wearer.

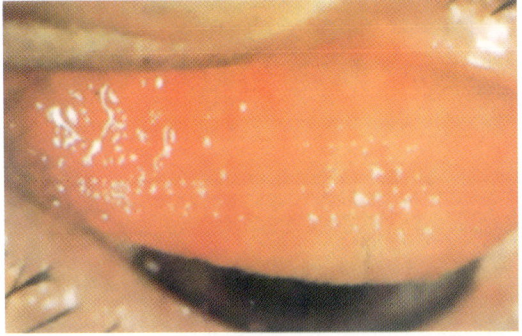

**Fig. 27.24.** Early giant papillary conjunctivitis.

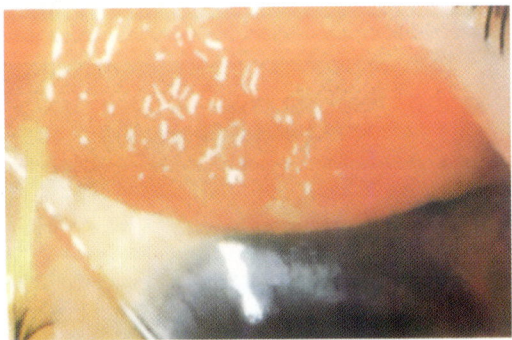

**Fig. 27.25.** An advanced case of giant papillary conjunctivitis.

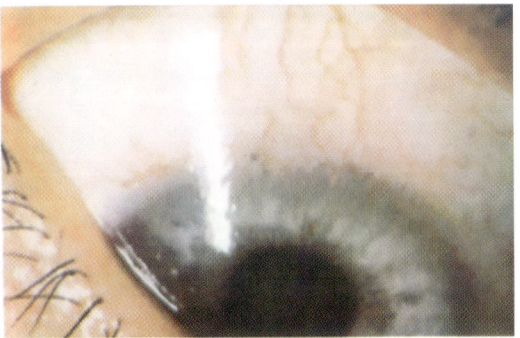

**Fig. 27.26.** Early thiomersal toxicity.

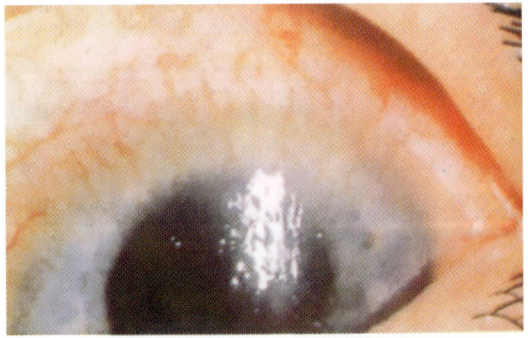

**Fig. 27.27.** Established thiomersal keratopathy.

# CHAPTER 28

# Low Vision Aids

## Basic definitions

Economic blindness is defined in visual performance terms

- as a distance visual acuity of 6/60 or less in the better eye with best ophthalmic correction or
- as a defect in the visual field so that the widest diameter of vision subtends an angle no greater than 20° in the better eye or
- as a distance visual acuity of 6/60 or less in one eye with the best optical correction and a defect in the visual field so that the widest diameter of vision subtends an angle no greater than 20° in the other eye.

Partially sighted child for educational purposes is the one who has a distance visual acuity between 6/24 to 6/60 in the better eye with best correction and who can use vision as his primary channel of learning.

The following are the limitations of these definitions :

- They do not consider reading or near vision.
- They do not consider scotomas.
- They do not judge visual performances in terms of usefulness.

## Low vision

Essentially it is the vision which interferes with the daily performance of the individual and aims at exploitation of the residual vision for the benefit of the individual to make him more useful to the society.

In the surveys held in India about 7% of the population is considered to be visually handicapped.

## Travel vision

This functional classification differentiates functionally sighted from functionally blind on the basis of their ability to read and write, recognise familiar objects and travel safely in unfamiliar environment.

The identification of patient for low vision services should be on visual efficiency based on performance and the felt needs of the patient, as such an approach is likely to give better results.

A case of functionally blind requires a careful assessment.

## Case history

- Duration of ocular pathology, diagnosis and prognosis.
- Present vision.
- Age and education status.
- Ability to move independently.
- Low vision aids including contact lenses or spectacles used till now.
- Does he prefer more light or less light?
- Is the vision good for near or distance or bad for both?
- What does he want to do?
- Psychological build up (to determine readiness for aid acceptance).

Answers to these questions give a fairly accurate idea about diagnosis, prognosis, and the psychological build up of the patient.

An idea about the extent of usefulness of residual vision can be made by noting the movements of the patient as he enters the clinic. A fairly accurate idea about his psychological set up can be had during the interrogation.

In the recently handicapped, hope to regain vision is the biggest hurdle in accepting any aid and may require psychologist's help to convince the patient. Exact requirements of the patient in terms of near, intermediate, or distance vision are asked.

Special observation by the patient as to better vision in dim light than bright indicates a central obstacle due to any cause. The patient may feel better with bright light. He may be able to see street signs, bus numbers, headlines of ordinary print newspaper. He may give history of seeing better at an angle (sensory obstacle). He reads with grandma's spectacles (high plus glass). It is better to know whether he can move independently indoors or outdoors. These specific observations or complaints give fairly accurate idea about the loss of vision and the extent of damage in a disease process.

**Duration :** A long-standing case may have deep-rooted amblyopia ex anopsia and, therefore, may take a long time to recognise words and read fluently.

Similarly, children who are not familiar with words present difficulty in the beginning.

Type of pathology can be assessed by a thorough clinical examination. Conditions which are favourable for low vision correction are chorioretinal and macular degenerations, optic atrophy, cataract, albinism, myopia, corneal irregularities. Unfavourable cases are diabetic and hypertensive retinopathy, optic atrophy due to intracranial lesions, glaucoma and retinitis pigmentosa.

As the expectancy of life is increasing patients in older age groups are seeking assistance due to macular pathology which is either myopic in origin or is an age-related disorder. Patients with retinitis pigmentosa, glaucoma, diabetic retinopathy, optic atrophy and even strabismus amblyopics are also roaming about to seek visual aid.

The patient's response to the same extent of improvement may differ significantly. Children and persons who have lost their sight for many years may make very little progress at the onset. A visual training is essential to make them familiar with the various words.

A practitioner may be able to anticipate the disease by the age of the patient. Common diseases encountered in children are congenital cataract, colobomas, nystagmus, myopia and microphthalmos.

In adult and adolescent age diabetes, macular degeneration, glaucoma, and trauma are common causes of diminished vision.

In old age cataract, senile macular degeneration, glaucoma, diabetes and retinopathies are common causes of visual handicap. A sense of resignation is often noted and aids are accepted only with great persuasion. Specific problems such as tremors on close reading distance must be dealt with accordingly.

After a good assessment of the case a decision has to be made on :

- Whether a low vision aid can be prescribed?
- What type of low vision aid will be most suitable?

## Guidelines for prescribing LVAs

In prescribing LVAs one should keep the following points in mind :

- The fundamental concept is to provide maximum possible visual acuity as well as mobility to the visually impaired.
- The person's visual acuity should be adequate with the aid given when the retinal image has been enlarged by the magnifier.
- As the magnification increases the visual field and working distance decrease.
- The aid needed may vary from person to person even though visual impairment may be caused by the same disease.
- The LVA provided should be simple, portable and flexible enough for use. Complicated and cumbersome aids are to be avoided as far as possible, unless it is strongly indicated.

Proper illumination of the object and a modified reading table may be helpful. Special adjustable lamps are available and may be used to advantage.

In prescribing low vision aid the basic principle is the exploitation of the residual vision to the best advantage of the patient with the best possible visual aid.

## Importance of lighting

Proper lighting is also important in low vision

management. With no eye disorder an old man may need twice the illumination than a younger person to perform the same job comfortably. Light requirement of a low vision person is much more. Light should be placed close to the reading material for better visibility.

## Low vision aid clinic

It is essential that each ophthalmic section in a hospital is provided with a low vision aid clinic. The following equipment will be necessary :

- A good trial frame
- Lensometer
- Snellen's or Bausch & Lomb's chart for distance, or Bailey-Lovie Logmar distance acuity and reading chart.
- Keeler's and Sloan's charts for near and distance
- Reading boards, chin rest, measuring rod, and a table lamp with rheostat
- A trial set which should have full aperture telescopes of 1.8, 2, 2.5 magnification with near caps and prism telescopes of 6, 8, 10 magnification for long and intermediate distances.

For near vision the trial case should have :

- Microscopic lenses 2 to 15.
- Stand magnifiers : Various types are used in assessment.
  - 1.8 × Visolett (thick plano-convex magnifiers)
  - 2 × of combined opticals 2 ×, 3 × and 5 ×, 7.5 × Igard type
  - 8 ×, 10 ×, 12 ×, and 15 × Keeler's illuminated magnifiers
  - Hand magnifiers
  - Pinhole
- Slits
- Filters
- Visors
- Typoscope

## Examination

The ophthalmologist may have to discard the conventional ideas about refractive results as in prescribing low vision aids subjective improve-

ment with no objective confirmation is the usual methodology employed.

### *Preliminary examination*

The low vision aids examination requires a longer time, more cooperation by the patient and more patience on the part of the examiner. Invariably more than one visit is required for full examination and proper prescription.

Basically, it follows a conventional pattern which includes :

- Recording of vision
- External and internal ocular examination
- Tonometry and slit-lamp examination
- Ophthalmometry, retinoscopy and ophthalmoscopy
- Field charting

Recording of vision of a visually handicapped is a special technique. Examination gives us the visual acuity magnification required and possible aids which can help the patient. It starts with recording of sight. Further improvement noted by verifying the power of sphere and cylinder and the axis of the latter. Visual acuity is recorded by a chart at 3 to $1\frac{1}{2}$ metre. Charts commonly used for distance are those of Bausch & Lomb, Sloan, Straub or Snellen or Bailey-Lovie Logmar distance acuity and reading chart (Fig. 28.1). Response is recorded for increased or decreased illumination both at the text and in the background. It is better to express the acuity in decimals. Acuity for near can be tested with Sloan's charts and Keeler's charts. Most popular are Sloan's charts. They are M cards, read at 40 cm and are constituted by the continuous test. Sizes vary from $M_1$ to $M_{20}$, and $M_1$ corresponds to news print. It directly gives the magnification required, i.e., if a patient reads $M_7$ that means he needs 7 times magnification to read. M charts give a better score than Keeler's charts. Recording of Sloan M chart at 40 cm can be converted into distance Snellen visual acuity at 20 feet. If a person can read $M_1$ at 40 cm then he would not require any addition of more than 2.50 D (Table 28.1).

*Keeler's charts :* These are a series of A charts starting from $A_1$ to $A_{20}$ and are made up of individual letters. $A_3$ represents an acuity of 80% of $A_2$ and 64% of $A_1$. The charts are read at 25

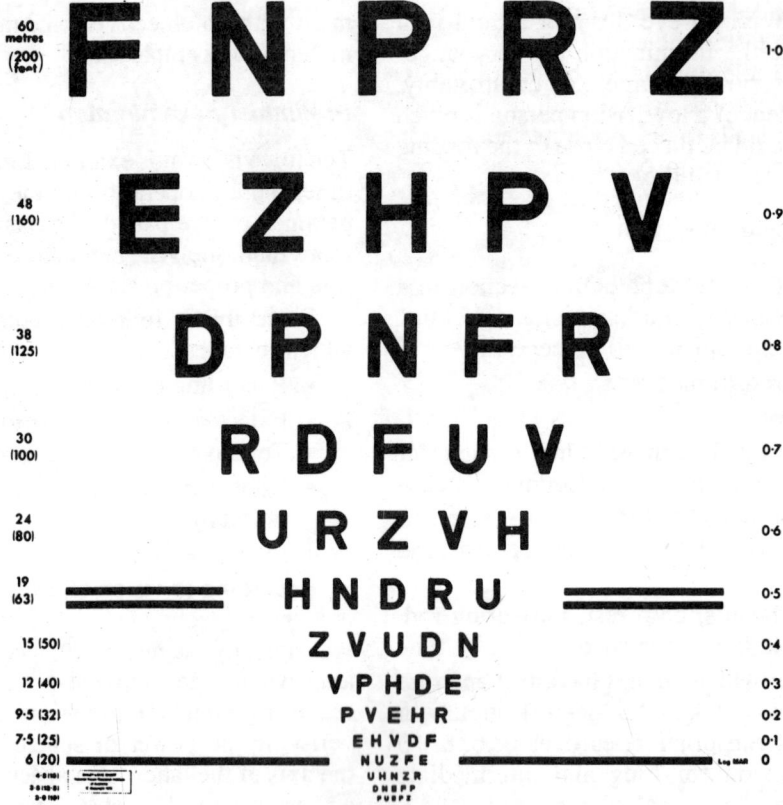

**Fig. 28.1.** Bailey-Lovie Logmar distance acuity and reading chart.

**Table 28.1. Sloan's system for determining visual acuity**

| Size of print in Sloan M units | Acuity required at 40 cm | Equivalent distance acuity | Dioptric power or reading addition required to read 1 M print (assuming emmetropia and zero accommodation) |
|---|---|---|---|
| 1.0 | 40/100 | 20/50 | +2.50 D |
| 1.5 | 40/150 | 20/75 | +3.75 D |
| 2.0 | 40/200 | 20/100 | +5.00 D |
| 2.5 | 40/250 | 20/125 | +6.25 D |
| 3.0 | 40/300 | 20/150 | +7.50 D |
| 4.0 | 40/400 | 20/200 | +10.00 D |
| 5.0 | 40/500 | 20/250 or 16/200 | +12.50 D |
| 7.0 | 40/700 | 20/350 or 11.5/200 | +15.00 D |
| 10.0 | 40/1000 | 20/500 or 8/200 | +25.00 D |
| 14.0 | 40/1400 | 20/700 or 5.8/200 | +30.00 D |
| 20.0 | 40/1000 | 20/1000 or 4/200 | +50.00 D |

cm and magnification required is noted from the chart. Despite the variation in distance and type of text the recording should be similar in all charts. However, discrepancies may creep in due to peripheral or centrally located opacities in the media or in cases of pendular nystagmus.

For distance, minimum magnification required for the task is noted by trying × 1.8, × 2, × 2.5 and × 3 telescopes. For higher magnifications prism telescopes are used. Since increase in magnification leads to reduction in fields, a compromise might have to be adopted. For near, a reading cap can be fitted over the telescope. Telescopes for near give almost double working distance compared to glasses of equivalent magnification.

For near, usually plus lenses are prescribed. Their power varies from +4 to +100 D though one rarely goes beyond +32 D. In lower and similar binocular additions as +6 D or +8 D binocularity should be tried by adding prisms.

Alternative magnifiers like the hand stand and the projection magnifiers may be tried. Lastly, a trial is given with filters, pinholes and typoscopes.

Illumination should vary from 60 to 110 watts. The bulb should be focused behind the patient. To cut down glare for higher magnification (× 12) a built-in illumination system should be provided.

Higher illumination is required by old persons and cases of fundus lesions, and a lower magnification for cases with opacities in the media. To add clarity and contrast a yellow filter is sometimes used.

**Definite examination :** After the preliminary investigation the patient is tried with aids. If possible the chosen aid is given on loan and the patient gives his decision on the next visit. Keeler and Sloan methods give a good starting point but clinically 50% of the patients may accept an entirely different prescription. Improvement for near vision or comparatively a better performance for near is noted especially in children because of utilisation of decreased working distance which magnifies the image. This distance is sustained by excessive accommodation at such short distances. It is an interesting observation that magnification required may be reduced with passage of time as performance of the patient improves.

### Prescription, visual re-education and rehabilitation

Lenses should be given another trial for the particular visual performance. Least magnifica-

tion and maximum working distance should be the aim. As far as possible conventional spectacles with a high addition should be prescribed. Both eyes should be corrected if the difference in magnification is insignificant, better eye should be used for acute vision and the worse eye for the general near vision. Should the patient experience diplopia or confusion, occlusion is tried. In the prescriptions avoid occlusion and try to prescribe a distance correction. Plane glass, or a balance glass are more suitable. If the job requires a greater working distance telescopic lenses should be given a trial.

In the old patient, keeping the print at a fixed focus may be a problem; a trial should be given with a stand magnifier in these cases.

Plastic lenses should be used in spectacles because they are light, safe and unbreakable. For children persuasion and understanding may be required to win them over. It may be necessary to defer prescribing of proper lens till the child is old enough to understand their value.

When the patient is one-eyed a telescope or high addition may be given without hesitation. Reversible glasses with different lenses are also useful in providing different magnification. If vision fails to improve with a small aperture telescope, a wider field telescope is tried. Balance telescopes are given on front of the other eye for better cosmetic appearance.

For momentary functions, prism monocular units are used with × 4 to × 8 magnification.

For emmetropes half frame spectacles can be tried and patient can view distant things by looking over these.

Should there be an unequal vision in both eyes, better eye is improved for distance and the worse for near.

In very high magnification, fixed focus housing, providing a constant distance of the object is used. It is most suitable for older patients with trembling hands.

Such fixed focus devices are usually not liked by patients who have incomplete scotomas because of the great to and fro movement of the print.

Visual training is necessary for successful acceptance of the prescription. This involves instruction on the correct way of handling, the working distance, the illumination and the limitations of each device. Before a definite prescription this training assures more success.

## Rehabilitation of individual

Individual reaction to the prescription may vary. Some feel easily fatigued to begin with, but later get adapted. New co-ordination reflexes develop. Older postures and methods of viewing may have to be left. If a patient is interested in a particular job he is trained for that job (as threading the needle and sewing is required for a tailor).

## Distance vision

Tremendous patience and perseverance is needed in the initial stages. Regarding a telescope, it should be explained that the best situation is to use it while sitting and observing stationary object. It is more difficult to watch a moving object and most difficult when both object and the subject are in motion.

Older patients may take a longer time and should be taught in more than one visit.

Wearing time should be gradually increased. Patient has to learn to move his head rather than his eyes.

## Near vision

Due to lack of practice, patient might have to acquire the habit of reading again. Correct posture, position of print and its angulation are all of importance. To avoid fatigue reading is gradually increased (10 to 15 minutes every day).

A patient should start by reading large prints for a short period but should eventually aim for small print at greater speed and for a longer duration.

Finally emphasis should be laid on the care of the lenses and placing them back in leather case when not in use.

## Optics of low vision aids

The specified magnifying powers of most of the commercially available aids are computed from a simple formula $M = D/4$ in which $D$ is the dioptric power. This conventional formula works on the arbitrary assumption that with the unaided eye the patient can sustain just enough accommodation to hold the matter at a distance of 25 cm. It assumes also that when magnification is used, the reading material is placed at the principal focal plane of the lens. Since neither of these assumptions is true in practice, this formula may not hold good. From optical considerations, magnification can be classified as "magnification in which the distance from the object to the lens can be varied."

This group includes spectacles, hand-held reading devices and head-borne loupes.

A general formula for these can be written as

$$M_{40} = \frac{D + A}{2.5} \qquad \ldots(1)$$

where $D$ is the dioptric strength of the lens, and $A$ is accommodation contributed by the patient's eye.

If the distance between eye and lens is appreciable then magnification is given by formula

$$M_{40} = \frac{D + A - hAD}{2.5}$$

where $h$ is the eye-lens distance in metres.

This formula clearly says that to get maximum benefit out of the focusable aid :

Eye should be kept close to the lens to reduce $h$.

Reading matter should be as close to the lens as patient's accommodation allows. There is one exception where any value of $h$ is immaterial. This situation is created when the print is at the focus of the lens; here as $A = 0$, so $hAD$ will also be zero.

Magnification in which the distance from the object to the lens is fixed.

These are stand magnifiers. Here the optical lens distance is predetermined, i.e., it is either just within the focus or much less than the focal length. Magnification can be found by the same formula, i.e.,

$$M_{40} = \frac{D + A - hAD}{2.5}$$

but more conveniently

$$M_{40} = \frac{1}{1 - Dh} \times \frac{A}{2.5} \qquad \ldots(2)$$

where $h$ is the object lens distance in metres. Here

again magnification depends upon increasing the value of $A$, i.e., decreasing the eye-lens distance.

If, for example, print is located at a fixed distance of 38.4 mm from 20 D lens, the light emerges with a divergence of 6 D, and the virtual image lies 167 mm behind the lens. The observer who can accommodate 6 D will bring his eye close to the lens. If he can accommodate only 3 D then he must place his eyes $333 - 167 = 166$ mm from the lens.

From the formula (1), magnification is :

$$\frac{20 + 6}{2.5} = 10.4$$

and

$$\frac{20 + 3 - 0.166\,(60)}{2.5} = 5.2$$

if he can sustain only 3 dioptres of accommodation.

In formula (2), if you substitute the same value :

$$M_{40} = \frac{1}{1 - Dh} \times \frac{A}{2.5}$$

$$= \frac{1}{1 - 20\,(0.384)} \times \frac{A}{2.5}$$

$$= \frac{4.3A}{2.5}$$

By substituting value of $A$ as 6 and 3 magnification is 10.4 and 5.2 as attained by formula (1). For projection, magnification formula is :

$$M_{40} = \frac{M_p A}{2.5}$$

$M_p$ is the ratio of the size of projected image to the size of the object.

### Classification of optical aids

The various types of optical aids have created much confusion in a field already complicated by advertising and publicity. The following classification of optical aids is presented for clarification and simplification :

### For distance

*Spectacles*

- Conventional spectacles (result of careful refraction).
- Telescopic spectacles (Fig. 28.2).
- Pinhole spectacles.

*Spectacles modification*

- Clip-on monocular telescopic spectacles, for example, Aloe monocular loupe.
- Behr loupe with +12 D sph. or 12 D segment cemented in upper outer part of lens used with 3 D sph. at distance of 10 inches.

*Contact lenses*

(Dealt in Chapter 27).

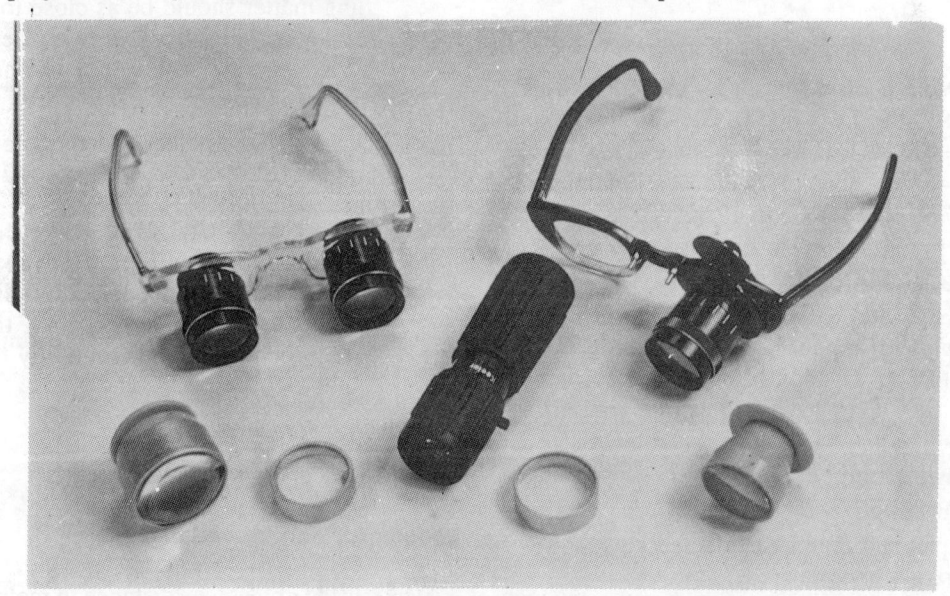

**Fig. 28.2.** Telescopic spectacles.

*Non-spectacle aids*

- Monocular and binocular field glasses, 3 ×, and prism telescopes, average power 6 ×.
- +4 D sph. held at 10 inches from uncorrected eye for aphakia, for dislocated lenses, and for high hyperopia.

## For near

*Spectacles*

A. Strong convex full size or half eye spectacles :

- Single vision lenses.
- Bifocal lenses.
  - Fused segments up to +7 D additions.
  - One-piece ground segment (Ultex) up to +20 D addition.
  - American optical magnification bifocal lenses +8 D and +12 D addition (distance correction can be ground on these additions).
  - High-power Ultex bifocal lenses : +5 D, +6 D, +7 D, +8 D, +10 D, +12 D, +16 D and +20 D additions (distance correction can be ground on these additions).
  - Cemented segments (epoxy resin).
  - High-add cataract bifocal lenses, Aolite plastic aspheric.

B. Best-form lenses : +16 D, +20 D and +24 D.

C. Specially designed lenses :

- Aspheric lenses
  - Volk conoid (glass) : +15 D, +40.00 D, +50.00 D, +60.00 D, +80.00 D and +100.00 D.
  - Aolite (plastic) magnification lenses : 7 ×, 8 ×, 10 × and 12 ×.
  - Hyperocular (plastic) : 4 ×, 6 × and 8 ×.
  - Keeler bifocal inserts.
  - High-add cataract bifocal lenses, Aolite plastic aspheric : 6.00 D, +12.00 D, +18.00 D additions (distant correction +8.00 D to +20.00 D can be ground).
- Doublet and triplet air-spaced lenses
  - Feinbloom.
  - Bechtold.
- Triplet and doublet cemented lenses.
  - Policoff (bifocal inserts).

- Doublet lenses : +28.00 D, +40.00 D and +64.00 D.

D. Telescopic spectacles with reading additions ranging from +2.00 D to +14.00 D.

- Single vision.
- Binocular vision (Keeler units; Feinbloom lenses).

*Spectacles modification*

- Binocular head-borne loupe, for example, Magnifocuser.
- Auxiliary convex lenses for sliding over one or both lenses (for example, Behr or Jeweller's monocular loupe which attaches to temple or frame).
- Monocular telescopic clip-on unit, for example, Aloe loupe.

*Non-spectacle magnifiers*

- Hand-held (greatest field of usefulness +12.00 D or less—Fig. 28.3.

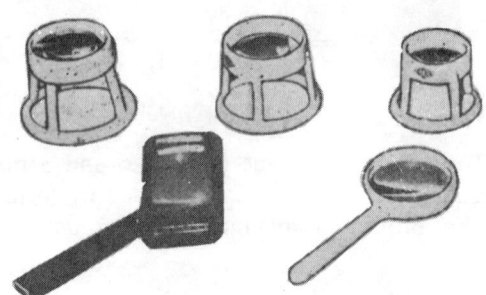

**Fig. 28.3.** Hand magnifier.

- Stand with fixed object-to-lens distance (for example, Keeler and Adisco) +29.00 D (Figs. 28.4 and 28.5).
- Focusable stand magnifier, for example, Sloan, Keeler and Tripod (Fig. 28.6).
- Paperweight or Visolett (Fig. 28.7).
- Non-magnifying reading aid, reading slit or typoscope.

*Projection magnifiers*

- Megascope : 12 × and 20 ×.

## Lenses for distant vision

Strong minus lenses –10.00 D to –20.00 D

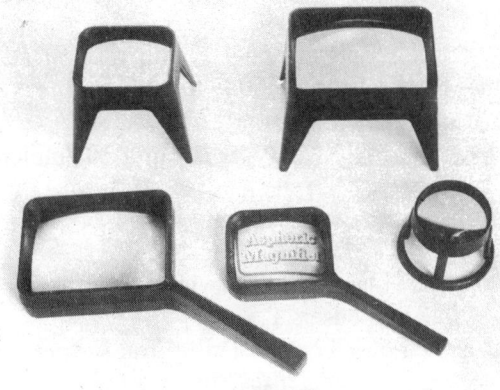

**Fig. 28.4.**

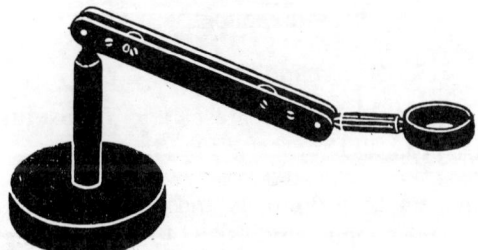

**Fig. 28.5.** Stand magnifier.

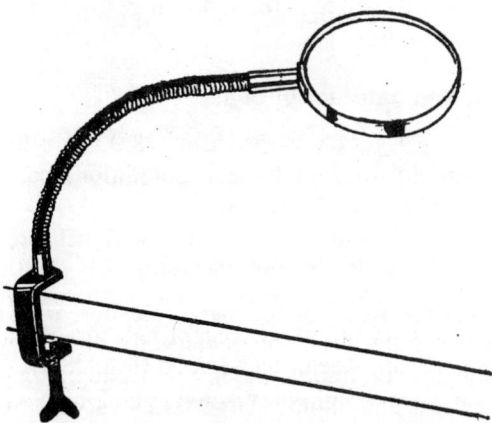

**Fig. 28.6.** Focusable stand magnifiers.

ground with plano on the outside. Higher minus appear thinner and, therefore, cosmetically more acceptable if they are ground biconcave. They are not equally biconcave but ocular surface –20.00 D and remaining number is ground on the outer surface. Lenticular lenses are used usually above –15.00 D.

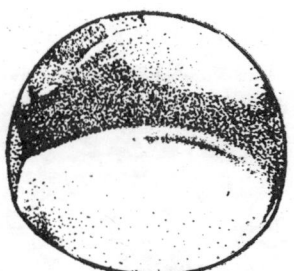

**Fig. 28.7.** Paper weight.

Strong plus lenses appear thinner when ocular surface is ground plano. For higher plus numbers +14.00 to +16.00 is ground on front surface and remainder is ground on the ocular surface.

Weight of the higher plus lenses can be reduced by using plastic lenses or Fresnel lenses.

## Lenses for near vision

As a general rule all plus lenses after +8.00 should be ground with plano ocular surface and biconvex after +14.00 on the front surface.

## High plus reading bifocals (Fig. 28.8)

Kestenbaum was the first to prescribe strong reading addition, calling them 'microlenses' because their diameter was small. He recommended decreasing the diameter of the reading spot with increase in number, i.e., +20.00 (30 mm) and +40.00 (15 mm).

## American Optical's Magnifying Bifocals (A.O.C.)

They are high adds varying between +8.00 to +32.00 and are ground on plano ocular surface. Height of segment varies with power +8.00 and +12.00 (30 mm) +16.00, +24.00 (25 mm) and +32.00 (20 mm).

## High power bifocal

Power of segment varies from +5.00 D to +20.00 D. Compared to American optical's ocular surface is –8.50 instead of plano. This helps to achieve more minus and less plus.

## Cemented bifocal

Cemented lenses are not permanent and must be

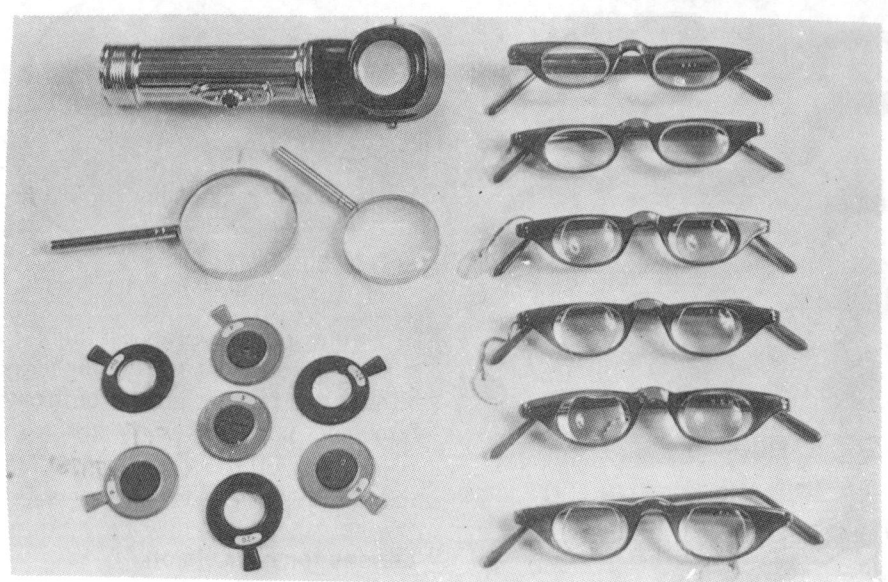

**Fig. 28.8.** High plus reading bifocals.

recommended for 6 to 12 months. Epoxy resin joins segment permanently but it is rarely used.

### Best form lenses

Best form lenses are ground on preferred coflexures and resulting shape gives maximum field of vision. For example, for +16.00, +20.00 and +24.00 ocular surface will be +2.00, +4.00 and +8.00 respectively, and the remainder will be ground on the front surface.

### Specially designed lenses

These include aspheric lenses, doublet and triplet air-spaced lenses, doublet and triplet cemented lenses, all of which reduce spherical and chromatic aberration, astigmatism of oblique incidence, curvature of field and distortion.

### Aspheric lenses

Here ocular surface is spheric and front surface is aspheric, i.e., the lens becomes weaker towards the periphery.

Allvar Gullstrand (1900) made the first aspheric lenses +15, +20, +25, +30, +40, +50, +60, +80 and +100 D. Last three are ground on both the surfaces. They remove aberrations, more

permanent than doublets and less conspicuous. Excessive weight, small size (40 mm) and higher expenses, constitute the disadvantages of Volk's lenses. Keeler's, Aolite and Igard are the other companies which are supplying high power aspheric lenses.

### High and cataract bifocals

Distant correction varies from +8.00 to +20.00 cylinder up to 5 and reading additions can be +6.00, +12.00 and +18.00.

### Doublet and triplet (air space)

Lenses are fitted in the same housing, with air separating the two. This reduces the aberrations. They are available under the trade name of Murvisors and another large series varying from +8.00 to +80.00 has been marketed by William, Feinbloom and Keeler. They are expensive, less permanent, conspicuous, bifocals impossible and cannot be fitted in any frame.

### Cemented doublet and triplet

They are usually cemented combination of crown and flint. Palicoff introduced them into a plastic distant lens. It has advantage of being bifocal,

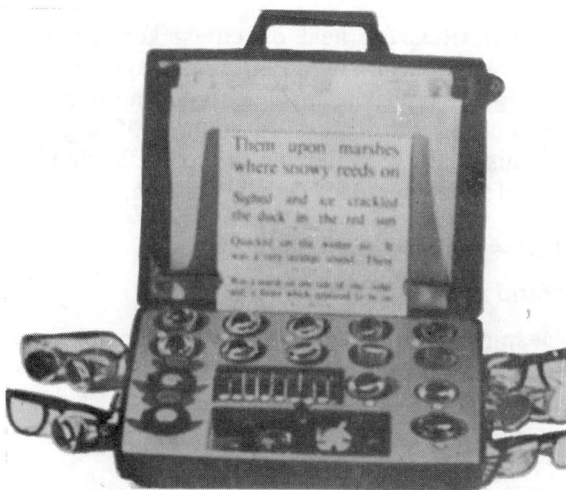

**Fig. 28.9.** Keeler telescopic trial set.

correction of aberration, simultaneous vision for distant and near. It remains conspicuous, becomes loose, restricts field of vision in stronger powers.

The higher the power, the lower the field, depth of focus and illumination. Depth of focus of +16.00 D is 4 mm and that of the +32.00 D is 1 mm. This makes spectacle unsuitable for those people whose hands are trembling. This is overcome by providing a housing which serves as a platform or a stop for preventing trembling of hand so that the book remains at a constant distance thereby keeping the print always at the focal length of the device. Disadvantages of illumination which is not provided and for that built-in illumination of Keelers (as in illuminated/ spectacle magnifier) is the best.

### Telescopes

Hans Lippershey, a spectacle maker of Holland, made three designs of telescopes based on Galilean principle (1608). The first had a minus ocular separated from the plus objective by air, the second was shaped like cork and made up of solid glass bounded by plus and minus surfaces on sides. The third had a concave mirror as ocular and convex mirror as objective. The system has never become popular due to a central scotoma.

Real development in telescope system was done by von Rohr. These days various companies are making the telescopic system for diagnostic purposes. These have magnification varying from 1.7 to 2.2 and are marketed under the name of Zeiss, Stigmat, 'Kollmorgen', Bier Fleming and Keeler (Figs. 28.9 and 28.10).

In the afocal telescope the more powerful minus eyepiece is placed within the focal length of the weaker plus objective. Separation between

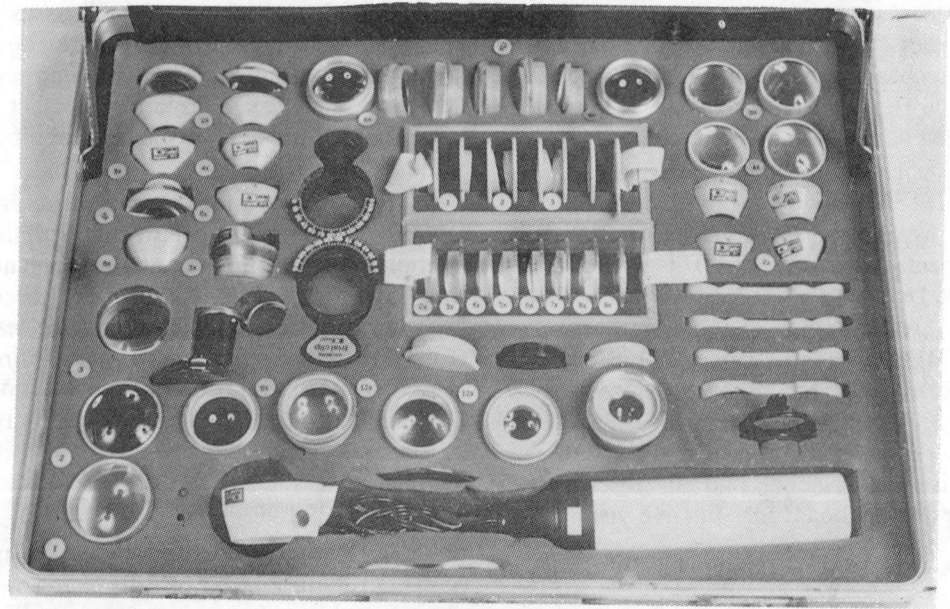

**Fig. 28.10.**

the two lenses is the difference between focal lengths of the two lenses. Parallel rays entering the objective will leave the eyepiece as parallel bundle. Addition of a near cap over the objective undoes the divergence from a near point. The ratio of the angle of the incident rays to angle of the rays emerging out of concave lens determines the magnification. Since both the incident and the emergent rays are parallel it is called an afocal system.

The need of a telescope is always intermittent because it reduces the fields considerably. 2.2 telescope reduces the fields to less than 14°. They cannot be used while moving and objects are magnified and hence appear near. For near vision a telescope gives double the working distance compared to glasses. There are certain advantages of spectacles, i.e.,

- Less conspicuous
- Larger fields
- Simultaneous vision for near and distance
- Less expensive
- More comfortable
- More conveniently used

Telescopes have limited value for intermediate distance. It is most valuable for surgeons who get magnification with a good working distance thereby avoiding instruments touching his spectacles. In actual practice one can have small telescopes fitted over the spectacles bearing prescription. This gives him advantage of corrected vision when he is not using the telescope.

For distant vision Fonda suggested to use a hand-held +3.00 D in conjunction with uncorrected hyperopia. Kestenbaum suggested to use a cemented segment of −20.00 D and hand-held +8.00 D.

For higher telescopic magnification. × 2 and × 4 magnification can be achieved by reducing the distance to one half and one fourth respectively. Children achieve magnification by keeping the book closer to the eye. Handicapped children and adult utilise this principle and sit closer to the television or blackboard for effective vision.

## Contact lenses and low vision

Contact lenses are of great value in low vision cases. They help by removing the anterior surface irregularities (corneal opacities, keratoconus, high astigmatism), by magnifying image with the fellow eye (aphakia, anisometropia, aniseikonia), by cutting the excessive amount of light in albinism, and by removing the cosmetic blemish in deformed eyes (for details, see Chapter 27).

## Non-spectacle magnifiers

### Hand and stand magnifiers

Despite the bigger field with spectacles of equivalent power hand and stand magnifiers are indicated in the following situations :

- When fields are reduced to 10° or more.
- As auxiliary lens for finer jobs.
- When final prescription is still undecided.
- In patients with tremors.
- Where patients insist, but pathology is hopeless.
- When patient has been using hand or stand magnifiers for many years.

## Management of patient

The management of a patient with a sight-threatening disease requires attention to all aspects of vision loss including his successful rehabilitation. It is important for ophthalmologists to help patients with sight-threatening diseases to deal with their fears about living with impaired vision at the time of diagnosis. Those needing additional assistance can then be referred to other professionals and agencies involved in rehabilitating the visually handicapped.

Various optical and non-optical aids are available for patients with impairment. With the introduction of microcomputers and video technology, the future of patients with low vision has brightened. The use of close circuit television (CCTV) as video magnifier has been in vogue for long time. The application of this technology as a mobile device is the latest addition in the field of low vision management.

## Video microcomputers in low vision

Video technology offers the advantages not only of high magnification but also the option of contrast enhancement and contrast reversal. Since the screen can be focused binocularly from a comfortable distance, there are fewer postural constraints even after its constant use for a long time. Newer and ongoing developments include smaller cameras that make the hand-held unit more feasible, a flat panel liquid crystal display (LCD) and miniature displays that can be hand monitored. These are particularly useful for students and others with voluminous reading work.

### Bright eyes

This is the first electronic portable reading system to incorporate a head-borne display. It combines a battery pack with a hand-held camera and a light emitting diode (LED) display mounted on a head band or a spectacle frame. The LED display is monocular and produces either a red on black or black on red image. Because the display is monocular, the user can easily switch visual attention between the display and environment. This display is unique because it can present an image (virtual) that appears to float in front of the observer. Two magnification levels are provided using a switch on the control box. The magnification depends on the setting used and the distance between the LED display and the wearer's eye. The battery pack provides operation for approximately 2 to 3 hours of continuous use. The display control box and battery weighs 37 oz. making it an extremely portable reading aid. In general, the magnification and field of view are similar to that of a 12-inch monitor viewed at the distance of 18 inches.

### Low vision enhancement system

This is a head-mounted video display device, developed at the Wilmer Eye Institute Low Vision Centre, at Johns Hopkins University, USA, and is worn like a visor or goggles over the eyes. The low vision enhancement system (LVES) is projected in front of the two eyes, two miniature video cameras for wide field viewing, one mounted in front of each eye and a third mounted in the centre of the device. The LVES is battery-powered and is designed to aid those having partial visual impairment with an visual acuity of 20/100 to 20/800 to their vision more effectively by magnifying images and enhancing contrast.

Like bright eyes, the LVES has a head-mounted display. However, the LVES display is binocular and uses LCD technology. As mentioned earlier, the input for LVES comes from three charged coupled device (CCD) cameras (two for distant vision and one for near vision) also mounted on the headset. Because the device uses CCD camera technology, it can also operate in conditions with less ambient lightning. This will benefit patients with night blindness. The most important advantage of LVES is the incorporation of enhancement for both travel and near vision within a single device.

**Features of LVES :** When wearing the LVES, the only view the patient sees is provided by the black and white video displays; all other light is blocked out. The field of view is 50 degrees horizontally and 40 degrees vertically as compared to 180 degrees normal field of vision. The apparent screen size is equivalent to 60 inches large screen TV at a distance of 4 feet. A switch on the control pack allows the user to select the wide field cameras or the centre mounted zoom camera. The latter provides magnification of 3 × to 4 × to see closer objects at a distance of ½-1 feet. An auxiliary close up lens must be flipped open in front of the zoom lens. Contrast enhancement and negative image options are also provided. Video in-out facility helps the patient to view from an external video source and others can also see through a monitor the images that the patient is seeing through the LVES. These images can also be recorded for demonstration. An auxiliary stand-mounted video camera, a hand-held scanner or an optical magnifier can also be used if required. While viewing a standard TV programme, the patient can still view the surroundings by switching on to wide field camera input, as the TV signals override the zoom camera output. Using a connector, the patient can use LVES as a computer display along with a print enlarging software.

**Limitations of LVES :** Walking and driving is not usually possible wearing the LVES. Prior mobility training is needed for its occasional limited use while walking.

The LVES weighs 1000 grams (35 oz.) and can be operated for 1½ to 2 hours with a 9 volt rechargeable battery. The option of using a 12 V adapter or a car cigarette lighter adapter is also available.

It is not possible to use this visual aid without training. A three-day training session helps the patient to learn its use and utility, supported by periodic follows-ups during which the progress of individual patients is noted.

## Electronic visual aids

Electronic visual aids offer many important and unusual features. The degree of magnification can be varied from $4 \times$ to $60 \times$ depending on the size of the screen and the brand. They can be used with a typewriter, enabling the person to see what is being typed. In addition they can also be helpful in allowing the visually impaired to write and easily see the script on the monitor. Most of these also have large print computer readout systems and talking software capabilities that are compatible with many computers.

### Reading machines (Fig. 28.11)

Reading machines require a scanner and compatible computer. The scanner sees a printed page and the 'reader' interprets the page which is stored in the computer. Any large print or speech software can be used in conjunction with the 'reader'. Once the document is scanned by the computer, the user may see or hear it. The 'reader' is compatible with variety of scanners and all popular word processors.

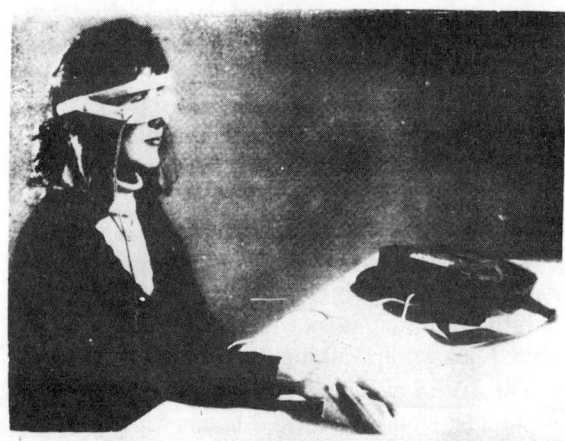

**Fig. 28.11.**

### Robotron text reading machine

This text reading machine reads matter in English language. It is suitable for schools, libraries, work places, or any place for visually-impaired people who may need access to printed documents. It can be connected to any cassette, tape recorder thereby enabling institutions to build a talking library on various subjects. It can also be connected to a Braille printer, working independently, without any additional equipment. It has 9 different voices to suit individual conveniences.

## Video magnifiers

Video magnifiers enable material to be magnified in either black and white or white on black background. Colour monitors also can be used. These devices allow patients to read mail, pay bills and correspondence with great ease. The major drawback of this system is its lack of portability and high expense. It is important, however, to demonstrate the devices to all patients so that they know that these are available.

Traditionally the video magnifier or the system CCTV consists of an X-Y table for moving the text, and CCD camera with a zoom lens and a CRT video display. A 19-inch monitor occupies a desk area of approximately $20 \times 25$ inches, while the 14-inch monitor occupies an area of approximately $14 \times 22$ inches. The advantages are not only high magnification but also the option of contrast enhancement and contrast reversal.

Consideration should be given to the patient's need for magnification, field of view, contrast and when appropriate, to eccentric viewing. Large print access software, screen magnifiers (Fresnel lens with $1.5 \times$ magnification), glare and polarizing filters, coloured screen filters, etc., can bring about a substantial improvement in the patient's ability to use microcomputers.

### Larger computer monitor (Fig. 28.12)

Monitors of 20 inches (51 cm) or larger provide large text and graphic images of $1.4 \times$. Greater magnification can be attained with a much larger monitor. Spectacle-mounted optical aids combined with monitor and stand facilitates a shorter viewing distance. For instance, moving the screen from 18

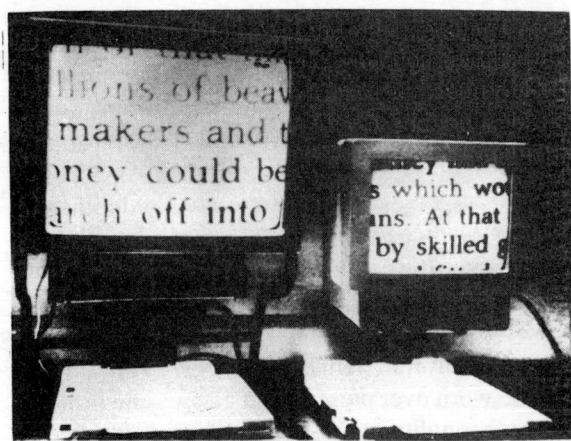

**Fig. 28.12.**

inches to 9 inches provides 2 × magnification. Moving it to 6 inches provides 3 × magnification without restricting the information visible on each screen.

**Large print software :** Large print software generally allows convenient accesses to the computer and allows projection of dark text on a light background (positive) or a light text on dark background (negative). The patient can take advantage of both the video magnifier's ability to magnify the source document and the access software's ability to magnify the computer text. Some computers present the text in single line after scanning. Reading single line text is easier for patients with a central scotoma.

### Voice output and combined access system

A combination of large print and synthesized speech offers the most effective computer access. A small external or internal speaker can be used or a headset can be employed to provide privacy to the visually impaired computer user to have the computer screen information read to him in synthesized speech.

### Scanning laser ophthalmoscope (SLO) : Role as a low vision aid

Low vision patients have disrupted central vision due to macular diseases and other ocular conditions. Evaluation of macular function traditionally has relied on measurement of visual acuity. This, however, does not provide the total picture of the macular function status. SLO macular perimetry provides information about the central visual field in patients with decreased visual acuity that is difficult to obtain in any other way. The SLO uses nearly invisible infrared laser (780 nm) and a modulated visible red light laser (633 nm). This technology involves projecting a fixation target on the macular area, asking the patient to look at it and performing a visual field test right on the retina. The area which the patient actually focuses is called the preferred retinal locus (PRL). With the SLO, one can determine the actual relationship between the PRL and the damaged retina. Macular scotomas can be mapped on the SLO with kinetic, static or hybrid testing techniques. SLO macular perimetry clearly identifies whether central scotomas are present and where the naturally chosen PRL is located relative to the scotoma. Thus it allows prediction of which activities of daily living are likely to be difficult by the visually impaired person.

## Miscellaneous aids and personal items for the visually impaired

### Lamps

Various models of specially designed lamps for table, floor, and bedside use are available with flexible, telescope or gooseneck stands. These are optically designed to intensify, direct and concentrate better quality penetrating light which reduces glare and eye fatigue. They are constructed to prevent undue heating of the lamp shade. Depending on the requirement, 25 W to 200 W cool-light long-lasting lamps can be used. An extra portable good light source worn around the neck is available for reading and working anywhere.

### Clocks

*Table clocks :* Talking table clocks are available now. Models with alarm and large LED display are both available.

*Pyramid clock :* This novel triangular clock speaks when one sets time and alarm so one can be sure of the correct settings. It also announces the alarm time when a push button is pressed. It can be set to announce time on the hour. It also speaks the correct time at the touch of large button at the peak of pyramid. The alarm either beeps or crows like a rooster. This is also available in pocket size travel model.

*Desktop alarm clock :* This is available with a large LED display, snoozer alarm and an optional talking device. It also announces the month and date on pressing a tiny button.

*Wrist watch with talking calculator :* This hand-held clock calculator automatically announces the time every hour on the hour and can also be set for use as an alarm clock. Other features includes a countdown timer and ability to announce the month and day on command. When used as calculator it announces each use of the button, i.e., add, subtract, etc.

*Low vision watch :* Low vision watches with a white face and large black numbers or white numbers on black background are nowadays available for visually handicapped individuals.

*Talking wrist watches :* Talking wrist watches with synthesised voice announcement and digital display are also available.

### Writing aids

These include heavy lined papers with wide lines of ⅝" thickness, narrow lines of ¼" thickness and fine and heavy line maker print that does not bleed, very black soft lead pencils, 3-D markers which consist of a plastic paste to apply on paper, cloth, wood or metal and are useful for marking appliances. Black thick felt pens are also helpful as writing aids for the visually handicapped.

*Signature guide :* This consists of a black plastic of a 3¼" × 2" with a ⅝" opening.

*Typoscope reading and writing guide :* This guide consists of a black plastic piece 5" × 3½" wide with a 4" wide by ½" deep opening. This serves to highlight the text being read.

*Cheque writing guide :* The cheque writing guide consists of a black plastic template for filling in necessary information on a standard 2¾" × 6" cheque.

*Envelope addressing guide :* The envelope addressing guide consists of a black plastic mask with cutout lines with a standard 'address to' and 'address from' area of 4⅛" × 7¾".

### Personal items

*Magnifying mirror with suction base :* This is so constructed that its angle with the object to be viewed is adjustable. The image of the object to be viewed appears on the mirror in a magnified form. It is helpful for combing hair, shaving and applying make-up, etc.

*Instant sunglasses :* These are flexible, light weight, shatter-proof and can be wrapped around the glass. It offers maximum UV and glare protection, and can be slipped in the back of the glasses.

*Super visors :* This sun goggle with shields can be worn over prescription glasses and is made of high quality, light weight, heavy plastic. It offers 100% UV protection and blocks 83% blue light. It has a universal size.

Needle threader, table glass holders, pocket purse with slots for different types of coins are other conveniences which help to facilitate the daily chores for a visually handicapped individual.

*Playing cards :* Special playing cards with a regular plastic with large numbers in red and blue black are available for visually handicapped people. These have red numbers outlined in black to help in identification by people who have problem in recognizing red colour.

*Talking scale :* This has five memory and automatic zero facility. At the touch of the button, the scale asks you to 'Please step on the scale'. Seconds later it announces your weight and tells you how much you have lost or gained from the last reading. After saying 'Goodbye' it turns itself off automatically. The machine also announces 'My battery is low' at the appropriate time.

*Thermometer :* These are available with colour coded and larger read-out or in bold digital display. No shaking is needed in the later model. Touching of a button clears the display for the next use.

*Magnifying syringe :* Easy loading syringes with built-in magnifiers are available for use by diabetics with visual handicap.

*Large print voice calculator :* An eight digit desktop calculator which announces every entry, has memory function, and is battery operated is available for use by visually handicapped individuals.

*Enlarged telephone dial :* This fits over the regular dial. It is made of white plastic and has numbers printed in black. Enlarged telephone dials are also available for push button phones, in black with white numbers.

*Big timer :* A big sixty minutes timer with bold letters can be used on counters, desks or can be mounted on a wall.

*Lightweight folding book holder :* This is used to hold large print oversized books. It is foldable and easy to carry.

*Large print books :* Reading materials, hand-work pattern (e.g. knitting, crochet) cross-word puzzles, world atlas and large print calendars are all available in large print for the visually handicapped.

*Mobility guides :* Various ultrasonic guides which are available for the visually impaired include ultrasonic canes, sonic guide, path finder, etc. These give auditory and/or tactile indications to the individual while walking.

Individuals with impaired vision must finally determine as to what type of visuals aids are best suited to them. Each person's ability to adjust to a particular degree of visual impairment is individual and each person's needs are different. Professional guidance must be sought before consideration is given to procuring sophisticated optical and non-optical aids. It is now obvious that there are many things that can be done to improve the quality of vision. With the available low vision aids for rehabilitation, a person can remain independent and productive in society to a very large extent.

# Ophthalmic Lenses, Making and Fitting of Spectacles

# CHAPTER 29

# Ophthalmic Lenses

Ophthalmic lenses are worn for one or more reasons as under :

- To correct or relieve refractive errors and anomalies of binocular vision.
- To improve subnormal visual acuity or to provide magnification when desired.
- To protect the eye from harmful radiations or from injury by agencies such as wind, dust, flying particles, etc.

The lenses are usually made from glass or organic plastics.

**Glass** : The most commonly used material for spectacles is white ophthalmic crown glass, which has a refractive index of 1.523. The glasses used are those annealed. Annealing is a process which allows the glass to cool very slowly over several days, thus preventing the outer portion of the slab cooling before the inner. The two opposite surfaces of the slab are finally flattened and polished and turned out in discs of the required size and thickness, either flat in shape or curved. These pieces are termed as blanks.

These blanks are subjected to a grinding process by which the surfaces are shaped by electrically driving the lens on tools of known curvature. These tools are of cast iron and finely grained. To produce the necessary effect abrasion is effected by a hard powder (carborundum or emery) of gradually increasing fineness till the lens is very smooth (surfacing) when it is polished with rouge (oxide of iron) and water. The process is finally completed by a process in which a covering cloth of wax is substituted for the powder.

Certain other glasses having a mean refractive index appreciably higher than ophthalmic crown glass are used in the manufacture of spectacle lenses, notably in the segments of fused bifocals

and multifocals. These are dense flint, extradense flint and dense barium crown glasses with a refractive index of over 1.62.

Optic plastics which are usually polymers of methyl methacrylate are used. Focalite which is basically a copolymer of acrylic resins or some polyesters like allyl diglycol carbonate are also used as optical lenses which are either compression moulded or 'casted' (polyesters).

All surfaces commonly employed in ophthalmic lens manufacture are surfaces of revolution and are grouped into two fundamental types :

## Surfaces having axial symmetry

They are :

- Spherical surface where the surface generated would be a portion of sphere with its centre coinciding with the centre of curvature of the surface.
- Plane surface, defined as a surface with zero curvature.
- Aspherical surface, e.g., a portion of an ellipse; though these are not spheres yet they have an axial symmetry.

## Astigmatic surfaces

They are either cylindrical or toroidal. Their characteristic feature is a gradual change of curvature from one meridian change or curvature from one meridian to another; the meridians of minimum curvature being always at right angles to each other.

In all designs of lenses the most important aberration to eliminate is the astigmatism of oblique pencils so that the patient wearing a spectacle is comfortable. There are two forms of lenses for each power by which this astigmatic error can be

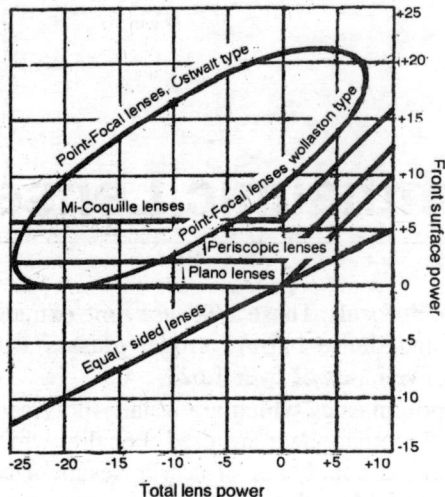

**Fig. 29.1.** Toric spectacle lens surfaces for correction of astigmatism.

eliminated—the shallow form of Ostwald and the deep form of Wollaston (Fig. 29.1). On this basis lower stigmatic lenses have been designed (point focals) and these allow the coalescence of the tangential and sagittal spheres. These lenses also minimize curvature distortion and chromatic aberrations so that they come within the tolerance range of the eye. It would be seen that for different dioptric powers of the lenses different form and base curve is needed. This is practically not possible as it would require a huge stock and become very costly. So in practice for plus lenses up to +3.00 D a base curve of –6.00 (back surface) is employed and for minus lenses up to –5 D to –9 D a base curve of +3 D (front surface) is employed; from –9 D sph. to –15 a base curve (front surface) +1.25 is used and from –1500 to –20.00 a plano front surface is needed. These figures indicate that minus base curve is ground on the back surface and is used in the making of plus prescribed lenses up to +7 D while a decreasing plus base curve is grounded on the front surface ranging from +6.00 to plano for the prescribed minus lenses up to –20.00 D. A lens with a base curve of 6 D is called a deep meniscus lens while one with a base curve of +1.25 D is called a periscopic lens. Beyond this range of +7.00 D and –20.00 D it is not possible to neutralize the oblique astigmatism of lenses. With the

advent of computers, which have enabled one to obtain quick mathematical calculations facilitating to determine the criteria of the design for a particular power and the case, it is possible to rapidly produce lenses of best forms and the services may become personalized.

## Astigmatic lenses

To a large extent astigmatic lenses have forms similar to spherical lenses. The only way to minimize the aberrations in astigmatic lenses is to harden the lens. When a sphero-cylindrical lens is bent it takes the form of a toric surface. It is generated by evolution of a circular arc of radius around the central axis which does not pass through its centre (Fig. 29.2). There are thus two curvatures of the surface (Fig. 29.3)—one meridional with the radius of curvature ($r_1$) and the other rotational ($r_2$). If $r_2$ is greater then $r_1$ a tyre-shaped toric surface results (Fig. 29.4) and if $r_2$ is less than $r_1$ a barrel-shaped surface results (Fig. 29.5).

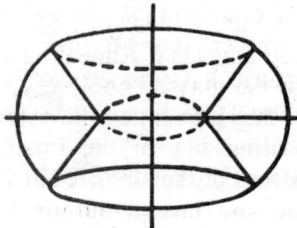

**Fig. 29.2.** Generation of a toric surface by revolution.

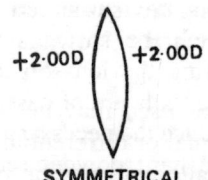

**Fig. 29.3.** Two symmetrical planes.

It is not possible to attain an equality of effective refractive powers of astigmatic lens over its entire area. A good astigmatic lens should aim at equalizing the circles of least confusion in the two meridians so as to lie in a sphere concentric with the centre of rotation of the eye.

The lenses used may be round or any other shape. The shape and size of lens be such as to

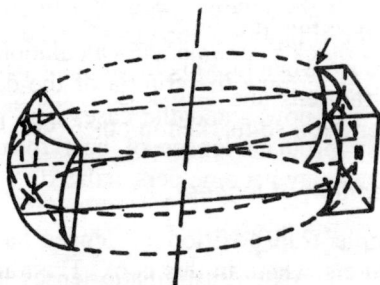

**Fig. 29.4.** Tyre-shaped toric surface.

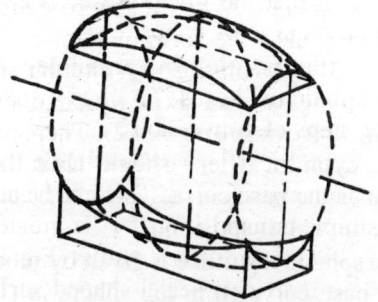

**Fig. 29.5.** Barrel-shaped toric surface.

+2·00D +2·00D   SYMMETRICAL

+1·00D +3·00   ASYMMETRICAL

+4·00D   PLANO

−1·2·D +5·25D   PERISCOPIC (BASE,+ 1.25D)

6·00D +10·00D   DEEP MENISCUS (BASE,− 6.00D)

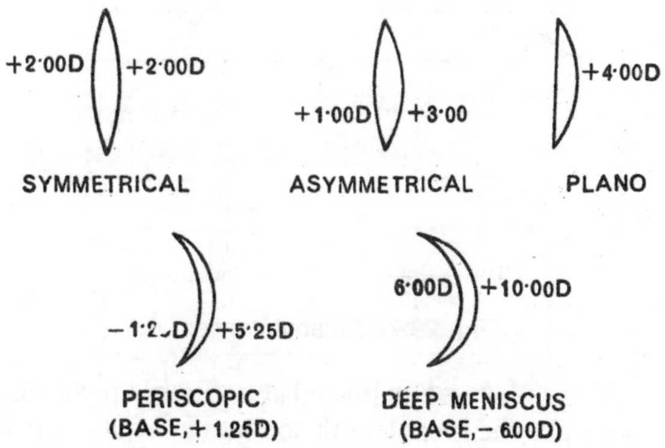

**Fig. 29.6.** Various types of lenses.

provide a full field of vision especially so in children who are prone to look over the lenses.

Symmetrical Asymmetrical Plano Periscopic Deep meniscus (Base +1.25 D) (Base –6.00 D)

The disadvantage of round shape in cylindrical lenses is that they rotate in the frame should they become loose. The rotation leads to a change in axis and discomfort to the patient. In other shapes this disadvantage is abolished. Even in round lenses, locking devices are known which prevent them from rotating. Nowadays round lenses are seldom used.

The lenses used may be biconvex or bicon-cave with equal or differential curvature on both surfaces, plano-concave or plano-convex or a meniscus. The lenses may be periscopic (a base curve of +1.25 D) or a deep meniscus (base curve –6 D). Different types of lenses are illustrated in Fig. 29.6. When cylindrical lenses are used a sphero-cylinder is bent and the lens is called toric lens. The spherical power of lens can be ground on one surface and the cylindrical on the other. The centre of pupil in primary position coincides with the centre of the lens.

When the eyes rotate and the head is kept still the lens does not shift and if the optical system is only accurate for the axial rays it will become inaccurate for the eccentric rays. It is well estab-lished that in the movements of the eye it moves round a centre of rotation which is about 13 mm behind the apex of the cornea. If the object moves concentric to the centre of rotation it will be brought to a sharp focus on the macula. If this is for near for which the eye accommodates it is called proximate sphere of sharp definition and if it is for the far point it is called a remote sphere. The space lying between the proximate sphere and the remote sphere contains all points at which an object can be seen clearly without moving the head. The aim of all refractions is to simulate an emmetropic eye as far as possible. The ophthal-mic lenses, therefore, likewise should reproduce conditions of naked eye as far as the spheres are concerned. This can be achieved by varying the radii of the two surfaces of the lens which at best can be regarded as compromise forms.

The rays of light passing through a lens, as described elsewhere, undergoes spherical aberra-tion but this can be overcome by making the more convex surface facing the incident light (Fig. 29.7) and the combination should be made as to produce approximately equal deviations at each surface of the lens. The guidelines have been described above.

Lenses other than symmetrical, biconvex or biconcave may cause displacement of principal planes and if focal length of these lenses is equal to that of symmetrical lens, they will have to be placed at different distances from the cornea to have the same effective refractive power. A

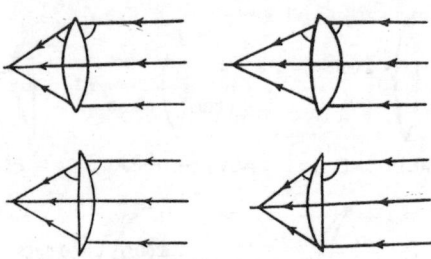

**Fig. 29.7.** Aplantic lenses.

correction lens when placed at a suitable position, must have the focal length so that its second focal point corresponds to the remote point of the eye and the image of the remote point is brought to the focus on the retina by the dioptric system of the eye. This focal length is termed 'back vertex power'. Having been given the back vertex power, the thickness and the base curve, it is to be determined what curve be given to the other surface of the lens. The usual formula is as under :

$$F_1 = \frac{F_{1u} - F_2}{1 + \dfrac{d}{n(F_{1v} - F_2)}}$$

where $F_1$ is the power of the front surface; $F_{1u}$ is the back vertex power; $d$ is the thickness of the lens; $F_2$ is the base curve; and $n$ is the refractive index of the material used.

The surface power is

$$F_1 = \frac{n-1}{r_1}$$

Thus the radius of curvature of the front surface is easily calculated.

To obviate these mathematical calculations and errors the ophthalmic lenses, used in all trial cases, in refracting instruments and in correction of refractive errors, are calibrated in vertex power. Vertex power is defined as the reciprocal of focal length from the surface nearest the eye. As elucidated earlier, they thus use the distance between the posterior surface and principal focus instead of focal length for calibration of these lenses. In these cases, periscopic, meniscus and toric lenses are preferred as they offer the following advantages :

- Keep the back focal length of the lens more nearly constant for different eye positions.

- Lessen the angular astigmatism produced by the obliquity of the visual axis to the lens surface when looking through the periphery of the lens and also lessens the spherical aberration so marked in other types.

**Transposition of lenses**

The simple transposition of lenses has been described elsewhere in this book. The transposition of spheres in deep meniscus and periscopic lenses one has simply to add algebraically with the provision that the given power is combined with the base curve of opposite sign.

In toric transposition the principles of transposition remain unaltered. To them be added the following steps of conversion :

1. The cylindrical lens should have the same sign as the base curve. This can be achieved by simple transposition.
2. The spherical surface is given by subtracting the base curve from the sphere in (1). This is written in the numerator fraction.
3. Fix the cylinder base curve with its axis at right angles to the cylinder in (1).
4. Add to the base curve one cylinder in (1) with its axis at right angles to the base curve.

Let the steps be explained by an example :

The prescription given is –2.00 D sph. with +3.00 D cyl. axis 90° in a base curve of –6.00 D.

*Step 1*

**Simple transposition :** Convert the cylinder into the same sign as the base curve. The prescription will read as +1.00 D sph. with –3.00 D cyl. axis 180°.

*Step 2*

Algebraically subtract base curve (–6 D) from the spherical prescription, i.e., +1 D sph. – (–6 D sph.) = +7.00 D sph. This becomes the numerator of the toric surface.

*Step 3*

Fix the cylinder of the base curve at right angles to the cylinder of the prescription, i.e., –6.00 D cyl. axis 90°.

*Step 4*

Fix the cylinder of the prescription by adding it to the base curve, i.e., –6.00 D cyl. + (–3.00 D cyl.) or –9.00 D cyl. and place it at right angles to the cylinder of the base curve, i.e., at 180°. The final prescription, therefore, can be written as :

+7.00 D sph.

–6.00 cyl. axis 90° – 9.00 D cyl. 180°

Let us take another example.

+1.00 D sph. with +4.00 D cyl. axis 180°

Simple transposition will mean

+5.00 D sph. with –4.00 D cyl. axis 90° and the final toric prescription will then be :

+11.00 D sph.

–6.00 D cyl. axis 180° – 10.00 D cyl. axis 90°

A third example may be taken

–1.00 D sph. with –4.00 D cyl. axis 90°

No simple transposition is required as the cylinder is already of the same sign as the base curve. The final toric prescription will read as :

+5.00 D sph.

–6.00 D cyl. axis 180° – 10.00 D cyl. axis 90°

In accurate vertex transposition the radius of curvature of the new lens should be found out by the formula already given. Once the radius of curvature is known the vertex power of the lens in relation to thickness of the lens can be determined and given.

### Combination of lenses (bifocals, trifocals and multifocals)

The patient who is to wear a different correction for distance and near can either keep two pairs of glasses, one for near and the other for distance, or keep a glass which can provide correction for different distances, which may be bifocals, trifocals or even multifocals. No doubt having a separate pair for near and distance is the ideal to be kept in mind from the optical point of view but it is very inconvenient to the patients who find changing and keeping of glasses rather irksome. A combination of lenses is, therefore, a practical solution to the problem and convenient. Other more elaborate designs have multiple optical focusing properties suitable for 3 or more distances.

**Bifocals :** Various forms of bifocal lenses

have been evolved but all of them have three optical requirements :

1. The two portions should provide equally clear vision free from aberration.
2. There should be no sudden change in the prismatic effect at the junction of the two segments so that, when the eye changes from one to the other, objects do not appear to 'jump'. This will require that the optical centres of both near and distant portions should be located at or near the junction of the two segments. Monocentric bifocals is the ideal wherein the centres for near and distance are coincident.
3. The centring of the two portions should be exact for their different purposes. It is rather difficult to achieve.

In distant vision the visual axis of the eye passes through the spectacle lens at a point referred to as the distant visual point (Fig. 28.8).

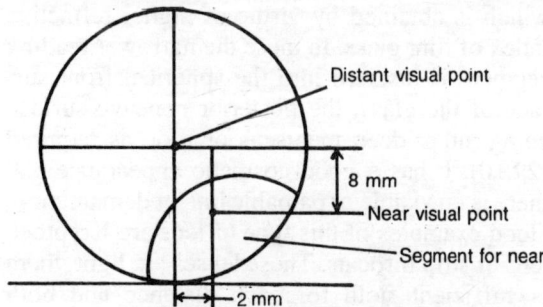

**Fig. 29.8.** A bifocal lens.

The prismatic effects, both vertical and horizontal, to which wearers of bifocals are subject are considerable and muscle balance in these cases assumes considerable importance. It should be carefully assessed and exercises prescribed if necessary. On the whole the aim should be to prescribe bifocals which are so designed as to reduce and minimize the optical disadvantages inherent in these lenses.

The tolerance of bifocals is by no means universal and in many individuals these are best avoided particularly in old age if they are being prescribed for the first time and the near correction added is considerable. There is considerable difficulty experienced while looking down. The objects are blurred which may be a source of danger while descending the stairs or stepping off a kerb. These should also not be prescribed in patients who suffer from vertigo. The difficulty in descending the stairs can be combated by leaving a small segment of distance correction underneath the near correction.

There are several types of bifocals :

**Split or two piece bifocals :** In which the dividing line is horizontal and very conspicuous. These are not used these days (Fig. 29.9).

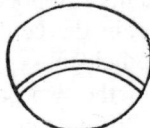

**Fig. 29.9.** Split bifocal lens.

**Fused bifocals :** The invisible bifocals are made by combining a lens of crown glass with a lens of flint glass of higher refractive power which is obtained by virtue of higher refractive index of flint glass. In these the narrower reading segment is inserted into the spherical front surface of the glass, the posterior concave surface being either deep meniscus or toric as required (29.10). It has a good cosmetic appearance and there is no visible or palpable line of demarcation. Good examples of this type of lens are Kryptoch lens or strip bifocals. These lenses are light, there is sufficient field for each distance and both elements are accurately centred and correctly tilted.

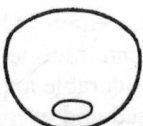

**Fig. 29.10.** Fused bifocals (Kryptoch).

**Cemented glasses :** In cemented bifocals a separate piece or a supplementary lens is cemented onto the surface of the main glass (Fig. 29.11). One surface is cemented onto the distance correction lens while the other surface provides the curvature for the near correction. This lens is cemented with Canada balsam which has the same refractive index as the glass.

**Other types :** A further improvement occurred

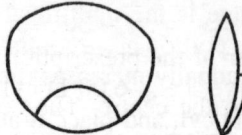

**Fig. 29.11.** Bifocal with supplementary wafer.

when supplementary lens was inserted into the middle of the lens of the distance correction which is split for the purpose (Fig. 29.12).

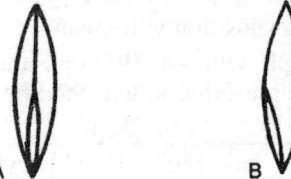

**Fig. 29.12.** Bifocal lenses with inserted or fused wafer.

Improvements went on till fused lenses were evolved. There is still room enough to achieve the ideal.

Some executives, office workers, lecturers and speakers are usually not satisfied with the bifocal lenses as they want to utilize their spectacles for varying distances. There are optically complex problems yet to a certain extent the needs can be met by trifocal or multifocal lenses.

Trifocal lenses (Fig. 29.13) have become both popular and practicable. These lenses are specially useful for persons who require a high additional

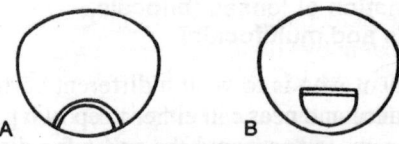

**Fig. 29.13.** Trifocal lenses.

correction for the near. The addition for intermediate correction varies in different designs but, within limits it is usually half that of correction for near vision. This addition is found to be effective and most useful. The trifocals have the advantage that the patient can see across the room while at the same time he is able to read and do the near work without change of glasses or discomfort. These are, however, very expensive and all do not find it easy to adjust with them.

A more complicated lens without any countervailing advantage is the multifocal lens. In this lens the reading portion has a continuous variable curve which gradually increases the power from the periphery to the centre. The central portion has the effective reading correction. This directly incorporates lens power for intermediate distances from infinity to the working distance eliminating the sharp 'jump' from near to a distant focus or from a distant to a near focus. These thus try and seem to provide multiple range stimulating a normal accommodative mechanism, but in practice, have not been found to be satisfactory for the continuously varying curve is effective only in the vertical central line. The distortion on either side of this line is considerable and often too much to tolerate which is the cause of discomfort to the patient.

### Lenses for special purposes

**Aphakia :** Aphakic glasses have several disadvantages if biconvex lenses are used :

- Peripheral aberrations and thus reducing the effective field of view.
- True restriction of field because of prismatic effect at the edge of the lens.
- Jack in the box phenomenon.
- Increase in the size of retinal image and also in view of high cylindrical correction a meridional disparity in the size of image.
- Excessive weight.
- Unsightliness.

These defects are sought to be corrected to a certain extent by adopting various types of lenses particularly the low aperture type.

**Lenticular lenses :** The optical portion of the lens is in the central position and the peripheral portion is eliminated. These are lighter and thinner. For near vision the patient should be prescribed a separate pair though bifocals can be given. Most of the bifocals are of lenticular type. The best amongst them is Volk conoid aphakic bifocal lens (Fig. 29.14).

The lenticular lenses may be of various types (Figs. 29.15 to 29.18) like solid, convex, uniseal, rotoid, alphakat.

### Lenses for high myopia

Full aperture lenses for higher myopia are usually

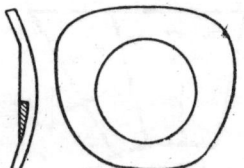

**Fig. 29.14.** Conoid aphakic bifocal.

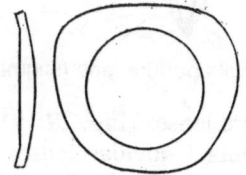

**Fig. 29.15.** Solid lenticular lens.

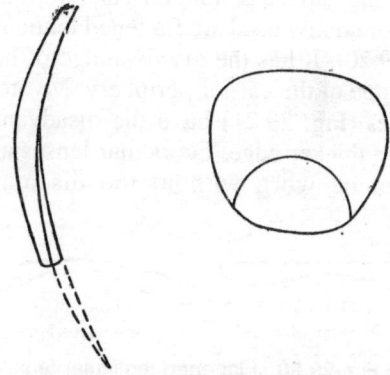

**Fig. 29.16.** Convex uniseal lenticular lens.

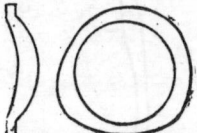

**Fig. 29.17.** Rotoid lens.

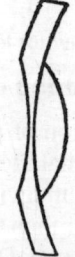

**Fig. 29.18.** Alphakat lens.

best in plano-concave form special glazing techniques for the edge can minimize the power rings

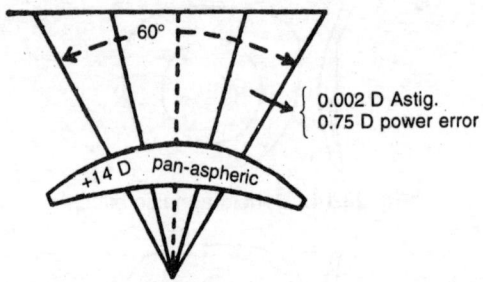

**Fig. 29.19.** Full aperture lens (stigmatic edge lens).

in full aperture lenses (Fig. 29.19). Like aphakia in high myopia lenticular lenses give the best optical results by eliminating some of the peripheral portion. While the central portion has the dioptric power, the carrier peripheral part is afocal. The types commonly used are flattened lenticular lens (Fig. 29.20). It has the disadvantage of having a sharp edge of the carrier periphery. Myotor types of lenses (Fig. 29.21) have the disadvantage of having a thicker edge. Lenticular lenses are light and can be worn without the discomfort of weight.

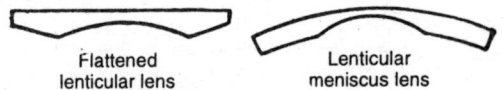

**Fig. 29.20.** Flattened lenticular lens.

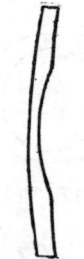

**Fig. 29.21.** Myotor lenticular lens.

### Centring and decentring of lenses

A lens is a combination of prisms which meet at the optical centre so that the rays passing through the optical centre go undeviated. If the rays meet the lens at points other than the optical centre they act as prisms. It is essential that the optical centre coincides with the visual axis of the wearer of the spectacles otherwise prismatic effects will give rise to strain. The non-coincidence of the optical centre with visual axis results in decentration

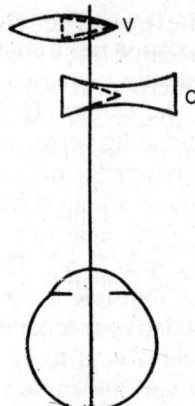

**Fig. 29.22.** Decentration and prismatic effort.

(Fig. 29.22) with prismatic effects. The lenses may sometimes be deliberately decentred. This is done specially for reading glasses. For near work the visual axes are directed downwards and are at the same time converged. If the lenses are not decentred the optical centre of the lens does not coincide with the visual axis or the centre of the pupil while the person is converging for the near. If the error is small, the prismatic error produced is negligible and the desire and capability to fuse overcomes the prismatic effect without undue strain. The patient, therefore, does not have the feeling of discomfort. If the error is large the prismatic effect is larger and considerable strain is produced to overcome the error. Sometimes the fusional reserve may be sufficient to overcome the prismatic error introduced by glasses leading to symptoms and signs of heterophoria.

The position of the optical centre of the lens can be calculated easily. In Fig. 29.23, let O and O′ be the centre of rotation of the eyes and OR and O′R′ be the visual axes when the patient is looking at a distant object. The visual axes are passing through the optical centres of the lenses

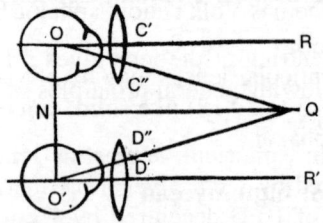

**Fig. 29.23.** Decentring for near work.

in front of the eye. The visual gaze is now directed to a near object situated at 25 cm from the eyes. The interpupillary distance of the patient is 60 mm. In order to see the object Q the visual axes are turned in the direction of OQ and O'Q. The visual axis OQ instead of passing through C' passes through C'' and the visual axis O'Q instead of passing through D' passes through D''. The position of C' and D' can be calculated as under :

$$\frac{ON}{NQ} = \tan OQN$$

$$= \tan C'OC''$$

$$= \frac{C'C''}{C'O}$$

$$C'C'' = C'O \times \frac{OW}{NQ}$$

NQ = distance of object from the eye + distance of glass from the centre of rotation (25 mm)

= 250 mm + 25 mm

= 275 mm

ON = 1/2 the interpupillary distance

= 30 mm

C'O = 25 mm

Hence      $C'C'' = 25 \times \dfrac{30}{275} = 2.75$ mm

Thus for a distance of 25 cm for a patient with an interpupillary distance of 60 mm the lenses should be decentred by about 2.75 mm for comfortable work.

The geometrical centre of a lens is a point in the middle of the lens. It is distinct from the optical centre which is the centre of the optical system formed by the lens and all rays passing through it are undeviated. In a symmetrical face the geometrical and the optical centre may coincide but not necessarily so. The lens may be displaced in any direction provided the optical centre coincides with the visual axis. The geometrical centre of the lens should lie opposite the pupillary centre.

Decentring of the lens gives prismatic effect. The following general principles should be borne in mind :

1. In spherical lenses, a lens of 1 D if decentred by 1 cm gives a prismatic effect 1 D. A lens of 10 D decentred by 1 cm gives a prismatic effect of 10 D. A 1 D prismatic effect in a

10 D lens is obtained by a decentring of the lens by 1 mm.

The dioptric strength of the prism may be calculated by the following formula :

$$C \times D = \Delta$$

where $\Delta$ is the dioptric strength of the prism; D the dioptric strength of the spherical lens to be decentred; and C the amount of decentring in centimetres.

2. The decentring of a cylindrical lens in its axis produces no prismatic effect. Decentring of cylindrical lenses at right angles to the axis of the cylinder produces the same effect as the decentring of a spherical lens. A cylindrical lens of +2 D at 90° axis if decentred vertically produces no effect but if it is decentred by 1 cm in the horizontal direction it produces an effect equal to 2 prism dioptres.

3. In compound lenses, i.e., a combination of spherical and a cylindrical lens a 1 cm decentring in the axis of the cylinder produces a prismatic effect equivalent to the dioptric power of the spherical lens and decentring at right angles to the axis of the cylinder produces a prismatic effect equivalent to the combined dioptric power of the cylindrical and the spherical lens. It may be illustrated by an example. Let $\dfrac{+2 \text{ D sph.}}{+1 \text{ D cyl. axis } 90°}$ be the strength of the compound lens then (a) 1 cm vertical decentring of this lens system produces a 2 $\Delta$ prismatic effect, and (b) 1 cm decentring in the horizontal direction produces a 3 $\Delta$ prismatic effect.

4. In compound lenses consisting of a combination of a spherical lens with a cylindrical lens of opposite denomination decentring produces the following results :

Let $\dfrac{+2 \text{ D sph.}}{-4 \text{ D cyl.}}$ be the strength of the compound lens then (a) 1 cm decentring at 180° produces a prismatic effect of 2 $\Delta$ (if the decentring is inwards it has a base out prismatic value), and (b) 1 cm upward decentring at 90° produces a prismatic effect of 2 $\Delta$ ($-4 + 2 = -2$) with a base up prismatic value, i.e., the base on the concave axis. Decentration is in the direction of decentration and on the convex axis it is opposite the direction of decentration.

5. Sometimes decentring may be required both in horizontal and vertical directions. In these cases decentration is done in an oblique direction (Fig. 29.24).

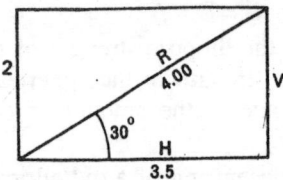

**Fig. 29.24.** To measure oblique decentration.

In this figure, let the vertical prismatic effect required be equal to 2 $\Delta$ and horizontal prismatic effect required be equal to 3.5 $\Delta$ in a spherical lens of 1 dioptre. Draw a vertical line of 2 cm and a horizontal line of 3.5 cm at right angles to the vertical line from the optical centre of the lens. Complete the rectangle and join the diagonal which will be about 4.03 cm. The point represents the point of the optical centre of the lens. This can be calculated as $R^2 = V^2 + H^2$ and the angular direction = tan $(V/H)$. If this is done in each eye so that there is a base up and in one eye and base down in the other eye it will produce 4 $\Delta$ hyperphoria and 7 $\Delta$ exophoria.

The decentring of lenses may be done in such a way that though the optical and geometrical centres coincide, the visual axis passes through a different point. This can be achieved by lengthening or shortening of the nose piece. This is not preferred due to cosmetic reasons. The lens may be displaced in a rim, the geometrical centres coincide with the centre of the pupil and the optical centre is displaced.

Decentring of lenses may be required for
- near work,
- to adopt the glasses for asymmetrical face,
- to correct heterophoria or to overcome a deficiency or excess of convergence as a relieving prism, and
- to give exercise to the muscles in phoric conditions.

## Verification of lenses

The lenses may be verified by
- neutralization,
- Geneva lens measure, or
- vertex refractionometer.

**Neutralisation :** It is the most practical method though not absolutely accurate. A distant object is viewed through an unknown lens and the lens is moved from side to side. If the image of the object moves in the opposite direction, the lens is convex; if the image moves in the same direction, the lens is concave. If the lens is rotated and there is a distortion of the image of the distant object, it has either a cylindrical or a prismatic component.

Having roughly determined the type and the nature of the lens, the lenses from the trial set of opposite sign and gradually increasing strength are held up in combination with the lens under examination in a way that their optical centres coincide and till there is no movement of the image of the distant object of regard. The lens, which in a combination with the lens under examination, gives no movement of the image gives the dioptric value of the spherical component of lens. The combination is now moved in a direction at right angles to the original axis; if there is still no movement the lens is spherical and the dioptric power has already been determined. If the image moves it is likewise neutralized. The dioptric power of the additional lens gives the power of the cylindric component. The axis of this component is the axis at which the first neutralization was done. The axes are marked with a glass pencil and the optical centre is the point where the two axes intersect. The point at which the visual axis cuts the lens is now marked. If the point coincides with the optical centre the lens is decentred and has a prismatic effect which can be determined by measurements.

**Geneva lens measure :** It is an adaptation of spherometer. It is widely used for determining the dioptric power of the lens. It is provided with two fixed supports on either side and a movable one in the centre so that when placed upon a lens the movable leg is deflected and the deflection can be measured on a dial (Fig. 29.25) of this instrument. The dioptric strength can be read directly. This is dependent upon curvature of the lens. It is graduated for glass of a refractive index of 1.523 so that if any other glass is employed a correction factor must be applied. The curvature

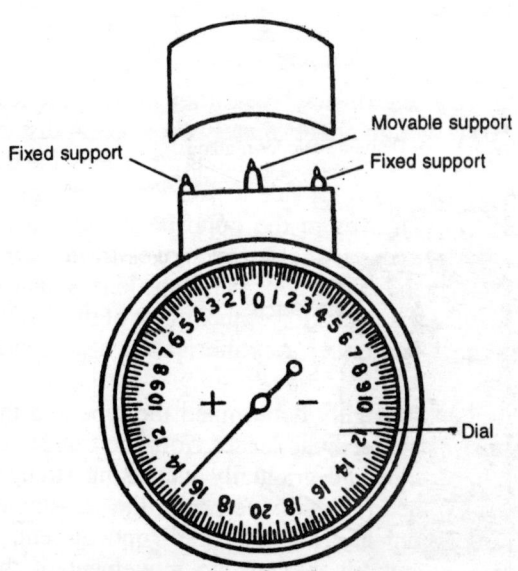

Fig. 29.25. Geneva lens measure.

of each surface is measured separately. The principal axis is first determined and the dioptric value of the lens is ascertained in this axis on both the surfaces. An algebraic summation of the two readings gives dioptric strength in the meridian of the principal axis. The process is repeated in an axis at right angles to the principal axis. The difference in dioptric power between the two axes, if any, gives the cylindric value, the axis of the cylinder is the axis of the lower dioptric value. The optical instrument for measuring the dioptric power of the lens, the correcting lenses and the trial case lenses are calibrated in the vertex power. The theory of the instrument is based on the calculation of lens sag.

In Fig. 29.26, let MON be the curvature of the lens surface of radius ($r$).

MN represents a chord of the circle of which

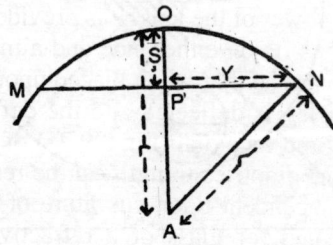

**Fig. 29.26.** Theory of calculation of Geneva-lens measure.

one-half PN = $y$. OP is the sag ($s$). The two fixed legs of the instrument are comparable to MN and the deflection of the movable leg is the sag OP ($s$).

Then

$$r^2 = y^2 + (r-s)^2$$

or

$$r^2 = y^2 + r^2 + s^2 - 2rs$$

or

$$2rs = y^2 + s^2$$

or

$$r = \frac{y^2 + s^2}{2s}$$

In most of the spectacle lenses $s^2$ is so small that it is neglected. For a given instrument $y$ is constant; hence

$$f = \frac{y^2}{2s}$$

It implies that the curvature is directly proportional to the sag. In modern instruments the sag can be directly read and converted into dioptric power of the lens.

### Vertex refractionometer (Fig. 29.27)

The image of the target is seen through a telescope and is focused by a standard lens. The unknown lens is inserted into the system and the target is focused once again (Figs. 29.28 and 29.29). The change in position of the target gives the measure of the dioptric strength. The instruments is versatile and capable of determining optical centre, locating cylindrical axes, measuring the power and locating the direction of prisms. The optical principle is as under :

In Fig. 29.30, a clear image of the target C is focused by a standard lens and is seen through the telescope T. The target C comes into focus only when it coincides with the focal point $F_1$ of the standard lens. The ray $F_1H$ passing through the focal point $F_1$ of the standard lens is refracted parallel to the axis $F_1F_2$ and meets the telescope T at T. The ray is focused by the telescope T in the aperture E and is seen through the eyepiece. This is the zero position. The combination of lenses or the lens whose dioptric strength is to be determined is inserted at D to make the whole a co-axial homocentric system of lenses. The back surface of the combination faces the standard lens. The homocentric system will now have the focal point at $F_2$ and the target C will be focused at the aperture E if C coincides with $F_2$. The

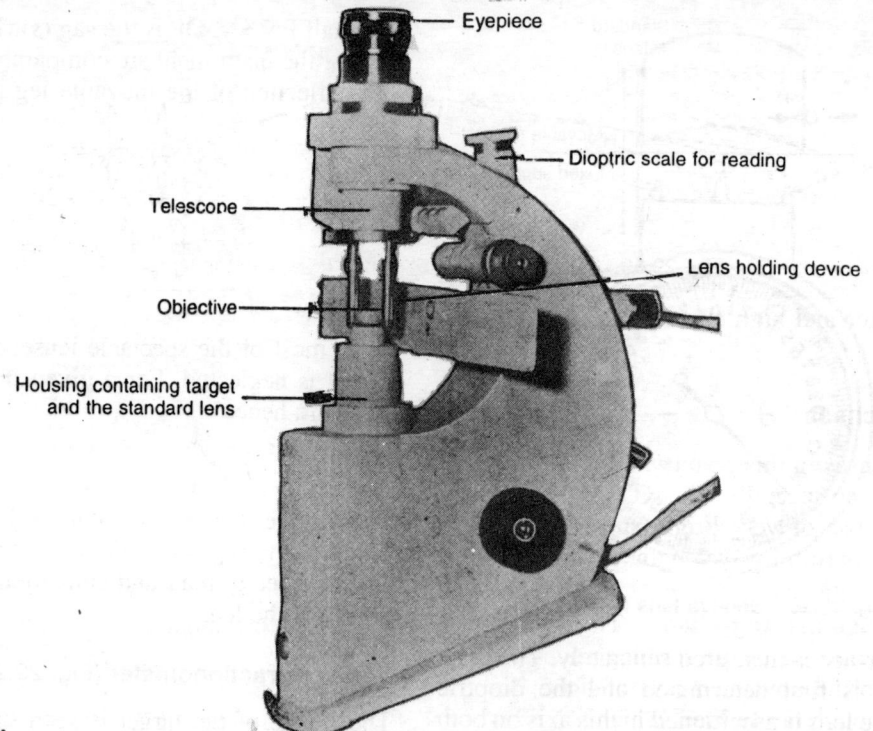

**Fig. 29.27. Vertex refractionometer.**

excursion of the target is calibrated and the reading of the excursion gives the dioptric strength. The position of $F_2$ varies according to whether the unknown lens is concave or convex. In concave lenses the shift from $F_1$ is away from the standard lens and in cases of convex lenses the shift from

$F_1$ is towards the standard lens. The instrument is so calibrated as to give direct readings of back vertex power and can be gainfully employed for measuring the back vertex power of the lens. The instrument, however, is unsuitable for measuring the back vertex power of meniscus lenses of

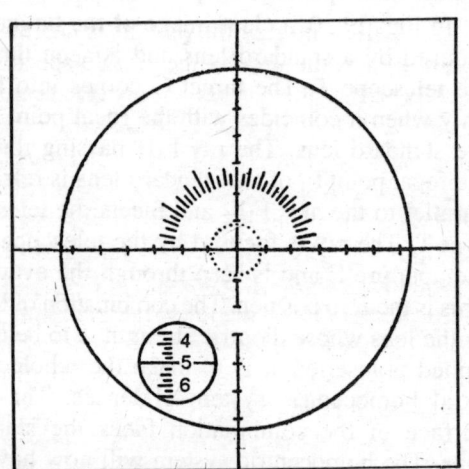

**Fig. 29.28.** Method of measurement by vertex refractionometer.

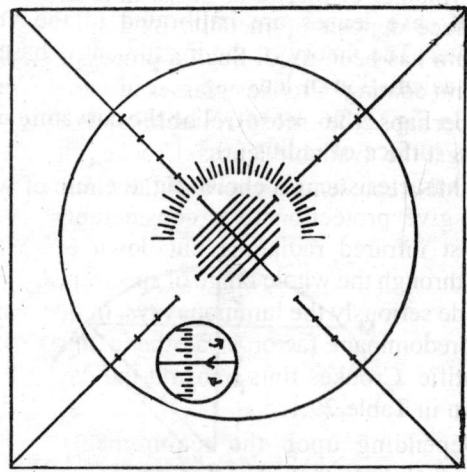

**Fig. 29.29.** Method of measurement by vertex refractionometer.

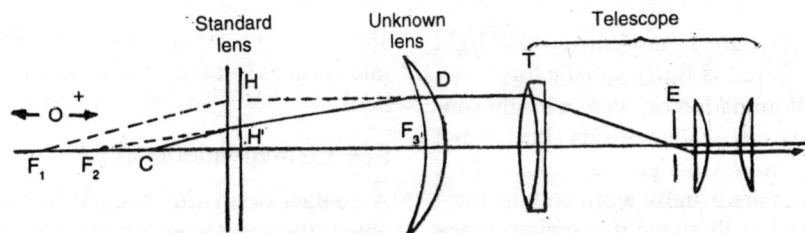

**Fig. 29.30.** Optical principle of vertex refractionometer.

small diameter and high curvature, e.g., contact lenses.

## Protective lenses

Protective lenses in this country are of considerable importance specially when it is industrialising and because of very bright sunshine which emits rays of harmful wavelength, particularly in the long and short wavelengths of the spectrum.

**Glasses against radiation :** This is most commonly achieved by prescribing such lenses which absorb the unwanted rays of light. There are lenses, though rarely used, which achieve the same end by reflecting the unwanted rays. Since all material used for absorption of rays are coloured, tinted glasses are made and used. The lenses can be technically made either by incorporating the substances in the material used for making the lenses or a thin layer of the protective material of uniform thickness may be cemented or fused onto the back surface of the spectacle lens, whether of plastic or glass. In recent years a surface deposit of metallic oxides in a high vacuum has been used. Such a process is called vacuum coating. Crookes glasses of various tints are perhaps the most reliable and efficient amongst the available lenses. Crookes B tint has the characteristic of excluding the ultraviolet rays, give protection to a considerable extent against infrared radiation, cut down excessive light through the whole range of spectrum and not impede seriously the luminous rays. In other tints the predominant factor is aesthetic rather than scientific. Crookes tints transmit the daylight as shown in Table 29.1.

Depending upon the requirements of the individual, tints should be chosen.

More recently photochromatic glass has been

**Table 29.1. Transmission of light**

| Type | % transmission of daylight | |
|------|:--------------:|:--------------:|
|      | 2 mm thickness | 3 mm thickness |
| $A_1$ | 81.50 | 77.00 |
| $A_2$ | 76.50 | 73.00 |
| $B_1$ | 47.00 | 34.00 |
| $B_2$ | 19.50 | 10.00 |

introduced. This alters its colour on exposure to ultraviolet rays light because of incorporation of submicroscopic crystals of silver iodides. The glasses are ingeniously conceived but require considerable improvement particularly so because the change in colour is a slow process.

As far as light is concerned tinted glasses are used for

- protection against visible wavelength,
- protection against infrared, and
- protection against ultraviolet rays.

In protection against visible rays, in cases where the eye is healthy, the ideal glass is the one which cuts off as little of the light as is necessary for comfort and throughout the visible spectrum uniformly so that there is hardly any interference with colour vision. However, tints like Crookes $A_1$ or $A_2$ may be necessary in some pathological states and also in some high degrees of myopia.

In protection against the infrared rays, e.g., in professions like glass blowers or metal smelters, a glass which cuts back infrared rays, even if it reduces some of the visible light, should be preferred. Crookes sage-green is such a glass which has the added advantage of cutting off the ultraviolet light also.

In protection against the ultraviolet light especially in occupations like electric welding arc where ultraviolet lamps are used, in high altitudes with snow, film studios and ultraviolet light clinics, Crookes B tint is fairly satisfactory.

In ordinary illumination or even in bright sunlight these glasses are unnecessary but in hot summers of the tropics do give a little cooling effect; dark shades are usually worn and the most preferable is Crookes $B_2$ shade if visual accuracy is not demanded at that time. Various shades of glasses are, however, extensively used as a measure of fashion, erroneous ideas about harmful action of bright sunlight on the eye or as part of neurasthenic syndrome. In the dusty plains or work fields of this country they may be necessary where the intensity is increased because of reflection of light by dust particles especially sandy particles.

Protection against mechanical injury side shields to ordinary spectacles or the goggles may be used to protect against dust, wind or flying particles. These are particularly useful in lagophthalmos and cases of diminished corneal sensitivity.

A large number of protective optical devices are used to protect against industrial hazards and microwaves but they are beyond the scope of this book.

## Spectacle dermatitis

A contact dermatitis excited by the materials of which the spectacles are made is not uncommon in sensitive persons. The condition was quite common when nickel frames were used but can still occasionally be seen. Eczematous dermatitis (vesicular, papular) can be seen on the nose bridge, the temple and behind the ear. It is most commonly seen behind the ear. In plastic frames no direct evidence of allergy has been produced and the belief is that such a condition depends upon constitutional predisposition.

In metallic frames the condition resembles the dermatitis of nickel plating workers in industry and is considered to be due to some alteration by the nickel ions in the tissue cells which thereafter become sensitized so that continued or subsequent contact leads to eczematous changes.

# Material for Further Reading

The literature on the subject of optics and refraction, contact lenses, correction of subnormal vision, orthoptic and squint is voluminous. The following additional reading material is suggested as it will be helpful to the students and practitioners.

Abrams David (1993) : Duke-Elder's Practice of Refraction, 10th ed., B.I. Churchill Livingstone, London.

Abraham SV (1951) : The Nature of Heterophorias. *Amer. J. Ophth.* 34 : 7.

Acharyajee S. (1995) : *VisiScan*, vol. 3 No. 2.

Adel NL (1966) : Electromyographic and entoptic studies suggesting a theory of action of the ciliary muscles in accommodation for near work and its influence on the development of myopia. *Arch. of the Amer. Acad. of Opt.* 43.

Adler E (1953) : Pathologic physiology of strabismus. *Arch. Ophth.* 50 : 1.

Adler F (1965) : Physiology of the Eye with Clinical Applications. Mosby & Sons, St. Louis.

Agarwal Lalit P : Agarwal's Eye Diseases. CBS Publishers, Delhi.

Alajmo A (1954) : Research in eikonometry : Contribution to the study of the frequency of aniseikonia and its clinical significance. *G. Ital. Oftal.* 7.

Allen MJ (1956) : The influence of age on the speed of accommodation. *Arch. of the Amer. Acad. of Opt.* 33.

Alpar John J, Fechner Paul U (1986) : Fechner's Intraocular Lenses. George Thieme Verlag, Stuttgart, New York.

Amano K (1958) : Measurement of the axial length in the living eye by X-ray photography. *Acta. Soc. Opht. Jap.* 62.

Askovitz SI (1956) : The circle of least confusion in Sturm's conoid of astigmatism. *Arch. Ophth.* 56.

Baldwin WR, West D, Jolley J, Reid W (1959) : Effect of contact lenses on refractive, corneal and axial length changes in young myopes. *Arch. of the Amer. Acad. of Opt.* 46 : 12.

Bannon RE (1949) : Aniseikonia and binocular vision. *Arch. of the Amer. Acad. of Opt.* 26 : 6.

Barfoed P (1953) : On the prognosis in excessive myopia. *Acta. Ophth.* 31.

Barnett AH (1964) : Contact lenses and myopia. 1st Int. Conf. on Myopia, New York.

Batra DV (1967) : Refraction in aphakia. *Indian J. Opt.* 1 : 1.

Bays JA (1966) : Heredity and myopia. *Arch. of the Amer. Acad. of Opt.* 37.

Bennet AG : Refraction by automation? New applications of Scheiner disc. *Optician*, 1960; 139 : 5.

Berens C, Bannon RE (1963) : Aniseikonia. *Arch. Ophth.* 70 : 2.

Berge HL (1956) : Myopia caused by prematurity. *Amer. J. Ophth.* 41.

Berti AP, Harwood KA (1961) : The clinical correction of aniseikonia. *Brit. J. Phys. Opt.* 18.

Bienfang DC (1975) : Crossing axons in third nerve nucleus. *Invest. Ophth.* 14/12 : 927.

Bier N (1960) : Correction of Subnormal Vision. Butterworths & Co. Ltd., London and Boston.

Bier N, Lowther GE (1977) : Contact Lens Correction. Butterworths & Co. Ltd., London and Boston.

Bitonte JL, Keates RH (1972) : Symposium on the Flexible Lens. The C.V. Mosby Company, St. Louis.

Blair WA (1960) : Photoelectric Keratoscopy Testing. *Contacto*; 4 : 7.

Boeder P (1961) : The cooperation of extraocular muscles. *Amer. J. Ophth.* 51.

Borish IM and The Division of Optometry (1970) : Indiana University. Clinical Refraction, 3th ed. The Professional Press, Inc., Chicago.

Bostrom C, Keller EL, Marg E (1978) : A consideration of visual evoked potentials for fast automated ophthalmic refractions. *Invest. Ophth.* 17/2 : 182.

Boyd FB : Highlights of ophthalmology, 1993, vol. 21, No. 12.

Brain VC (1960) : The pathogenesis of congenital myopia. *A.M.A. Sect. Ophth. Trans.*

Brubaker RF, Reinecke RD, Copeland JC : Meridional refractometry. 1. Derivation of equations. *Arch. Ophthalmol.* 1969; 81 : 849.

Bucklers M (1953) : Changes in refraction during life. *Brit. J. Ophth.* 37.

Burian H (1945) : Sensorial retinal relationship in concomitant strabismus. *Trans. Amer. Acad. Ophth.* 43.

Burian HW (1939) : Fusional movements. *Arch. Ophth.* 21 : 3.

Burton TCE, Herron BE, Ossoining KC (1977) : Axial length changes. *Amer. J. Ophth.* 83 : 59.

Campbell CJ, Koester CJ, Rittler MC, Tackaberry RB (1974) : Physiological Optics. Harper & Row, New York.

Chin MB, Breinen GM (1967) : Ratio of accommodative convergence to accommodation. *Arch. Ophth.* 77 : 6.

Colenbrander A : Low vision rehabilitation. *Ophthal. Cl. North Amer.* 1993; 6 (4) : 581-587.

Constenbader FD (1964) : Symposium : The 'A' and 'V' patterns in strabismus. *Trans. Amer. Acad. Ophth.* 68.

Cushman B (1955) : Hyperphoria and some of its problems. *Amer. J. Ophth.* 39.

De Lacey AD (1956) : Routine refraction : A commentary. *Opt. Oct.* 20.

Dolman NG (1950) : Use of cross-cylinders in retinoscopy. *Opt.* July 7.

Duke-Elder W (1949) : Textbook of Ophthalmology. C.V. Mosby & Co., St. Louis.

Duke-Elder W : The Practice of Refraction, 8th ed. J. & A. Churchill Ltd., London.

Duke-Elder W, Abrams D (i970) : System of Ophthalmology, vol. V. The C. V. Mosby & Co., St. Louis.

Ehlers H (1953) : Clinical testing of visual acuity. *Arch. Ophth.* 49 : 4.

Ellerbrock VJ (1960) : Partial Vision and Optical Aids. Vision of the Ageing Patient. Hirsch MJ, Wick RE. Chilton Books.

Fink WH (1962) : Surgery of the Vertical Muscles of the Eye, 2nd ed. Charles C. Thomas, Springfield.

Fonda G (1970) : Management of Patients with Subnormal Vision, 2nd ed. The C.V. Mosby Co., St. Louis.

Fonda GE et al. : Evaluation of CCTV as LVA. *Trans. Amer. Acad. Ophthalmol. Otolaryngol.* 1973; 79 : 1-468.

Fonseca Caddison JA (1961) : Importance of keratometry in measurement of total astigmatism. *Arch. Bras. Oftal.* 24.

Foster RS, Paul TO, Jampolsky R (1976) : Infantile esotropia. *Amer. J. Ophth.* 82 : 291.

Fry GA (1960) : Lens prescription and order for eye wear. *Arch. of the Amer. Acad. of Opt.* 37 : 3.

Gardiner PA (1956) : Observation of food habits of myopic children. *Trans. Oph. Soc.*, U.K. 76.

Gasset AR, Lobo L, Houde W (1977) : Permanent-wear aphakic lenses. *Amer. J. Ophth.* 83 : 115.

Goodrich GL : Applying video and microcomputer technology on a low vision setting. *Ophthal. Cl. North Amer.* 1994; 7 (2) : 177-185.

Gorman JJ, Cogan DG, Gelles SS (1957) : An apparatus for grading visual acuity of infants on the basis of optokinetic nystagmus. *Pediatrics,* 19.

Grolman B : Apparatus for measuring and recording refractive errors of a patient's eye. US Patent No. 1981; 3,572,908.

Haine C, Long W, Reading R : Laser meridional refractometry. *Am. J. Optom. Physical Opt.* 1976; 53 : 194.

Hartstein J (1982) : Extended wear contact lenses for aphakia and myopia. C.V. Mosby Co., St. Louis.

Havenaar WH (1958) : Schepen's binocular indirect ophthalmoscope. *Amer. J. Ophth.* 45.

Helveston EM (1973) : Atlas of Strabismus Surgery. The C.V. Mosby Co., St. Louis.

Hirsch MJ (1965a) : The prevention and/or cure of myopia. *Arch. of the Amer. Acad. of Opt.* 42.

Hirsch MJ (1966b) : Summary of current research in refractive anomalies. *Arch. of the Amer. Acad. of Opt.* 43 : 4.

Hodd FAB (1955) : Working method retinoscopy. *Brit. J. Phys. Opt.* 12.

Howland HC, Howland B : Photorefraction : A technique for study of refractive state at a distance. *J. Opt. Soc. Am.* 1974; 64 : 240.

Hurtt S, Resicovici A, Windsor CE (1977) : Comprehensive Review of Orthoptics and Ocular Motility, 2nd ed. The C.V. Mosby Co, St. Louis.

International Ophthalmology Clinics Intraocular Lens Implantation. Langston, Roger, HS : Little Brown and Company, Boston, 1982.

Jalie M, Wray L (1974) : Practical Ophthalmic Lenses. Butterworths & Co. Ltd., London.

Johns Hopkins Wilmer Eye Institute, Johns Hopkins University, USA, 1994. LVES and comprehensive vision rehabilitation programme.

Karlin DB, Curtin BJ (1976) : Myopia and choroidal lesions. *Amer. J. Ophth.* 81 : 625.

Keiner ECJF (1967) : Pathogenesis of eccentric fixation. *Amer. J. Ophth.* 63 : 1.

Keith Lyle T, Wybar KC (1967) : Practical Orthoptics in the Treatment of Squint. H.K. Lewis & Co. Ltd., London.

Knoll HA : Measuring ametropia with a gas laser : A preliminary report. *Am. J. Optom.* 1966; 43 : 415.

Kumar D : Contact Lens Practice. CBS Publishers, New Delhi.

Kuria Kose MP (1967) : Incidence of myopia. *Indian J. Opt.* I, 1.

Leary GA, Sorsby A, Richards JM, Chaston J (1963) : Ultrasonic measurements of the components of ocular refraction in life : Technical consideration. *Vision Research*; 3.

Lenkins FA, White HE (1937) : Fundamentals of Physical Optics. McGraw Hill Book Co. Inc., New York and London.

Levi DM, Harwerth RS (1978) : Contrast evoked potentials in strabismic and anisometropic amblyopia. *Invest. Ophth.* 17/6 : 571.

Lowe RF (1968) : Time amplitude ultrasonography for ocular biometry. *Amer. J. Ophth.* 66 : 5.

Lyle TK : Practical Orthoptics in the Treatment of Squint. H.K. Lewis & Co. Ltd., London (UK).

Marg E, Johnson DE, Anderson KW, Baker Neroth CC : Computer assisted eye examination. V. Preliminary evaluation of the Refractor III system for subjective examination. *Am. J. Physical Opt.* 1977; 54 : 2.

Miles PW (1953) : Annual Review Physiologic Optics. *Arch. Ophth.* 53 : 6.

Miles PW (1955) : Annual Review Refraction. *Arch. Ophth.* 53 : 6.

Nadell MC, Weymouth FW, Hirsch MJ (1957) : The relationship of frequency of use of the eyes in close work to the distribution of refractive error in a selected sample. *Arch. of the Amer. Acad. of Opt.* 34.

National Association for Visually Handicapped, New York. Visual Aids an tuation material, 8th ed., 1991-92.

Parsons' Diseases of the Eye (1990), 18th ed. Stephen J. Muller, Churchill Livingstone, London (UK).

Peyman-Saunders-Goldberg (1985) : Principles and Practice of Ophthalmology. W.B. Saunders Co., Philadelphia (USA).

Phillips DE, Mclarter GS, Dwyer WO : Validity of the laser refraction technique for meridional measurement. *Am. J. Optom. Physical Opt.* 1976; 53 : 447.

Porterfield W : A treatise on the eye. Hamilton and Balfour, Edinburgh, 1959, vol. 1, p. 423.

Rambo VC (1957) : The first graph of accommodation of the people of India. *J. All India Oph. Soc.*

Rakow Phyllis R : Ophthalmic Contact Lenses. Slack Incorporate Ohio, USA.

Regan D : Rapid objective refraction using evoked beam potentials. *Invest. Ophthalmol.* 1973; 12 : 669.

Robb RM (1977) : Refractive errors with haemangiomas. *Amer. J. Ophth.* 83 : 52.

Ruben M (1975) : Contact Lens Practice. Bailliers Tindall, London.

Schor C, Hallmark W (1978) : Slow control of eye position in strabismic amblyopia. *Invest. Ophth.* 17/6 : 582.

Seth RK (1983) : Ophthalmic News & Views, vol. 1, New Delhi.

Snider MT (1967) : Refractive error and accommodative amplitude in pre- and early presbyopes. *The Ind. Opt.* 37 : 2.

Sharma Namrata : VisiScan, Dec. 1995, vol. 3, No. 2, 131-135.

Soper JW (1974) : Contact Lens, Advances is Design, Fitting Application. Stratton Intercontinental Medical Book Corporation, New York.

Stein HA, Slatt BJ, Stein RM : Ophthalmic Assistant (1988), 5th ed. C.V. Mosby Company, Washington DC (USA).

Timbertake GT et al. : Retinal localization of scotomata by scanning laser ophthalmoscopy. Invest. *Ophthal. Va. Sci.* 1982; 22 : 91-92.

Volk D (1965) : Aspheric ophthalmic lenses. *Refraction* 5 : 2.

Von Noorden GK (1967) : Classification of amblyopia. *Amer. J. Ophth.* 63 : 2.

Von Noorden GK (1976) : Nystagmus compensation syndrome. *Amer. J. Ophth.* 82 : 283.

Von Noorden G, Maumence A (1967) : Atlas of Strabismus. The C.V. Mosby Co., St. Louis.

Welsh RC (1967) : Defects of vision through aphakic lenses. *Brit. J. Opt.* 51.

Westheimer G (1966) : Focusing response of the human eye. *Arch. of the Amer. Acad. of Opt.* 43.

Zee DS, Yee RD (1977) : Abnormal saccades. *Amer. J. Ophth.* 13 : 112.

# Appendix

## VISUAL STANDARDS FOR CENTRAL SERVICES

1. The existing classification into technical and non-technical services given below should continue and to meet their special requirements, separate standards should be prescribed for different categories :

A. *Technical*

1. Railway Engineering Service (Civil, Electrical, Mechanical and Signal), Transportation (Traffic) and Commercial Department and Watch and Ward Department and post on the Marine Establishment.

2. Central Engineering, Classes I and II, Telegraph Engineering, Classes I and II, Survey of India, Classes I and II and Class I and II posts in the Engineering Branch of the Overseas Communication Services, Technical Officers, Class I and II, of the Inspection Wing of the Directorate General of Supplies and Disposals.

B. *Non-Technical*

1. I.A.S., Indian Customs Service, Indian Railway Accounts Service, Indian Defence Accounts Service, Medical Stores and Establishment, Department of the Indian Railways and other posts, Income Tax Officers (Class I Grade II and Class II Service), India Postal Service (Class I) and Military Lands and Cantonments Service, Classes I and II, Geological Survey of India, Class I and II, and other Central Civil Services, Class I and II, Technical Officers of Wireless Plan-

ning and Co-ordination Organisation, Classes I and II.

2. Indian Police Service.

2. It is not necessary to lay down any limit for minimum naked eye vision but it is desirable that the naked eye vision of the candidates should be recorded by the Medical Board or other medical authority in every case as it will furnish basic information with regard to the condition of the eye.

3. The following standards are prescribed for distant vision and near vision with or without glasses for different types of services.

| Class of service | Distant vision | | Near vision | |
|---|---|---|---|---|
| | Better eye | Worse eye | Better eye | Worse eye |
| Class I and II both technical and non-technical | 6/9 or 6/6 | 6/9 6/12 | 0.6 | 0.8 |
| Class III | 6/6 or 6/12 or 6/9 | Nil 6/12 6/18 | 0.6 | 0.8 |
| Class IV | 6/9 or 6/18 or 6/12 | Nil 6/18 6/24 | No standards | No standards |

4. Subject to the visual standards as laid down

in paragraph 3 above being satisfied, the amount of refractive error allowed in respect of Class I and II services shall be as follows :

## (i) All Technical Services and Indian Police Services

Total amount of myopia (including the cylinder) shall not exceed –4.00 D.

## (ii) Non-technical Services other than Indian Police Service

### (a) For candidates up to the age of 20 years

Total amount of myopia shall not exceed – 6.00 D. Total hypermetropia shall not exceed +6.00 D.

### (b) For candidates above the age of 20 years

Total amount of myopia shall not exceed – 8.00 D. Total hypermetropia shall not exceed +6.00 D.

## (iii) Class III and IV Services

No limit for the amount of refractive error in respect of Class III and Class IV services is prescribed provided their visual acuity is in accordance with the standards mentioned under para 3 above.

## (iv) Fundus examination

Wherever possible fundus examination should be carried out and results recorded. The necessity for carrying out such examination, may however, be left to the discretion of the Medical Board.

## (v) Colour vision

1. The testing of colour vision shall be essential in respect of the following Class I and Class II services.
   A. All technical services.
   B. Indian Police Service.
   C. Medical Officers employed under the Ministry of Railways.
2. In respect of Class III and Class IV services under the Ministry of Railways the existing practice of testing colour vision followed by that ministry for their employees should be continued. In respect of other Class III and IV services a test for colour perception shall be carried out only when specifically asked by the department concerned.
3. Colour perception should be graded into a higher and a lower grade depending upon the size of the aperture in the lantern as described in the table below :

| Grade | Higher grade of colour perception | Lower grade of colour perception |
|---|---|---|
| 1. Distance between the lamp and candidates | 16′ | 16′ |
| 2. Size of aperture | 1.3 mm | 13 mm |
| 3. Time of exposure | 5 sec | 5 sec |

For the Services concerned with the safety of the public, e.g., Pilots, Drivers, Guards, etc., the higher grade of colour vision is essential but for others the lower grade of colour vision should be considered sufficient. The same standards of colour vision should be applicable in respect of all engineering personnel in whose case colour perception is considered essential irrespective of the fact whether their duties involve field work or not.

4. Satisfactory colour vision constitutes recognition with ease and without hesitation of signal red, signal green and white colours. The use of Ishihara's plates, shown in good light and a suitable lantern like Edridge Green's shall be considered quite dependable for testing colour vision. While either of the two tests may ordinarily be considered sufficient, in respect of the services concerned with road, rail and air traffic, it is essential to carry out the lantern test. In doubtful cases or where a candidate fails to qualify when tested by only one of the two tests, both the tests should be employed.

## (vi) Field of vision

The field of vision should be tested in respect of all Class I and II services by the confrontation method. Where such test gives unsatisfactory or doubtful results the field of vision should be determined on the perimeter.

### (vii) Night-blindness

Night-blindness need not be tested as a routine, but only in special cases. No standard test for the testing of night-blindness or dark adaptation is prescribed. The Medical Board should be given the discretion to improvise such rough test, e.g., recording of visual acuity with reduced illumination or by making the candidate recognise various objects in a dark-room after he/she has been there for 20 to 30 minutes. Candidates' own statements should not always be relied upon, but they should be given due consideration.

### (vii) Ocular condition other than visual acuity

The ocular conditions or diseases which should be considered as a disqualification are as follows :

(a) Any organic disease or a progressive refractive error which is likely to result in lowering the visual acuity should be considered as a disqualification.

(b) Trachoma : Trachoma, unless complicated, shall ordinarily be not a cause for disqualification.

(c) Squint : For all Class I and II, Technical Services and the Indian Police Service where the presence of binocular vision is essential, squint, even if the visual acuity is of the prescribed standard should be considered as a disqualification. For other services the presence of squint should not be considered as a disqualification if the visual acuity is of the prescribed standard.

(d) One-eyed persons : The employment of one-eyed individuals in regular Class I and II services is not recommended but this need not be a disqualification in respect of Class III and Class IV services provided the prognosis about the functioning eye is good and its vision is not likely to be endangered by the condition of the worse eye and the visual standards mentioned under para (3) above are fully satisfied.

However, one-eyed individuals should not be altogether excluded from employ-ment in Class I and Class II services on a contract basis provided visual acuity in the functioning eye is 6/6 for distant vision and 0.6 for near vision and the refractive error is not more than + or − 4.00 D.

5. The standards prescribed above should be rigidly adhered to in respect of the regular service under the Government. Relaxation of these standards may, however, be allowed when the age of the candidate at the time of the first appointment is 35 years or more. In such cases the standards for corrected vision should be reduced by one step.

| Class of service | Corrected vision | |
|---|---|---|
| | Better eye | Worse eye |
| Class I and II services | 6/12 | 6/12 |
| | or | |
| | 6/9 | 6/18 |
| Class III services | 6/9 | Nil |
| | or | |
| | 6/18 | 6/18 |
| | or | |
| | 6/12 | 6/24 |
| Class IV services | 6/12 | Nil |
| | or | |
| | 6/24 | 6/24 |
| | or | |
| | 6/18 | 6/36 |

6. When a candidate is declared medically unfit on account of visual acuity any appeal preferred by him/her should be dealt with by a Special Medical Board, the composition of which should include two ophthalmologists. Ordinarily, the findings of this Special Medical Board should be considered as final but a second appeal should be permissible in doubtful cases and under special circumstances.

7. The above standards are not intended for the Defence Services Personnel. For the international Civil Aviation Organisation, Medical Standards shall apply to Assistant Aerodrome Officers and Aerodrome Operation Selection Grade.

8. It shall be open to Government to relax any

one of the conditions is favour of any candidate for special reasons.

9. All cases as have not finally been disposed of should be covered by these orders and should be dealt with accordingly.

10. In so far the persons serving in the Indian Audit and Accounts Department are concerned, these orders are issued after consultation with the Comptroller and Auditor General of India.

## VISUAL STANDARDS FOR NATIONAL DEFENCE ACADEMY, ARMY, NAVY & AIR FORCE IN INDIA

(a) **Visual acuity :**

|  | Better eye | Worse eye |
|---|---|---|
| Standard I | | |
| Distant vision | V = 6/6 | V = 6/9 Correctable to 6/6 |
| Near vision | Reads 0.5 or J₁ | Reads 0.5 or J₁ |
| Standard II | | |
| Distant vision | V = 6/12 Correctable to 6/6 | V = 6/18 Correctable to 6/9 |
| Near vision | Reads 0.5 or J₁ | Reads 0.5 or J₁ |
| Standard III | | |
| Distant vision | V = 6/24 Correctable to 6/6 | V = 6/24 Correctable to 6/12 |
| Near vision | Reads 0.5 or J₁ | Reads 0.5 or J₁ |

(b) **Colour vision :** Safe or defective safe

(c) **Field of vision :** Normal in each eye assessed by confrontation test

(d) **Binocular vision :** Candidates must possess good binocular vision

(e) **Requirement for the services :**

**ARMY :** Visual standard III (minimum standard)

**NAVY :**

(i) Visual standard I except that it is not essential for the vision in the worse eye to be correctable to 6/6.

(ii) Special requirements

Night vision standard : Candidates who fail to secure Grade II are to be rejected.

Heterophoria : Must not exceed

| Exophoria ⎫ Esophoria ⎭ | 6 prism dioptres |
|---|---|
| Hyperphoria | 1 prism dioptre |

Limits of hypermetropia (under homatropine) :

| *Better eye* | |
|---|---|
| Hypermetropia | +0.50 dioptres |
| Simple hypermetropic astigmatism | +0.75 dioptres |
| Compound hyper-metropic astigmatism | The error in the more hypermetropic meridian must not exceed +1.5 dioptres of which not more than +0.75 dioptre may be due to astigmatism. |
| *Worse eye* | |
| Hypermetropia | +2.5 dioptres |
| Simple hypermetropic astigmatism | +1.5 dioptres |
| Compound hyper-metropic astigmatism | The error in the more hypermetropic meridian must not exceed +2.5 dioptres of which not more than +1.00 dioptre may be due to astigmatism. |

Colour perception : Standard I

**AIR FORCE :**

(i) Visual standard I : No glasses will be worn.

(ii) Special requirements :

Ocular muscle balance : Heterophoria must not exceed :

| Exophoria | 6 prism dioptres |
|---|---|
| Esophoria | 6 prism dioptres |
| Hyperphoria | 1 prism dioptre |

Binocular vision : Normal as tested on Red Green test and Bishop Harman test.

If 2.5 prism dioptres of esophoria is present on the Red Green test together with 2.25 D hypermetropia, it will be a cause for rejection.

# Index

289